Recent Developments in Veterinary Medicine

Recent Developments in Veterinary Medicine

Edited by Gerardo Bailey

MURPHY & MOORE
www.murphy-moorepublishing.com

Published by Murphy & Moore Publishing,
1 Rockefeller Plaza,
New York City, NY 10020, USA
www.murphy-moorepublishing.com

Recent Developments in Veterinary Medicine
Edited by Gerardo Bailey

International Standard Book Number: 978-1-63987-481-1 (Hardback)

Cataloging-in-Publication Data

Recent developments in veterinary medicine / edited by Gerardo Bailey.
p. cm.
Includes bibliographical references and index.
ISBN 978-1-63987-481-1
1. Veterinary medicine. 2. Animals--Diseases. 3. Animal health. I. Bailey, Gerardo.
SF745 .R43 2022
636.089--dc23

TABLE OF CONTENTS

PREFACE

Veterinary medicine is a subfield of medicine that is concerned with the diagnosis, treatment, control and prevention of diseases in animals. The field is responsible for providing animal drug and medicated feeds for the treatment of diseases, disorders and injuries in animals. These diseases can be transmissible or non-transmissible. Drugs are therefore primarily produced to control and prevent zoonotic diseases. They are manufactured and designed to cover a large variety of prophylactic and therapeutic purposes, Veterinary medicine deals with household pets, exotic species, food producing animals and wild animals. This book is a valuable compilation of topics, ranging from the basic to the most complex advancements in the field of veterinary medicine. The aim of this book is to present researches that have transformed this discipline and aided its advancement. Through this book, we attempt to further enlighten the readers about the new concepts in this field.

After months of intensive research and writing, this book is the end result of all who devoted their time and efforts in the initiation and progress of this book. It will surely be a source of reference in enhancing the required knowledge of the new developments in the area. During the course of developing this book, certain measures such as accuracy, authenticity and research focused analytical studies were given preference in order to produce a comprehensive book in the area of study.

This book would not have been possible without the efforts of the authors and the publisher. I extend my sincere thanks to them. Secondly, I express my gratitude to my family and well-wishers. And most importantly, I thank my students for constantly expressing their willingness and curiosity in enhancing their knowledge in the field, which encourages me to take up further research projects for the advancement of the area.

Editor

1

The effect of miscellaneous oral dosage forms on the environmental pollution of sulfonamides in pig holdings

Jessica Stahl[1*†], Katrin Zessel[1†], Jochen Schulz[2], Jan Henrik Finke[3], Christel Charlotte Müller-Goymann[3] and Manfred Kietzmann[1]

Abstract

Background: Due to antibiotic treatment of humans and animals, the prevalence of bacterial resistances increases worldwide. Especially in livestock farming, large quantities of faeces contaminated with antibiotics pose a risk of the carryover of the active ingredient to the environment. Accordingly, the aim of the present study was the evaluation of the benefit of different oral dosage forms (powder, pellets, granula) in pigs concerning the environmental pollution of sulfadiazine. Two subtherapeutic dosages were evaluated in powder mixtures to gain information about their potential to pollute the pig barn. Furthermore, a new group of pigs was kept in the stable after powder feeding of another pig group to determine the possible absorption of environmentally distributed antibiotics.
Pigs were orally treated with three dosage forms. Simultaneously, sedimentation and airborne dust were collected and plasma and urine levels were determined.

Results: All formulations result in comparable plasma and urine levels, but massive differences in environmental pollution (powder > pellets, granula). Pigs housing in a contaminated barn exhibit traces of sulfadiazine in plasma and urine.

Conclusion: Using pharmaceutical formulations like pellets or granula, the environmental pollution of sulfonamides can significantly be diminished due to massive dust reduction during feeding.

Keywords: Dust, Sulfonamides, Environmental pollution, Antibiotic residues, Pigs

Background

To achieve an efficient treatment of animals and humans suffering from bacterial disease, an adequate antibiotic treatment is often required. A closer look into the antibacterial treatment of animals in Europe demonstrates that sulfonamides, tetracyclines and ß-lactam antibiotics are the most frequently used antibacterial agents [1–3]. Sulfonamides can be used in the treatment against gram-positive and gram-negative bacteria, as well as several rickettsia and protozoa (*Toxoplasma, Coccidia*) [4]. Active metabolites of sulfonamide excreted in urine or feces may pollute the environment [5–9]. Contamination from animal husbandry primarily affects soil and water, with pig, poultry and cattle manure, slurry and liquid dung, hospital waste water and sewage being the main sources [8, 10, 11]. Moreover, it has been demonstrated that sulfonamides contaminate ground water in particular by surface run off or sediment of shrimp ponds [12–15]. These antibiotic residues in the environment deriving from the antibiotic drug itself or its antibiotic metabolites pose the risk of the development of bacterial resistance due to subinhibitory concentrations (concentrations beyond the minimal inhibitory concentration) [16]. The antibiotic substance may be inhaled and swallowed. Furthermore, it can contaminate the skin of individuals and thus gets in contact with the normal skin flora, or it can orally be incorporated into the body, due to the contamination of food products. Tetracyclines and sulfonamides for example have been found in agricultural crops after

* Correspondence: jessica.stahl@tiho-hannover.de
†Equal contributors
[1]Department of Pharmacology, Toxicology and Pharmacy, University of Veterinary Medicine Hannover, Foundation, Buenteweg 17, 30559 Hannover, Germany
Full list of author information is available at the end of the article

distribution of antibiotic containing manure [17, 18]. Consequently, intestinal bacteria can be affected, as well. Another risk is, that antibiotics in stable dust can be distributed into the environment of the stable via emission [19–21].

Concerning the current problems of antibacterial resistances in both human and veterinary medicine and the associated problems of the inability of healing seriously ill individuals, it is of high importance to reduce the dissemination of antibacterial agents into the environment. Hamscher et al. (2003) demonstrated that antibiotic residues can be determined in stable dust for a long time [22]. Therefore, the present study was conducted to investigate the ability of different pharmaceutical formulations of antibiotics (sulfonamides) in the treatment of pigs to reduce environmental contaminations. Sulfonamide application was performed via powder, pellets and granula in order to test the absorption of the antibiotic agent in the oral dosage forms with various firmnesses (powder < pellets < granula). Environmental contamination was examined by collecting sedimentation dust in the stable and aerosol. Furthermore, untreated pigs (sentinels) were housed in a dry-cleaned stable after treatment of another pig group with sulfadiazine powder for several days to examine the effect of sulfonamide residues on plasma and urine samples of these untreated animals.

Methods

Sulfadiazine formulations

For powder manufacturing, usual pig feed (powder, Scharnebecker Muehle, Germany, comprising corn, wheat, barley, peas, oat and sorghum) was supplemented with sulfadiazine in the relevant concentrations (2.5 mg/kg body weight (BW), 5 mg/kg BW and 25 mg/kg BW) during a mixing process. Such sulfadiazine containing powder was also used for producing pellets in a pelletising machine under high pressure.

A granular formulation of sulfadiazine was produced via fluidized-bed spray-granulation. Potato starch was used as a binder in the granulation liquid consisting of 6 %(w/w) potato starch, 0.1 %(w/w) sulfadiazine and 93.9 %(w/w) deionized water. The granulation liquid was boiled for starch gelation. 4000 g of pig feed were placed in a fluidized-bed spray-granulator (WSG U5, Glatt GmbH) and sprayed at a spray rate of 40 rpm. After the spraying process, the granules were recovered and dried to a humidity of 7 % before filling and further application.

Animals

24 female piglets of a hybrid breed (db. Viktoria × db.77), all of which weighing 10–15 kg at the beginning of the experiment, were obtained from the Lehr- und Forschungsgut Ruthe, Germany. The pigs were kept under the same conditions in groups of 6 animals and had free access to tap water from drinking nipples. The pen measured 23.52^2, with 6 animals in bays of 8.8^2. A ventilation system maintained a constant temperature of 19-20 ° C in the stable, which was verified by random measurements.

All pigs were clinically healthy (determined via visual examination) during the study. The study was approved by the LAVES File number 33.12-42502-04-11/0338.

Experimental procedure

Pharmacokinetic studies were carried out in 4 groups of 6 pigs to determine the plasma and urine concentrations of sulfadiazine as well as the environmental pollution. Therefore, sulfadiazine was supplemented to the feed (powder mixing, pelletisation, granulation), which was given twice a day for four days. Events like feeding and cleaning were standardized. Sulfadiazine contamination of the stable was excluded before starting the experiment.

The whole experiment was performed in three different parts:

The first group of 6 pigs was treated via powder feeding (recommended formulation type) as follows: After 1 week of acclimatisation, the pigs were weight and received sulfadiazine (Trimosulf®, WDT, Garbsen, Germany) in powder in three different concentrations (two subtherapeutic concentrations) on 4 consecutive days. Between all treatments a washout-phase of three days was inserted (determined by a separate experiment). The first treatment was 2.5 mg/kg (subtherapeutic dosage) BW (body weight) for 4 days, followed by a washout-phase of three days. Afterwards, each pig received 5.0 mg/kg BW (subtherapeutic dosage) sulfadiazine for 4 days, followed by three non-medicated days. Finally, 25 mg/kg BW sulfadiazine (recommended dosage according to the package leaflet) was orally administered to the pigs for four days. Afterwards, the pigs were removed from the stable, which underwent a dry cleaning process and 6 untreated piglets moved into the stable in order to simulate a carry-over of sulfadiazine of a polluted stable. These untreated pigs were kept in the stable for 6 days and were fed with powder feed without antibiotic supplementation.

The second and third group of pigs was treated with sulfadiazine incorporated into pellets or granula in order to determine formulations of sulfadiazine with a high biocompatibility and low environmental contamination. The animals were treated with sulfadiazine (25 mg/kg BW) via pellets or granula over 4 days each. The sulfadiazine concentration in the feed was as followed: 94 mg/kg (powder; 2.5 mg/kg BW), 151 mg/kg (powder; 5 mg/kg BW), 820 mg/kg (powder, pellets, granula; 25 mg/kg BW).

Chemicals

Sulfadiazine and sulfamerazine were purchased from Sigma-Aldrich (Steinheim, Germany) and were of the highest purity available. Methanol (HPLC-grade) was obtained from Applichem, Darmstadt, Germany.

Determination of plasma concentrations

Plasma samples were taken immediately before antibiotic medication and after 3 h. Therefore, blood was collected from the jugular vein of each pig and was collected in EDTA-containing plastic tubes. After centrifugation for 10 min (3000 × g) the plasma was collected and stored at −20 °C until extraction procedure. Blood of untreated pigs (sentinel pigs) was collected once a day 30 min after feeding.

Determination of urine concentrations Urine samples were collected spontaneously once a day of each pig and were stored at −20 ° C until analysis.

Collection of sedimentation dust

Sedimentation dust was collected at five different localisations in the stable and was stored at−20 ° C until extraction. Therefore a card sheet was used to collect the dust from a predefined surface area and the dust was weight before extraction to determine the amount of sulfadiazine in μg/mg dust. The localisations are shown in Fig. 1.

The different areas are presented in Table 1, as well as height of the sampling area and the distance to the feeding area.

Aerosol collection

Air samples were taken simultaneously at two locations in the animal house (Fig. 1). Therefore SKC pumps with IOM samplers were used (PCWR (SKC INC., Eighty Four, P.A. USA). The air flow of the pumps was adjusted to 3 l/min. Dust was sampled on polycarbonate filters (0.8 μm diameter of the pores; Whatman, Dassel, Germany) over a time period of 9 h. The filters were weight before and after usage to determine the amount of collected dust.

Extraction procedures

Sulfadiazine was extracted from plasma, urine, and stable dust according to van Duijkeren (1994) [23]. Sulfamerazine was used as internal standard for extraction procedure.

Analytical methodology

High performance liquid chromatography (HPLC) was used to determine the amount of sulfadiazine and sulfamerazine consisting of the following parts (all Beckmann, Muenchen, Germany) according to Zessel et al. 2013 [24]. A 508-autosampler was used to inject 100 μl of the samples into the HPLC-system and a 126 Solvent System Pump maintained a constant flow of 1 ml/min. Separation was achieved on a Rp-18 LiChroCart 250-4-column (5 μm, 25 cm, Merck, Darmstadt, Germany) at 41 ° C. Detection was performed at 264 nm by a UV–VIS-166-Detector. The mobile phase consisted of 15 % methanol

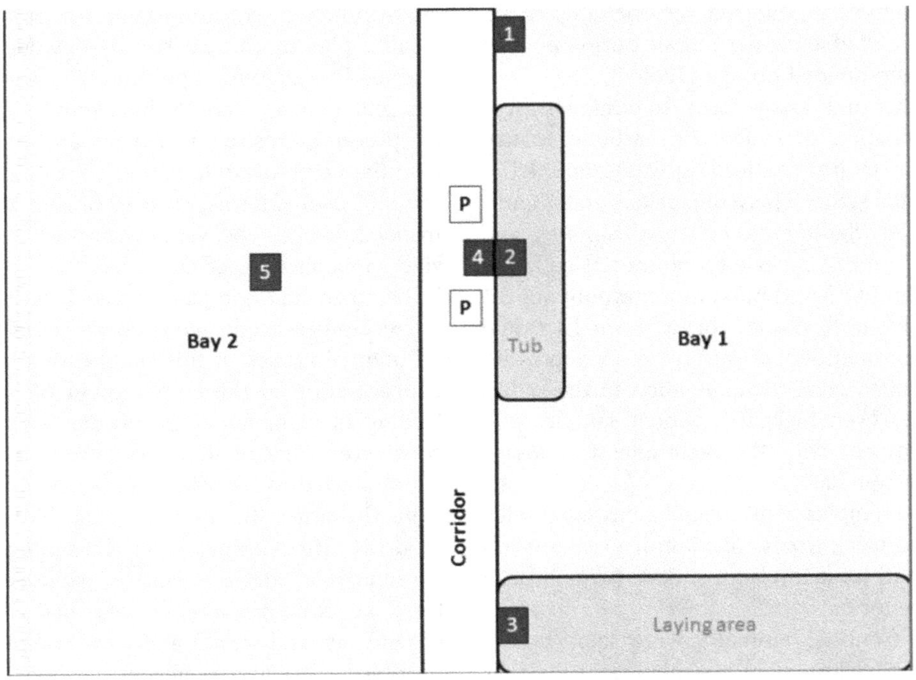

Fig. 1 Scheme of the pig stable. The numbers indicate the 5 areas of sedimentation dust sample withdrawal (1. window sill, 2. grid above the tub, 3. grid above the lying area, 4. gutters in front of the tub and 5. bay barrier on the other side of the stable), and "P" shows the positions of air samplings. Bay 1 was used for all experimental setups

Table 1 Locations of the sedimentation dust samples withdrawal in the stable with distance to the tub and height of sampling area

No.	Location of the sampling areas	Vertical distance to the feeding tub (m)	Height of the sampling area (m)
1	window sill	2	2.1
2	grid above the tub	0.0	1.4
3	grid above the lying area	2	1.4
4	gutters in front of the tub	0.6	0.0
5	bay barrier in bay 2	2.5	1.1

and 85 % McIlvaine-citrate buffer (pH 2.2). The limit of quantification (LOQ) was 0.1 μg/ml, the limit of detection was 0.09 μg/ml.

Statistics

Statistical analyses were carried out with the GraphPad Prism program (version 6.05, GraphPad Software Inc., San Diego, CA, USA). A two way ANOVA was used to gain information about significance, which was defined as $p < 0.05$.

Results

Sulfadiazine treatment via powder resulted in dust contaminations at all localisations in the stable with the highest amounts at the bay barrier in bay 2, followed by the tub (up to 1.7 μg/mg dust), the windowsill, the lying area, and the gutters in front of the tub (maximum 0.7 μg/mg dust, Table 2). Collected aerosol samples exhibited up to 8 μg sulfadiazine per m3 air during powder feeding of the recommended dosage (Table 3).

The ability of other oral dosage forms to diminish environmental contamination of sulfadiazine around treated pigs in comparison to powder feeding was examined in another experimental setup. Therefore, pellets and granula were manufactured. Sedimentation dust samples and aerosols (Tables 2 and 3) revealed amounts of sulfadiazine lower than the LOQ and maximum amounts of 0.1 to 0.2 μg/m3 air for both dosage forms. Even 10 % and 20 % of the recommended dosage given via powder feed, resulted in sulfadiazine contamination of the stable, that are sometimes even higher than dust samples collected during treatment with the recommended dosage given via pellets or granula.

Plasma and urine samples of all treated animals revealed similar plasma and urine levels (maximum plasma levels up to 14.2 μg/ml and urine levels up to 393 mg/ml, Figs. 2 and 3) of all dosage forms.

Untreated pigs (sentinel animals) were kept in the stable after powder treatment of six other pigs for four days. Analysis of the plasma demonstrates that only small amounts of sulfadiazine are detectable in plasma (day 1 and 4 < LOQ) (Fig. 2), but with concentrations in the urine up to 3.5 μg/ml on the first day of housing in the stable (Fig. 4).

Discussion

One aim of the present study was to examine the amount of environmental pollution of a commonly used oral dosage form (powder) of the test substance sulfadiazine in a pig stable during a four-day treatment in comparison to two other dosage forms. This general understanding is necessary since examinations of Hamscher et al. (2003) demonstrated that antibiotic residues (parent or metabolites) can be determined in stable dust during two decades [22]. Therefore, sulfadiazine powder was added to the powder feed, was mixed and was directly given to the pigs in a tub. The results of the dust samples demonstrate the importance of dust reduction in the stable of antibacterially treated animals, since sulfadiazine treatment via powder resulted in dust contaminations at all localisations in the stable. The difference in the degree of contamination in the different areas shows no satisfying correlation to the distance to the feeding area but may be explained by the air movement in the stable. Consequently, air movement resulting from the air conditioning has to be considered to reduce antibiotic contamination of untreated animals, but also the animals itself may be the reason for this differences, since trouble in the tub during feeding may lead to swirl up small dust particles containing sulfadiazine [21, 25].

The ability of other oral dosage forms to diminish environmental contamination of sulfadiazine around treated pigs in comparison to powder feeding was examined in a second experimental setup. Therefore, pellets and granula were manufactured. Sedimentation dust samples and aerosols revealed amounts of sulfadiazine lower than the LOQ (maximum amounts of 0.1 to 0.2 μg/m3 air) for both dosage forms. Even 10 % and 20 % of the recommended dosage given via powder feed, resulted in sulfadiazine contamination of the stable, that are sometimes even higher than dust samples collected during treatment with the recommended dosage given via pellets or granula.

Potential causes of this significantly lower sulfadiazine concentration in the environment of pellet and granula feeding in comparison to powder treatment have to be considered. First of all, the origin of dust has to be elucidated, since dust represents a mixture of particles deriving from the litter, the animals (skin, hair, faeces), and the food [21, 26]. The litter was the same in all experimental setups, so that this can be excluded as main reason for dust reduction. The animals had all the same background, age and weight and were housed under the same conditions, but since sulfadiazine is excreted mainly via the urine, the excretion rates caused by differences in the bioavailability of the different dosage forms had to be investigated. Therefore, plasma and urine samples of all

Table 2 Amount of sulfadiazine in µg/mg sedimentation dust at 5 localizations on 4 days

Localization	Treatment		µg sulfadiazine per mg sedimentation dust			
			Day 1	Day 2	Day 3	Day 4
1: Distance to the tub 2 m, height 2.10 m	Powder	2.5 mg/kg BW	< LOQ	< LOQ	< LOQ	< LOQ
		5.0 mg/kg BW	< LOQ	< LOQ	< LOQ	< LOQ
		25 mg/kg BW	0.8	1.2	1.1	1.3
	Pellets	25 mg/kg BW	< LOQ**	< LOQ**	< LOQ**	< LOQ**
	Granula	25 mg/kg BW	< LOQ**	< LOQ**	< LOQ**	< LOQ**
	Sentinels	untreated	1.3	1.9	1.0	1.1
2: Distance to the tub 0 m, height 1.40 m	Powder	2.5 mg/kg BW	< LOQ	< LOQ	< LOQ	< LOQ
		5.0 mg/kg BW	< LOQ	0.3	0.2	0.4
		25 mg/kg BW	0.6	1.3	1.8	1.7
	Pellets	25 mg/kg BW	< LOQ	< LOQ	< LOQ*	< LOQ*
	Granula	25 mg/kg BW	< LOQ	< LOQ	< LOQ*	< LOQ*
	Sentinels	untreated	1.3	1.3	1.3	1.4
3: Distance to the tub 2 m, height 1.40 m	Powder	2.5 mg/kg BW	< LOQ	< LOQ	< LOQ	< LOQ
		5.0 mg/kg BW	< LOQ	n.d.	0.1	0.1
		25 mg/kg BW	0.2	0.5	0.7	0.8
	Pellets	25 mg/kg BW	< LOQ	< LOQ	< LOQ*	< LOQ*
	Granula	25 mg/kg BW	< LOQ	< LOQ	< LOQ*	< LOQ*
	Sentinels	untreated	0.8	0.7	0.6	0.6
4: Distance to the tub 0.6 m, height 0 m	Powder	2.5 mg/kg BW	n.d.	< LOQ	< LOQ	n.d.
		5.0 mg/kg BW	0.1	0.2	0.1	0.1
		25 mg/kg BW	0.2	0.5	0.7	0.5
	Pellets	25 mg/kg BW	< LOQ	< LOQ	< LOQ*	< LOQ
	Granula	25 mg/kg BW	< LOQ	< LOQ	< LOQ*	< LOQ
	Sentinels	untreated	0.8	0.9	0.9	0.8
5: Distance to the tub 2.5 m, height 1.10 m	Powder	2.5 mg/kg BW	< LOQ	< LOQ	< LOQ	< LOQ
		5.0 mg/kg BW	< LOQ	< LOQ	< LOQ	0.1
		25 mg/kg BW	0.2	n.d.	0.9	2.8
	Pellets	25 mg/kg BW	< LOQ	< LOQ	< LOQ	< LOQ
	Granula	25 mg/kg BW	< LOQ	< LOQ	< LOQ	< LOQ
	Sentinels	untreated	0.9	1.1	1.0	1.0

BW body weight, *LOQ* limit of quantification; * = $p < 0.05$ (vs. pellets), ** = $p < 0.01$ (vs. pellets)

Table 3 Amount of sulfadiazine per m3 air (aerosol) measured on 4 days during the experiment

Aerosol		µg sulfadiazine per m3 air			
		Day 1	Day 2	Day 3	Day 4
Powder	2.5 mg/kg BW	< LOQ	< LOQ	< LOQ	< LOQ
	5.0 mg/kg BW	0.1	< LOQ	0.3	0.4
	25 mg/kg BW	2.7	8.0	5.7	3.2
Pellets	25 mg/kg BW	< LOQ	< LOQ*	< LOQ	0.2
Granula	25 mg/kg BW	< LOQ	0.2*	0.1	< LOQ
Sentinels	untreated	1.6	1.2	0.3	0.4

BW body weight, *LOQ* limit of quantification; * = $p < 0.05$ (vs. powder)

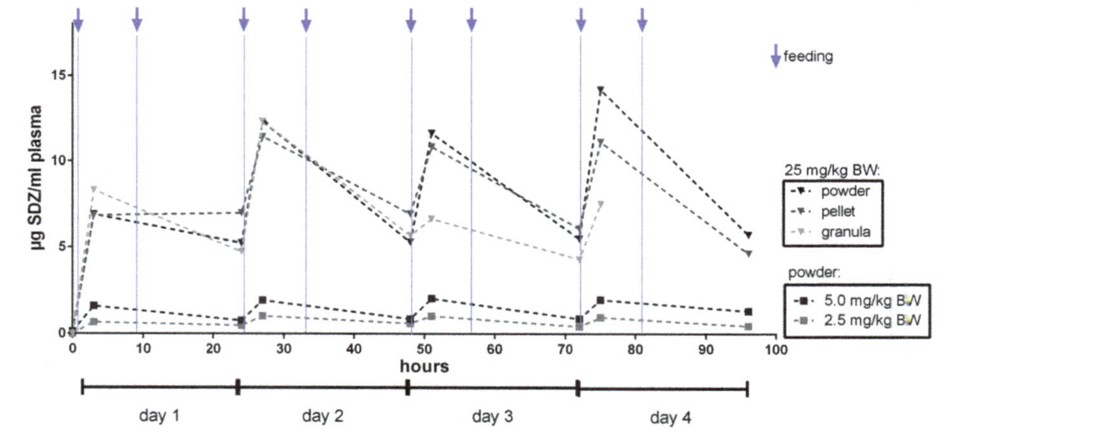

Fig. 2 Plasma concentration of sulfadiazine (SDZ; mean) in six pigs after powder feeding of sulfadiazine in three dosages: 2.5 mg/kg BW (body weight; grey box), 5 mg/kg BW (black box) and 25 mg/kg BW (black triangle) and after pellet (dark grey triangle) and granula (bright grey triangle) feeding in a concentration of 25 mg/kg BW; feeding was performed twice daily (asterisks)

treated animals were determined during the experiment and revealed similar plasma and urine levels for all dosage forms. Since all dosage forms exhibited nearly the same bioavailability, it can be concluded that the sulfadiazine distribution took place during the feeding process in dependence to the dosage form.

The possibility to absorb antibiotic residues from the environment was shown by Kietzmann et al. (1995) and raised the question if the detected sulfadiazine concentration in the environment during powder feeding is high enough to affect untreated animals in the dry cleaned stable. Therefore, untreated pigs (sentinel animals) were kept in the stable after powder treatment of six other pigs for four days. Analysis of the plasma demonstrates that only small amounts of sulfadiazine are detectable in plasma (day 1 and 4 < LOQ), but with concentrations in the urine up to 3.5 μg/ml on the first day of housing in the stable. This is not astonishing, since the stable was only dry cleaned and in sedimentation dust and aerosol samples exhibited sulfadiazine concentrations up to 1.9 μg/mg sedimentation dust and 1.6 μg/m3 air. To get knowledge about the magnitude of absorption, the comparison of the sentinel animals with the subtherapeutic dosages treated animals demonstrates that urine concentrations of the sentinel animals were 3–8 times lower than the sulfadiazine concentration in urine of the animals treated with 10 % of the recommended dosage.

The sentinel animals were exposed to a mean sedimentation dust concentration of 1.0 μg/mg (Table 2) and reached blood concentrations just below the limit of quantification (approximately 0.05-0.07 μg/ml, data not shown). To reach such a low plasma concentration the animals (body weight of 10–15 kg) had to orally adsorb 19–71 mg sedimentation dust (assuming a total blood volume of 4-7 % of the BW, [27] and 100 % oral bioavailability) from the environment. Since the aerosol exhibited mean sulfadiazine concentrations of 0.87 μg/m3 air (Table 3), a pig with a body weight of 10–15 kg and a blood concentration of 0.05-0.07 mg/ml

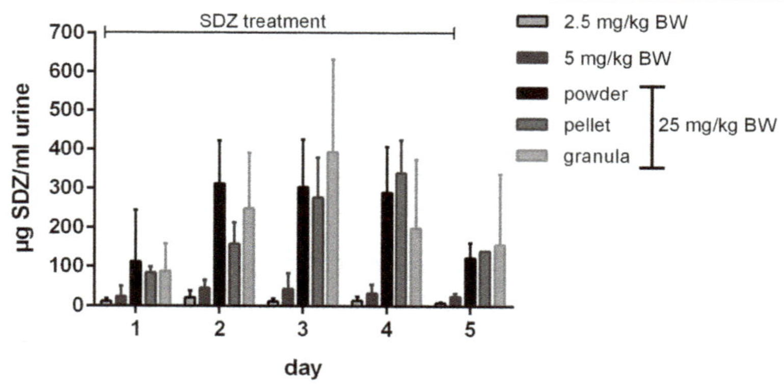

Fig. 3 Urine concentration of sulfadiazine (SDZ; mean ± standard deviation) in six pigs after powder feeding of sulfadiazine in three dosages (2.5 mg/kg BW (body weight), 5 mg/kg BW and 25 mg/kg BW) and after pellet and granula feeding; feeding was performed twice daily on day 1–4

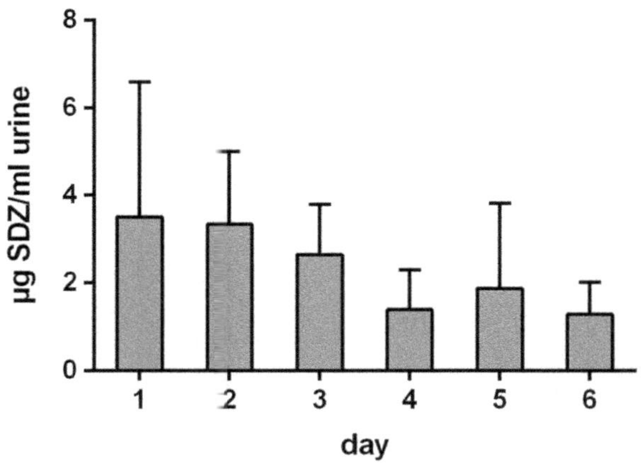

Fig. 4 Urine concentration of sulfadiazine (SDZ) in six untreated pig, all of which were housed in the stable after removing orally treated pigs (25 mg/kg BW over four days) and after dry cleaning; data are shown as mean + standard deviation; LOQ = 0.1 µg/ml

had to absorb 20–73.5 µg sulfadiazine, which in turn is inhaled via 23–84 m3 air. Assuming a lung ventilation of 4–5.6 l/min. [28], with a bioavailability via the lungs of 100 %, 128–704 h would be necessary to absorb this amount of sulfadiazine via aerosol. Therefore, it can be concluded that the oral uptake of dust sedimentation from the stable represents the main source of absorption and may be slightly completed via the lungs.

Conclusion

The present study demonstrates the importance of the pharmaceutical formulation on the entry of antibiotic residues into the environment of orally treated pigs. Pellets and granula produced lower concentrations of environmental contamination with sulfadiazine.

Abbreviations

EDTA: ethylenediaminetetraacetic acid; HPLC: high performance liquid chromatography; SDZ: sulfadiazine; SMR: sulfamerazine.

Competing interests

The authors declare that they have no competing interests.

Authors' contributions

KAZ performed, analysed and evaluated the experiments with the powder and the pellets. JS planned the study together with MK. JS coordinated the granulate experiments, performed the analysis and the evaluations of the results and created the manuscript. JOS helped in performing the stable dust experiments. JHF and CCM-G planned, coordinated and supervised the granulate development and production. All authors have read and approved the manuscript.

Acknowledgements

The Institute of Animal Nutrition, University of Veterinary Medicine Hannover is acknowledged for the manufacture and the supply of the pellets. Ursula Jahn, Markus Immer, Gesa Petter, and Michaela Schulze are acknowledged for their assistance in granulate development and production at the Department for Pharmaceutics. Furthermore, the technical help of Alina Narten and Dr. Isabell Roth is acknowledged.

Funding

This study was supported by the "Deutsche Bundesstiftung Umwelt DBU".

Author details

[1]Department of Pharmacology, Toxicology and Pharmacy, University of Veterinary Medicine Hannover, Foundation, Buenteweg 17, 30559 Hannover, Germany. [2]Institute for Animal Hygiene, Animal Welfare and Farm Animal Behaviour, Bischofsholer Damm 15, 30173 Hannover, Germany. [3]Institut Pharmazeutische Technologie, Technische Universität Braunschweig, Mendelssohnstr. 1, 38106 Braunschweig, Germany.

References

1. Kratz W, Abbas B, Linke I. Arzneimittelwirkstoffe in der Umwelt. Landesumweltamt Brandenburg, Abteilung: Okologie und Umweltanalytik; 2000.
2. Broll SK M, Bettin U, Kreienbrock L. Use of medicated feedingstuff in animal production in Schleswig-Holstein. Tierarztl Prax. 2002;30:357–61.
3. Kreienbrock L. Erfassung des Antibiotikaverbrauchs als Grundlage von Verminderungsstrategien in der Veterinärmedizin. Dresden: Statusseminar »Arzneistoffe in der Umwelt« am 7 und 8; 2011.
4. Plumb DC. Plumb's Veterinary Drug Handbook. 7th ed. Ames, Iowa: Wiley; 2011.
5. Nouws JF, Vree TB, Hekster YA. In vitro antimicrobial activity of hydroxy and N4-acetyl sulphonamide metabolites. Vet Q. 1985;7(1):70–2.
6. Nouws JF, Firth EC, Vree TB, Baakman M. Pharmacokinetics and renal clearance of sulfamethazine, sulfamerazine, and sulfadiazine and their N4-acetyl and hydroxy metabolites in horses. Am J Vet Res. 1987;48(3):392–402.
7. Nouws JF, Mevius D, Vree TB, Baakman M, Degen M. Pharmacokinetics, metabolism, and renal clearance of sulfadiazine, sulfamerazine, and sulfamethazine and of their N4-acetyl and hydroxy metabolites in calves and cows. Am J Vet Res. 1988;49(7):1059–65.
8. Hruska K, Franek M. Sulfonamides in the environment: a review and case report. Vet Med. 2012;57(1):1–35.
9. Baran W, Adamek E, Ziemianska J, Sobczak A. Effects of the presence of sulfonamides in the environment and their influence on human health. J Hazard Mater. 2011;196:1–15.
10. Tamtam F, Mercier F, Le Bot B, Eurin J, Tuc Dinh Q, Clement M, Chevreuil M. Occurrence and fate of antibiotics in the Seine River in various hydrological conditions. Sci Total Environ. 2008;393(1):84–95.
11. Luo Y, Xu L, Rysz M, Wang Y, Zhang H, Alvarez PJ. Occurrence and transport of tetracycline, sulfonamide, quinolone, and macrolide antibiotics in the Haihe River Basin, China. Environ Sci Technol. 2011;45(5):1827–33.
12. Le TX, Munekage Y. Residues of selected antibiotics in water and mud from shrimp ponds in mangrove areas in Viet Nam. Mar Pollut Bull. 2004;49(11–12):922–9.
13. Le TX, Munekage Y, Kato S. Antibiotic resistance in bacteria from shrimp farming in mangrove areas. Sci Total Environ. 2005;349(1–3):95–105.
14. Kay P, Blackwell PA, Boxall AB. Transport of veterinary antibiotics in overland flow following the application of slurry to arable land. Chemosphere. 2005;59(7):951–9.
15. Hamscher G. Different behavior of tetracyclines and sulfonamides in sandy soils after repeated fertilization with liquid manure. Environ Toxicol Chem. 2005;24:8.
16. Kümmerer K. Resistance in the environment. J Antimicrob Chemother. 2004;54(2):311–20.
17. Kumar K, Gupta SC, Baidoo SK, Chander Y, Rosen CJ. Antibiotic uptake by plants from soil fertilized with animal manure. J Environ Qual. 2005;34(6):2082–5.
18. Grote M, Schwake-Anduschus C, Michel R, Stevens H, Heyser W, Langenkämper G, Betsche T, Freitag M. Incorporation of veterinary

antibiotics into crops from manured soil. Landbauforschung Völkenrode 1. 2007;57:25–32.
19. Seedorf J, Hartung J. Emission of Airborne Particulates from Animal Production. Dtsch Tierarztl Wochenschr. 1995;102(7):283–8.
20. Hartung J, Seedorf J, Trickl T, Gronauer H. Emission of particulates from a pig farm with central air exhaust in the pig stall. Dtsch Tierarztl Wochenschr. 1998;105(6):244–5.
21. Pedersen S, Nonnenmann M, Rautiainen R, Demmers TG, Banhazi T, Lyngbye M. Dust in pig buildings. J Agric Saf Health. 2000;6(4):261–74.
22. Hamscher G, Pawelzick HT, Sczesny S, Nau H, Hartung J. Antibiotics in dust originating from a pig-fattening farm: a new source of health hazard for farmers? Environ Health Perspect. 2003;111(13):1590–4.
23. Van Duijkeren E, Vulto AG, Van Oldruitenborghoosterbaan MM S, Mevius DJ, Kessels BG, Breukink HJ, Van Miert AS. A comparative study of the pharmacokinetics of intravenous and oral trimethoprim/sulfadiazine formulations in the horse. J Vet Pharmacol Ther. 1994;17(6):440–6.
24. Zessel K. Decreased entry of veterinary drug residues into the environment by improved degradability of sulphonamides/Verringerung des Eintrags von Tierarzneimittelrückständen in die Umwelt mit besser abbaubaren Sulfonamiden. Hannover: University of Veterinary Medicine Hannover, Foundation; 2012.
25. Takai H, Pedersen S, Johnsen JO, Metz JHM, Groot Koerkamp PWG, Uenk GH, Phillips VR, Holden MR, Sneath RW, Short JL, et al. Concentrations and Emissions of Airborne Dust in Livestock Buildings in Northern Europe. J agric Engng Res. 1998;70(1):19.
26. Seedorf J, Hartung J. Dust and microorganisms in animal housing. 2002.
27. Rinderer R. Mini-Schweine: BOOKS ON DEMAND GMBH. 2010.
28. Von Engelhardt W. Physiologie der Haustiere. Stuttgart: Enke; 2005.

2

Sample size and number of outcome measures of veterinary randomised controlled trials of pharmaceutical interventions funded by different sources

K. J. Wareham[1], R. M. Hyde[1], D. Grindlay[2], M. L. Brennan[1] and R. S. Dean[1*]

Abstract

Background: Randomised controlled trials (RCTs) are a key component of the veterinary evidence base. Sample sizes and defined outcome measures are crucial components of RCTs.
To describe the sample size and number of outcome measures of veterinary RCTs either funded by the pharmaceutical industry or not, published in 2011.

Methods: A structured search of PubMed identified RCTs examining the efficacy of pharmaceutical interventions. Number of outcome measures, number of animals enrolled per trial, whether a primary outcome was identified, and the presence of a sample size calculation were extracted from the RCTs. The source of funding was identified for each trial and groups compared on the above parameters.

Results: Literature searches returned 972 papers; 86 papers comprising 126 individual trials were analysed. The median number of outcomes per trial was 5.0; there were no significant differences across funding groups ($p = 0.133$). The median number of animals enrolled per trial was 30.0; this was similar across funding groups ($p = 0.302$). A primary outcome was identified in 40.5% of trials and was significantly more likely to be stated in trials funded by a pharmaceutical company. A very low percentage of trials reported a sample size calculation (14.3%).

Conclusions: Failure to report primary outcomes, justify sample sizes and the reporting of multiple outcome measures was a common feature in all of the clinical trials examined in this study. It is possible some of these factors may be affected by the source of funding of the studies, but the influence of funding needs to be explored with a larger number of trials. Some veterinary RCTs provide a weak evidence base and targeted strategies are required to improve the quality of veterinary RCTs to ensure there is reliable evidence on which to base clinical decisions.

Keywords: Quality, Primary outcome, Study design and data analysis, Clinical trials, Evidence based medicine

* Correspondence: Rachel.Dean@nottingham.ac.uk
[1]Centre for Evidence-based Veterinary Medicine, School of Veterinary Medicine and Science, The University of Nottingham, Sutton Bonington campus, Loughborough LE12 5RD, UK
Full list of author information is available at the end of the article

Background

Randomised controlled trials (RCTs) are one of the main sources of evidence that can be directly used for clinical decision-making around treatment choice. They do however vary in quality, both in conduct and reporting, a problem which can reduce their reliability and usefulness to decision-makers. One important feature of trials is which, and how many, outcomes (or endpoints) are used to assess the effectiveness of an intervention. An outcome can be defined as:

> *"A component of a participant's clinical and functional status after an intervention has been applied, that is used to assess the effectiveness of an intervention."* (www.cochrane.org/glossary)

All outcomes should be relevant and specific to the question of interest being addressed, and, in almost all cases, should be pre-specified prior to the trial starting and reported in the trial protocol. Any post hoc outcome measures should have a clear rationale for their inclusion. Ideally, one single primary outcome (the outcome considered to be the most important to relevant stakeholders, and which the study is powered for) should be identified, with other outcomes of interest being clearly identified as secondary [1, 2]. Previous assessments of the veterinary clinical trials literature, based on a number of sampling strategies for trial selection, have demonstrated varied reporting standards of outcome measures and identification of primary outcomes. The proportion of trials that identify a primary outcome in previous studies of veterinary RCTs vary from 2% to 83% [3–7]. Understanding the current state of, and potential deficiencies in, outcome reporting is crucial to improve trial design, execution, and reporting and therefore increase the reliability of clinical trial results. The factors that affect the quality of outcome reporting need to be identified if improvements are to be made.

Another crucial factor in the reliability of RCT results is whether the study was adequately powered to detect a difference between two or more variables of interest within the study. Reporting guidelines for RCTs advocate reporting of a sample size calculation to determine the number of subjects required to detect a clinically relevant difference in a specified (primary) outcome between two trial groups [1, 2]. Sample size calculations have been shown in the past to be vastly underreported in the veterinary trials literature [3–7].

In a recent study, we reported that the source of funding (pharmaceutical company or other) has an effect on positive outcome reporting (sponsorship bias) in veterinary clinical trials [8]. The impact of funding on the size of trials and whether a sample size calculation has been undertaken remains unclear in medical RCTs [9–11]. To date, there has been no report of the influence of funding source on the size of veterinary RCTs and whether primary outcomes are stated or a sample size calculation has been undertaken. This study was done concurrently with Wareham et al. [8] to examine further whether funding source has an effect on other aspects of trial design and delivery.

The aim of this study is to describe the number of outcome measures reported, the animals included, whether primary outcome measures are stated and sample size calculations are performed in a sample of veterinary pharmaceutical single dose efficacy RCTs either funded by the pharmaceutical industry or not, published in a single calendar year (2011). The effect of funding source on these aspects of trial design and delivery was then explored.

Methods

A cross-sectional study of RCTs was conducted. The target population was feline, canine, equine, bovine and ovine RCTs where a pharmaceutical agent was the intervention of interest and efficacy was assessed. The sample population was feline, canine, equine, bovine and ovine RCTs published in 2011 within journals indexed in PubMed. This study was conducted in parallel with Wareham et al. [8] and the search strategy and literature filtering processes reported in full in that manuscript also apply to this study The same sample of literature was used for data extraction in both studies [8].

Search strategy and filtering of results

A structured search of PubMed was conducted in June 2013 using the "clinical trial" Publication Type combined with the relevant species MeSH heading e.g. "clinical trial" [publication type] AND cats [mh]. This was done for each of the 5 species studied: cats, dogs, horses, cattle and sheep. The search was limited to one calendar year with a PubMed filter: 01/01/11 – 31/12/11. Search results were exported into EndNote® software for filtering. Papers indexed as RCTs by PubMed ("randomised controlled trials" [publication type]) were extracted and confirmed if, when reviewed by the authors, they were RCTs according to the Cochrane definition below (http://www.cochrane.org/glossary/):

> "An experiment in which two or more interventions, possibly including a control intervention or no intervention, are compared by being randomly allocated to participants. In most trials one intervention is assigned to each individual but sometimes assignment is to defined groups of individuals (for example, in a household) or interventions are assigned within individuals (for example, in different orders or to different parts of the body)."

All publications containing RCTs, published in 2011, and relevant to the species of interest were then categorised into four intervention subcategories based on the main intervention of interest of the study (Table 1 - Level 1 exclusion criteria):

1. Pharmaceutical – consisting of an active pharmaceutical ingredient
2. Nutritional
3. Para-pharmaceutical – including probiotics, prebiotics, synbiotics, nutraceuticals and supplements/ vitamins/minerals if not considered part of the total dietary ration
4. Other – including surgical interventions, management/husbandry interventions, non-medicinal shampoos, studies relating to diagnostic tests.

Only publications within the 'Pharmaceutical intervention' subcategory were included in this study; these were assessed for further eligibility for analysis according to the second level of inclusion and exclusion criteria in Table 1.

Publications included in the analysis were therefore single dose efficacy studies of pharmaceutical interventions in cats, dogs, horses, cattle or sheep published in 2011. The single dose trials were selected for analysis as it was then possible to be certain an outcome was assigned to a single treatment. The trials included animals with naturally occurring and experimentally induced disease. A single calendar year was chosen to ensure it was feasible to complete this work within the timeframe of the funding in a situation where the total number of veterinary RCTs published per year is unknown. The year 2011 was chosen, as it was hoped that by the time the searching was done (June 2013) the 2011 trials would be fully indexed therefore possible to locate in PubMed and any erratum reported. In the case of a publication containing more than one trial, each trial was included independently in the analysis if it met all inclusion criteria.

Table 1 Two levels of inclusion and exclusion criteria applied to the search results

Level 1: Inclusion criteria for publications	Level 1: Exclusion criteria for publications
Species of interest is cats, dogs, horses, cattle or sheep	Not about cats, dogs, horses, cattle or sheep
Published in 2011	E published only in 2011 if full publication occurred in a different calendar year
RCT according to PubMed publication types and the Cochrane definition	Not an RCT (not indexed as an RCT by PubMed or not fulfilling Cochrane definition of an RCT)
Treatment of interest is a pharmaceutical intervention	Treatment of interest is not a pharmaceutical agent e.g. nutritional, surgical, animal husbandry etc
Level 2: Inclusion criteria for analysis of pharmaceutical RCTs	Level 2: Exclusion criteria for analysis of pharmaceutical RCTs
Primary aim is to assess efficacy	Primary aim was not to assess efficacy (pharmacokinetic/ dynamic studies, safety studies, physiological effects, resistance testing, testing routes of administration only, testing timing of administration only)
Identifiable treatment or protocol of interest	Treatment or protocol of interest could not be identified
Single dose of the treatment of interest used	Multiple doses of the treatment of interest used/dose finding studies
Published in English	Not available in English

Sources of funding

For each included trial the source of funding was categorised as one of the following:

1. Pharmaceutical company funding stated or pharmaceutical company involvement (e.g. drug donated by a pharmaceutical company or authors associated with a pharmaceutical company) (P)
2. Non-pharmaceutical company funding stated (NP)
3. No funding source stated (NF)

Outcome recording

A data extraction form (Additional file 1) was used by the authors. Outcomes mentioned in the materials and methods section of the manuscripts were included in the analysis; outcomes that were reported as results but not mentioned in the methods were not included. Outcomes that had multiple components (e.g. complete blood count, serum biochemistry, and meat yield and meat quality grade assessments) were classed as a single outcome each unless specific features were relevant to the disease, in which case these were extracted as individual outcomes.

The following information was extracted:

1) **Total number of outcome results:** Every result for each unique outcome measure is included in this total. Where multiple treatment and control groups were used, each group containing the treatment of interest (either alone or in combination) was compared to its relevant control group for each outcome measure i.e. each unique outcome measure could actually be recorded more than once within this total. For example, a trial measuring heart rate and respiratory rate, which compared two different treatment groups to a control group, would have a total number of 4 outcome results.

2) **Number of unique outcome measures:** The number of individual outcome measures mentioned in the methods section of the manuscripts, i.e. each mentioned outcome measure included only once in this total. For example, a trial measuring heart rate and respiratory rate would have a unique number of 2 outcome measures.
3) **Primary outcome measure:** If the primary outcome measure was stated this was recorded. Trials reporting only one outcome measure, or completing a sample size calculation for one specific outcome measure were automatically categorised as having identified a primary outcome.
4) **Number of animals:** The number of animals enrolled in each trial was recorded.
5) **Sample size calculation:** Reporting of a sample size calculation was recorded as 'yes' or 'no'. Post-hoc power calculations were recorded as 'no'.

All assessments made throughout the study were agreed upon by two authors (KW and RH/RD) with any disputes resolved by a third author (RD/RH). The authors who undertook the assessments of the studies are all veterinary surgeons with methodological expertise in study design and critical appraisal.

Statistical analysis

Categorical data were presented descriptively as raw numbers and percentages. Numerical discrete data that were not normally distributed were presented as median, inter-quartile range (IQR) and range (R). Within a data set, if some subsets of data were non-normally distributed, all were presented as median, IQR and R. Statistical comparisons between funding categories for the number of outcomes measured, number of unique outcome measures, and the number of animals in the trials, were made using an independent samples Kruskal-Wallis test with a significance level of 0.05. Statistical comparisons between funding categories for whether a primary outcome was stated or not and whether a sample size calculation was done or not were made using Fishers Exact test with a significance level of 0.05. The NP and NF groups were sometimes combined and compared to the P group (the group od interest) as there were far more trials stated to be funded by pharmaceutical companies than other sources, Results for different species are described only and were not compared statistically due to small group sizes. All statistical analyses were conducted in IBM SPSS Version 21.

Results

Study numbers

Initial searches returned 972 papers across the five species studied. Following application of the two levels of exclusion criteria (Table 1), 86 papers reporting 126 individual trials remained for data extraction and analysis (Table 2, Additional file 2; for full details see 20). Of the 126 trials, 86 (68%) were in the pharmaceutical funding category, 19 (15%) were in the non-pharmaceutical funding category and the remaining 21 (17%) were in the 'no funding source stated' category.

Number of outcomes reported

Total number of outcome results

The median total number of outcome results reported per trial was 5.0, with a large overall range (IQR = 3.0–11.0, Range = 1.0–36.0, N = 126, Table 3). For individual funding categories, the highest number of outcomes reported per trial (N = 9.0) occurred in the non-pharmaceutical funding category (IQR = 3.0–16.0, Range = 2.0–24.0) compared to 5.0 (IQR = 3.0–9.3, Range = 1.0-36.0) in the pharmaceutical category and 6.0 (IQR = 2.5–14.5, Range = 1.0–26.0) in the 'no

Table 2 Number and funding source of papers and individual trials following level 2 exclusion criteria application

	Number of cat papers (trials)	Number of dog papers (trials)	Number of horse papers (trials)	Number of cattle papers (trials)	Number of sheep papers (trials)	Total number of papers (trials, % of total trials)
Papers including pharmaceutical agent RCTs	17	49	28	61	17	172
Papers excluded from analysis	9	21	17	29	10	86
Papers analysed	8 (9 trials)	28 (44 trials)	11 (11 trials)	32 (36 trials)	7 (26 trials)	86 (126 trials)
Funding sources of analysed papers						
Pharmaceutical company funded/ pharmaceutical company involvement	4 (5 trials)	17 (33 trials)	4 (4 trials)	20 (23 trials)	2 (21 trials)	47 (86 trials; 68%)
Non pharmaceutical funding stated	3 (3 trials)	4 (4 trials)	2 (2 trials)	6 (7 trials)	3 (3 trials)	18 (19 trials; 15%)
No funding stated	1 (1 trial)	7 (7 trials)	5 (5 trials)	6 (6 trials)	2 (2 trials)	21 (21 trials; 17%)

Included studies are the pharmaceutical agent RCTs. Table reproduced from REF companion manuscript

Table 3 Number of outcomes reported per trial for funding categories and individual species

		Median	Interquartile range	Range
Species	Cats (*N* = 9)	10.0	5.5–14.0	2.0–24.0
	Dogs (*N* = 44)	4.5	2.0–5.0	1.0–36.0
	Horses (*N* = 11)	12.0	7.0–14.0	1.0–26.0
	Cattle (*N* = 36)	5.5	3.0–11.8	1.0–36.0
	Sheep (*N* = 26)	5.0	3.0–8.5	1.0–18.0
Funding category	Trials with pharmaceutical funding/ involvement (*N* = 86)	5.0	3.0–9.3	1.0–36.0
	Trials with non-pharmaceutical funding stated (*N* = 19)	9.0	3.0–16.0	2.0–24.0
	Trials with no funding source stated (*N* = 21)	6.0	2.5–14.5	1.0–26.0
All funding categories and species combined	All trials (*N* = 126)	5.0	3.0–11.0	1.0–36.0

funding source declared' category. The differences between funding categories were not significant (p = 0.133).

Number of unique outcome measures

Overall, the median number of unique outcome measures per trial (discounting instances where the same outcome measure was recorded more than once) were lower but largely similar to the results for the total number of outcomes reported (Median = 5.0, IQR = 3.0–8.0, Range = 1.0–36.0, Additional file 2: Table S1). The differences between funding categories were not significant (p = 0.26).

Primary outcome identification

Overall, 51 out of the 126 trials (40.5%) defined a primary outcome (Table 4). A significantly larger proportion of all trials within the pharmaceutical funding category identified a primary outcome compared to the other funding groups (P = 42/86, 48.8%; NP = 4/19, 21.1%; NF = 5/21, 23.8%; p = 0.01). The proportions of trials defining a primary outcome did vary from this pattern across the different species, with sheep having the largest proportion of trials identifying a primary outcome, and horses the lowest (Table 4).

Number of animals per trial

Overall the median number of animals enrolled per trial was 30, with a large associated range (IQR = 17.5–98.8, Range = 5–5996, Table 5). The median number of animals enrolled per trial was broadly similar and not significantly different between all the funding categories (*P* = 30.0, NP = 24.0, NF = 42.0, p = 0.302; Table 5). The number of animals enrolled per trial was similar across all the species examined except for cattle where it was noticeably higher (cats = 32.0, dogs = 27.5, horses = 26.0, cattle = 233.0 and sheep = 20.0; Table 5).

Sample size calculations

Within the 126 trials, only 18 (14.3%) reported performing a sample size calculation. The proportions of trials across the funding groups reporting a sample size calculation were low and very similar, with no statistical difference across the funding groups (PH = 12/86, 14.0%; NP = 3/19, 15.8%; NF = 3/21, 14.3%, p = 0.9). Again, there were differences across the species in the proportions within each category ranging from 0% of sheep trials, to 27.8% of cattle trials reporting a sample size calculation (Table 6).

Discussion

This sample of 126 veterinary RCTs reported multiple outcomes (median of 5 per trial) assessed on a relatively

Table 4 Number and percentages of trials identifying a primary outcome for individual species and funding categories

	Trials with pharmaceutical funding/ involvement	Trials with non-pharmaceutical funding stated	Trials with no funding source stated	All trials
Cats	2/5 (40%)	1/3 (33.3%)	1/1 (100%)	4/9 (44.4%)
Dogs	8/33 (24.2%)	2/4 (50%)	1/7 (14.3%)	11/44 (25%)
Horses	2/4 (50%)	0/2 (0%)	0/5 (0%)	2/11 (18.2%)
Cattle	11/23 (47.8%)	1/7 (14.3%)	2/6 (33.3%)	14/36 (38.9%)
Sheep	19/21 (90.5%)	0/3 (0%)	1/2 (50%)	20/26 (76.9%)
All species	42/86 (48.8%)	4/19 (21.1%)	5/21 (23.8%)	51/126 (40.5%)

Table 5 Numbers of animals enrolled per trial for individual species and funding categories

		Median	Interquartile range	Range
Species	Cats (*N* = 9)	32.0	21.5–93.0	16.0–121.0
	Dogs (*N* = 44)	27.5	16.0–43.0	5.0–316.0
	Horses (*N* = 11)	26.0	15.0 – 61.0	6.0–373.0
	Cattle (*N* = 36)	233.0	35.0–943.0	8.0–5996.0
	Sheep (*N* = 26)	20.0	19.0–24.8	10.0–655.0
Funding category	Trials with pharmaceutical funding/ involvement (*N* = 86)	30.0	19.8–125.8	7.0–5996.0
	Trials with non-pharmaceutical funding stated (*N* = 19)	24.0	14.0–69.0	8.0–369.0
	Trials with no funding source stated (*N* = 21)	42.0	16.0–75.0	5.0–1031.0
All funding categories and species combined	All trials (*N* = 126)	30.0	17.5–98.8	5.0–5996.0

small number of (median 30) animals per trial. Less than half of the trials specified a primary outcome in their materials and methods and sample size calculations were rarely performed. Of these measures only whether a primary outcome measure was defined or not was significantly affected by the source of funding.

The influence that the source of funding has on the reporting of RCTs was recently reported in a related manuscript [8] and it was found that trials with pharmaceutical company involvement were more likely to have positive outcomes of treatment (sponsorship bias) Wareham et al. found that across all trials, regardless of funding, it was found that due to poor reporting and/or conduct of the trials an unclear risk of bias was highly prevalent [8]. In the current study only whether a primary outcome was reported or not seemed to be significantly affected by funding source. However the current study is a descriptive hypothesis generating study and the number of trials in some of the funding categories may be subject to both Type I and Type II errors. The reasons behind why funding source may affect how outcomes are measured and reported and the size of trials are unclear. In medical RCTs, there has been some suggestion that funding source may influence the size of trials across a number of different pharmaceutical, surgical and nursing interventions, so further investigation in the veterinary field may be warranted [9–11].

A median value of 5 outcomes per trial is lower than has been previously reported in similar studies of veterinary clinical trials. Other reports include a mean of 10.8 outcomes per trial in a study examining dog and cat clinical trials [5], and a median of 8.5 outcomes per trial in livestock clinical trials [3]. These studies were published in 2010 and 2009 respectively and a comparison of their results with the ones in this study could be interpreted as a general reduction in the number of outcomes reported per trial over time. Alternatively, methodological differences between the previous studies and this one could explain the findings. For example, the studies all include differing subsets of literature (e.g. clinical trials versus RCTs, any intervention versus pharmaceutical interventions only, different ranges of species included) and employ different data extraction methods. Interestingly, the non-pharmaceutical funding group in the current study had a similar median number of outcomes per trial (9.0) to these previous studies, with the pharmaceutical funding group having a lower median (5.0), although the ranges are wide and differences not significant within this sample. The maximum number of outcomes reported per trial was 36. One concern with having large numbers of outcomes in a trial is that statistically, the ability to accurately detect a difference between two groups diminishes as an increasing number of statistical tests are performed on a limited amount of

Table 6 Numbers and percentages of trials reporting sample size calculations for individual species and funding categories

	Trials with pharmaceutical funding/ involvement	Trials with non-pharmaceutical funding stated	Trials with no funding source stated	All trials
Cats	1/5 (20%)	0/3 (0%)	1/1 (100%)	2/9 (22.2%)
Dogs	2/33 (6.1%)	2/4 (50%)	1/7 (14.3%)	5/44 (11.4%)
Horses	0/4 (0%)	0/2 (0%)	1/5 (20%)	1/11 (9.1%)
Cattle	9/23 (39.1%)	1/7 (14.3%)	0/6 (0%)	10/36 (27.8%)
Sheep	0/21 (0%)	0/3 (0%)	0/2 (0%)	0/26 (0%)
All	12/86 (14.0%)	3/19 (15.8%)	3/21 (14.3%)	18/126 (14.3%)

data (and number of subjects), that is, the chance of introducing 'error' into the results increases [12]. However, if a trial is well designed and adequately powered a primary outcome and a number of secondary outcomes can be investigated if the sample size, statistical analysis are appropriate. In this study, trials involving cats and horses appeared to have a higher median number of outcomes per trial compared to the other species; however the small sample sizes make drawing conclusions from this problematic.

Selecting and properly defining a primary outcome (in advance of conducting a trial) is extremely important, and is outlined in the CONSORT RCT reporting guideline and the adapted livestock version REFLECT [1, 13, 14]. In the current study, 40% of trials specified a primary outcome and trials in the pharmaceutical funding category more frequently identified a primary outcome compared to the other groups. Previous studies have reported extremely varied findings on this topic with the number of trials defining a primary outcome varying from 86% of small animal RCTs [4] to 7% in dog and cat clinical trials [5]. If primary and secondary outcomes are not pre-specified and adhered to, there is the risk that throughout a trial, the most 'interesting' results can be reported rather than those the trial was designed to address. On the other hand, outcomes that prove to be 'negative' in respect to the treatment of interest may not be reported, biasing the evidence base. Such 'outcome switching' is currently being tracked in human trials literature by the COMPARE initiative [15]. Without a trials registry, where protocols can be made available before a trial begins, it is extremely difficult to track and address this issue.

Primary outcomes are also important as they are the measures used to determine the number of animals required for the trial, via a sample size calculation. The low percentage of authors reporting that they have undertaken a sample size calculation in this study is actually higher than previously found; reports have varied from 0 to 18% [3–7] which again could reflect a genuine improvement over time, or a difference in the sample of literature studied. The number of animals actually enrolled per trial encompassed a very large range (5-5996) with noticeably higher numbers of animals enrolled in cattle trials compared to the other species potentially reflecting the easier recruitment of large numbers of animals within herds to a trial. When a sample size calculation is not reported, the reader cannot easily identify if the number of subjects in the trial was sufficient to detect a difference between two intervention groups, even if such a difference exists [16], or if the identification of a difference between two groups is reliable. Conversely, excessively large sample sizes are an ethical concern as more participants are exposed to potential risks than is necessary [2, 16]. Whilst an adequately powered study is the ideal situation, there are advocates of the theory that some evidence is better than no evidence, and smaller trials can be performed and later combined in evidence syntheses to contribute substantially to the evidence base. There are certain caveats to this approach, which are that trials must be of sound methodological design to eliminate bias, and it is extremely important that all trials are published so they are available for evidence synthesis [17].

The proportions of trials defining a primary outcome, and particularly those reporting a sample size calculation, were vastly lower in the current study, and others in the veterinary literature, compared to those in the medical literature [18]. There are still huge improvements to be made; one way of improving how well veterinary RCTs are reported is through the endorsement and increased awareness of relevant reporting guidelines (e.g. CONSORT, REFLECT) by both authors and journals. Another approach to improve trial conduct, increase the transparency of RCTs, and reduce publication bias, is through compulsory registration of trial protocols, as advocated by the 'All-Trials' and 'Veterinary All-Trials' campaigns (www.alltrials.net), [19]. A veterinary clinical trials unit comprising a large network of practices would also be of huge benefit to the veterinary profession. It would enable access to large numbers of patients, records and provide centralised expertise and advice allowing the generation of high quality, relevant evidence. A cross-discipline approach where academia and industry work more closely together could also be beneficial for raising the overall standards of veterinary trials.

Strengths and limitations

To the authors knowledge, in veterinary medicine no-one has yet investigated the role of funding on the reporting of outcomes and size of RCTs involving veterinary species. This unique manuscript compliments Wareham et al. [12] and describes the potential role of funding in study design. The manuscript also provides further insight into outcome reporting and size of trials on a different sample of veterinary RCTs compared to those already published [3–7].

One major limitation of this study is the imbalance in trial numbers across the funding categories due to the large proportion of trials in the pharmaceutical funding group, resulting in the number of trials in the non-pharmaceutical funding group and the 'no funding source declared' group being relatively small. Of particular concern is that studies encompassing more than one trial (for example, one sheep study comprised 19 individual trials) tended to be in the pharmaceutical funding category and could have caused clustering of the data. Another limitation is that authors were not blinded to manuscript details while extracting data. Time and financial constraints limited this study to one calendar year of publications, which did not yield enough trials to rule exclude the possibility of Type II errors hence this is primarily a descriptive report of these RCTs. Hence a larger study, powered using the data from this study incorporating more years of publications would be beneficial; in particular this could allow potential species specific differences to be explored. In addition, only Medline was searched and it has been shown previously that Medline does not include all clinical veterinary literature [20] however, it does have functionality that enables RCTs to be identified. This does mean that not all trials in 2011 that met our inclusion criteria would have been found. An inherent problem for all studies investigating the quality of veterinary RCTs is the reliance on good reporting to enable the investigators to adequately analyse the trials.

Conclusions

The results of this study are important to those who use the results of pharmaceutical trials to inform practice and to researchers undertaking RCTs with veterinary species. The findings contribute to the body of knowledge indicating that veterinary clinical trials could be substantially improved in terms of reporting, and almost certainly design and execution, irrespective of funding source. It is difficult to accurately assess the true strength of trial conduct when they are poorly reported. Ultimately, the low quantity and quality of evidence available to veterinary practitioners severely inhibits our ability to practice in an evidence-based way; improvements are essential to ensure the veterinary profession has a sound scientific knowledge base on which to make clinical decisions, ensuring the best care for patients.

Abbreviations

CONSORT: Consolidated Standards for Reporting Trials; IQR: Interquartile range; NF: Group of trials for which no funding source was stated; NP: Group of trials for which non-pharmaceutical funding was stated; P: Group of trials for which pharmaceutical funding/involvement was stated; R: Range; RCT: Randomised controlled trial; REFLECT: Reporting guidelines for randomised control trials for livestock and food safety

Acknowledgements

Not applicable.

Funding

This work was supported by an unrestrictive grant from Elanco Animal Health and The University of Nottingham. The topic of study, study design, statistical analysis, interpretation of the results, decision to publish and writing of the manuscript were undertaken independently of all funders of the CEVM.

Authors' contributions

All authors were involved in the design of the research project. DG, KW and RH designed the searching strategies. KW, RH and RD extracted and analysed the data. All authors were involved in interpreting the analysed data. KW wrote the draft manuscript. All authors contributed to editing the manuscript. All authors read and approved the final manuscript.

Consent for publication

Not applicable.

Competing interests

The Centre for Evidence-based Veterinary Medicine (CEVM) is supported by an unrestrictive grant from Elanco Animal Health and The University of Nottingham. Three of the authors (KW, DG and RD) were funded by this grant, MB by the University of Nottingham and RH was an undergraduate veterinary student at the University Of Nottingham and then worked in private practice during the completion of this work. KW is currently funded by a grant from Elanco Animal Health.

Author details

[1]Centre for Evidence-based Veterinary Medicine, School of Veterinary Medicine and Science, The University of Nottingham, Sutton Bonington campus, Loughborough LE12 5RD, UK. [2]Centre of Evidence Based Dermatology, The University of Nottingham King's Meadow Campus Lenton Lane, Nottingham NG7 2NR, UK.

References

1. Moher D, Hopewell S, Schulz KF, Montori V, Gotzsche PC, Devereaux PJ, Elbourne D, Egger M, Altman DG: CONSORT 2010 Explanation and elaboration: updated guidelines for reporting parallel group randomised trials. Int J Surg 2012; 10(1):28-55.
2. Sargeant JM, O'Connor AM, Gardner IA, Dickson JS, Torrence ME, Dohoo IR, Lefebvre SL, Morley PS, Ramirez A, Snedeker K. The REFLECT statement: reporting guidelines for randomized controlled trials in livestock and food safety: explanation and elaboration. J Food Protection. 2010;73(3):579–603.
3. Di Girolamo N, Reynders RM. Deficiencies of effectiveness of intervention studies in veterinary medicine: a cross-sectional survey of ten leading veterinary and medical journals. PeerJ. 2016;4:e1649.
4. Giuffrida MA. Type II error and statistical power in reports of small animal clinical trials. J Am Vet Med Assoc. 2014;244(9):1075–80.
5. Sargeant JM, Elgie R, Valcour J, Saint-Onge J, Thompson A, Marcynuk P, Snedeker K. Methodological quality and completeness of reporting in clinical trials conducted in livestock species. Prev Vet Med. 2009;91(2-4):107–15.
6. Lund EM, James KM, Neaton JD. Veterinary randomized clinical trial reporting: a review of the small animal literature. J Vet Intern Med. 1998;12(2):57–60.
7. Sargeant JM, Thompson A, Valcour J, Elgie R, Saint-Onge J, Marcynuk P, Snedeker K. Quality of reporting of clinical trials of dogs and cats and associations with treatment effects. J Vet Intern Med. 2010;24(1):44–50.
8. Wareham KJ, Hyde RM, Grindlay D, Brennan ML, Dean RS. Sponsorship bias and quality of randomised controlled trials in veterinary medicine. BMC Vet Res. 2017;13:234.
9. Vaduganathan M, Samman-Tahhan A, Patel RB, Kelkar A, Papadimitriou L, Georgiopoulou VV, Greene SJ, Kalogeropoulos AP, Peterson E, Fonarow GC, Gheorghiade M. Association between funding sources and the scope and outcomes of cardiovascular clinical trials: a systematic review. Int J Cardiol. 2016;22.

10. Hodgson R, Allen R, Broderick E, Bland JM, Dumville JC, Ashby R, Bell-Syer S, Foxlee R, Hall J, Lamb S, Madden M. Funding source and the quality of reports of chronic wounds trials: 2004 to 2011. Trials. 2014 Jan 14;15(1):19.
11. Jefferson T, Di Pietrantonj C, Debalini MG, Rivetti A, Demicheli V. Relation of study quality, concordance, take home message, funding, and impact in studies of influenza vaccines: systematic review. BMJ. 2009;338:b354.
12. Tukey JW: Some thoughts on clinical trials, especially problems of multiplicity. Science (New York, NY) 1977;198(4318):679–684.
13. Begg C, Cho M, Eastwood S, Horton R, Moher D, Olkin I, Pitkin R, Rennie D, Schulz KF, Simel D, Stroup DF: Improving the quality of reporting of randomized controlled trials. The CONSORT statement. JAMA 1996; 276(8):637-639.
14. O'Connor AM, Sargeant JM, Gardner IA, Dickson JS, Torrence ME, Dewey CE, Dohoo IR, Evans RB, Gray JT, Greiner M, Keefe G, Lefebvre SL, Morley PS, Ramirez A, Sischo W, Smith DR, Snedeker K, Sofos J, Ward MP, Wills R. The REFLECT statement: methods and processes of creating reporting guidelines for randomized controlled trials for livestock and food safety. Prev Vet Med. 2010;93(1):11–8.
15. COMPARE: http://compare-trials.org/.
16. McKeown A, Gewandter JS, McDermott MP, Pawlowski JR, Poli JJ, Rothstein D, Farrar JT, Gilron I, Katz NP, Lin AH, Rappaport BA, Rowbotham MC, Turk DC, Dworkin RH, Smith SM. Reporting of sample size calculations in analgesic clinical trials: ACTTION systematic review. J Pain. 2015;16(3):199–206.e197.
17. Schulz KF, Grimes DA. Sample size calculations in randomised trials: mandatory and mystical. Lancet. 2005;365(9467):1348–53.
18. Hopewell S, Dutton S, Yu LM, Chan AW, Altman DG. The quality of reports of randomised trials in 2000 and 2006: comparative study of articles indexed in PubMed. BMJ. 2010;340:c723.
19. Dean R, Royle N, Boulton C, Turner S, McKenzie B, O'Connor A, Budsberg S, Pion P, Lambert A, Jarvis S, Reynolds S. Veterinary all trials initiative. Vet Rec. 2015;177(5):131–2.
20. Grindlay DJ, Brennan ML, Dean RS. Searching the veterinary literature: a comparison of the coverage of veterinary journals by nine bibliographic databases. Journal of veterinary medical education. 2012;39(4):404–12.

3

Patterns and predictors of antimicrobial resistance among *Staphylococcus* spp. from canine clinical cases presented at a veterinary academic hospital in South Africa

Daniel N. Qekwana[1], James W. Oguttu[2], Fortune Sithole[1,3] and Agricola Odoi[1,4*]

Abstract

Background: Antimicrobial resistance in staphylococci, often associated with treatment failure, is increasingly reported in veterinary medicine. The aim of this study was to investigate patterns and predictors of antimicrobial resistance among *Staphylococcus* spp. isolates from canine samples submitted to the bacteriology laboratory at the University of Pretoria academic veterinary hospital between 2007 and 2012. Retrospective data of 334 *Staphylococcus* isolates were used to calculate the proportion of samples resistant to 15 antimicrobial agents. The Cochran-Armitage trend test was used to investigate temporal trends and logistic regression models were used to investigate predictors of antimicrobial resistance in *Staphylococcus aureus* and *Staphylococcus pseudintermedius*.

Results: Results show that 98.2% (55/56) of the *S. aureus* isolates were resistant to at least one drug while 42.9% were multidrug resistant. Seventy-seven percent (214/278) of the *S. pseudintermedius* isolates were resistant to at least one drug and 25.9% (72/278) were multidrug resistant. Resistance to lincospectin was more common among *S. aureus* (64.3%) than *S. pseudintermedius* (38.9%). Similarly, resistance to clindamycin was higher in *S. aureus* (51.8%) than *S. pseudintermedius* (31.7%) isolates. There was a significant ($p = 0.005$) increase in *S. aureus* resistance to enrofloxacin over the study period. Similarly, *S. pseudintermedius* exhibited significant increasing temporal trend in resistance to trimethoprim-sulphamethoxazole ($p = 0.004$), clindamycin ($p = 0.022$) and orbifloxacin ($p = 0.042$). However, there was a significant decreasing temporal trend in the proportion of isolates resistant to doxycycline ($p = 0.041$), tylosin ($p = 0.008$), kanamycin ($p = 0.017$) and amoxicillin/clavulanic acid ($p = 0.032$).

Conclusions: High levels of multidrug resistance and the increasing levels of resistance to sulphonamides, lincosamides and fluoroquinolones among *Staphylococcus* spp. isolates in this study are concerning. Future studies will need to investigate local drivers of antimicrobial resistance to better guide control efforts to address the problem.

Keywords: *Staphylococcus aureus*, *Staphylococcus pseudintermedius*, multidrug resistance, MDR, Antimicrobial resistance, AMR, dogs, canine, predictors, risk factors

* Correspondence: aodoi@utk.edu
[1]Section of Veterinary Public Health, Department of Paraclinical Sciences, Faculty of Veterinary Science, University of Pretoria, Pretoria, South Africa
[4]Biomedical and Diagnostic Sciences, College of Veterinary Medicine, University of Tennessee, Knoxville, USA
Full list of author information is available at the end of the article

Background

Resistance of *Staphylococcus* spp. organisms to antimicrobial agents used in dogs may complicate treatments and result in increased morbidity, mortality and financial burdens to the owners [1]. According to Werckenthin et al. [2], the prevalence of antimicrobial drug resistance in staphylococcal infections in dogs, cattle and pigs is on the rise. Prescott et al. [3], in their study conducted in Canada, observed that the majority of *S. intermedius* isolates were resistant to enrofloxacin and gentamycin. In another study by Hauschild and Wójcik [4] carried out in Poland, it was reported that 41% and 35% of *S. intermedius* isolates tested were resistant to erythromycin and clindamycin, respectively. In both studies, the authors attributed the high levels of resistance to changes in the pattern of antimicrobial use for treatment of staphylococcal infections. Moreover, Hauschild and Wójcik [4] as well as Pellerin et al. [5] suggest that rapid introduction and the over prescription of new antimicrobial drugs in companion animals may also be contributing to the increased antimicrobial resistance seen in staphylococcal organisms. Hoekstra and Paulton [6] also reported that the type of organism, site of isolation, sex and age of the dogs is associated with the risk of resistance.

In South Africa, 269,794 kg of parenteral antimicrobials were sold between 2002 and 2004, with penicillins being the most commonly (60%) sold antimicrobial followed by tetracyclines (32%) [7]. A study by Kudakwashe [8] on antimicrobial usage patterns among companion animal veterinarians in South Africa reported that the most commonly used antimicrobials by the respondents were cephalosporins (100%), followed by penicillins (98%), quinolones (95%), and lincosamides (52%). In addition, 28% of the respondents indicated that they did not undertake routine antibiograms in cases of therapeutic failures. This is surprising considering 8.% of the respondents indicated that patients returned to the clinic due to treatment failures following use of the prescribed antimicrobials [8].

Although, several studies have reported increased antimicrobial resistance among *S. intermedius* isolates to ampicillin, penicillin and tetracycline [5, 9], not much information is available on antimicrobial resistance trends in *Staphylococcus* spp. in South Africa. Moreover, no work has been done to investigate the predictors of resistance among *Staphylococcus* spp. isolates from clinical cases. Therefore, the aim of this study was to investigate patterns and predictors of antimicrobial resistance among *Staphylococcus* spp. isolates from canine samples submitted to the bacteriology laboratory at the University of Pretoria academic veterinary hospital between 2007 and 2012.

Methods

Data collection and preparation

This was a retrospective study of *Staphylococcus* spp. isolates from canine clinical samples submitted to the University of Pretoria bacteriology laboratory as part of the routine diagnostic evaluation of cases presented to the university veterinary academic hospital between January 2007 and December 2012. All samples originated from cases treated at the university hospital. The bacteriology laboratory does not process samples from other sites/clinics/hospitals implying that samples included in the study are all from animals that were treated at the academic hospital. The data were assessed for duplicate entries, mixed infections (i.e. more than one isolate per sample), and if any animals were sampled multiple times during the study period. No duplicates were identified. Moreover, there were no samples with mixed infections (i.e. no samples with more than one isolate). Additionally, the dataset did not contain multiple tests from the same patient. The analyses were performed at isolate-level. However, since each sample had only one isolate, it implies that the results of isolate-level analysis are the same as sample level analysis (i.e. no problem of clustering arises).

A total of 334 confirmed *Staphylococcus* isolates consisting of *S. aureus* or *S. pseudintermedius* isolates were included in this study. Each case included in the analysis had data on the following variables: site of collection, breed, sex, age, date of submission and the antimicrobial agents tested. The American Kennel Club (AKC) breed classification was modified and used to classify breeds of dogs into the following categories: working, sporting, herding, hound, toy, terrier, nonsporting and mix-breed (http://www.akc.org/dog-breeds/). *Staphylococcus* species were identified based on the phenotypic characteristics including colony characteristics, catalase, D-mannitol, deoxyribonuclease (DNase) tests, and Gram-staining as described by Quinn et al. [10].

Antimicrobial susceptibility testing

Staphylococcus isolates were subjected to antimicrobial susceptibility testing against a panel of 15 drugs using the disc diffusion method. The following antimicrobials were included in the panel: 30 μg amikacin (AK), 30 μg doxycycline (DOX30), 5 μg enrofloxacin (ENR), 10 μg gentamicin (CN), 10 μg ampicillin (AM) 10 μg penicillin G (P), 25 μg trimethoprim-sulphamethoxazole (co-trimoxazole) (SXT), 30 μg chloramphenicol (C), 30 μg cephalothin (KF), 30 μg kanamycin (K), 2 μg clindamycin (MY), 100 μg lincospectin (LS100), 5 μg orbifloxacin (OBX5), 20/10 μg amoxicillin/clavulanic acid (AMC20/10) and 15 μg tylosin (TY). Unfortunately, since the laboratory does not routinely assess for methicillin susceptibility, the panel did not include this drug and therefore this study was not able to investigate the resistance of *Staphylococcus* spp. to methicillin. The laboratory from where the data were obtained, follows the Clinical and Laboratory Standards Institute (CLSI) procedures

[11–17] for isolation, testing and classification to determine the susceptibility profile (Susceptible, Intermediate or Resistant) of *Staphylococcus* isolates. The original raw data with exact diameter measurements of the inhibition zones were not available for this retrospective study. Thus, only interpretations of the susceptibility test results (i.e., Susceptible, Intermediate or Resistant) were available. Therefore, although a newer version of the CLSI document [18] is currently available it was not possible to interpret the susceptibility profile of isolates using this newer version of the document. For the purposes of the study, intermediate susceptibility was considered as susceptible and therefore re-coded as such for all subsequent analyses.

Data analysis

All the statistical analyses were performed using SAS 9.4 (SAS Institute Inc., Cary, NC, USA) statistical package. The data were assessed for missing data and inconsistencies such as improbable values. Age was categorised into <2 years, 2–4 years, 4–6 years, 6–8 years and >8 years. The frequencies and proportions of all categorical variables together with their 95% confidence intervals were calculated. Associations between categorical variables were assessed using the Chi-square or Fishers Exact tests where appropriate. The Cochran–Armitage trend tests were used to assess temporal trends in the proportion of samples resistant to each antimicrobial agent between 2007 and 2012. Statistical significance was assessed at 5% level of significance for all the above tests.

Investigation of the predictors of antimicrobial resistance (resistance to at least one antimicrobial) was performed in two steps. In the first step simple binary logistic regression models were fitted with antimicrobial resistance status (yes/no) as the outcome and each of the suspected predictors available in the dataset (age, sex, breed) as the explanatory variables. For each of the simple binary logistic regression models, the predictor variables with p-values less than 0.20 were considered for inclusion in the multivariable logistic regression model fit in the second step of the modeling effort. In this second step, a multivariable logistic regression model using manual backwards selection was fitted containing all variables that had potential univariate associations ($p < 0.2$) with the outcome. Confounding was assessed by comparing the change in parameter estimate of the variables in the model with and without the suspected confounding variable. If there was a 20% change in the estimate, the variable of interest was considered to be a significant confounder and was retained in the final model. The odds ratios and their corresponding 95% confidence intervals were computed for all variables included in the final model. The predictor variables with p-values <0.05 were considered to be statistically significant based on the Wald Chi-Squared Test. Steps 1 and 2 above were repeated with binary (yes/no) multidrug resistance (resistance to three or more antimicrobial classes) as the outcome variable. Goodness of fit of the final models was assessed using the Hosmer-Lemeshow goodness of fit test.

Results

Antimicrobial resistance patterns

Of the 1497 samples tested, 26.5% (396/1497) were *Staphylococcus* positive and included *S. aureus* (n = 57), *S. epidermidis* (n = 11), *S. pseudintermedius* (n = 284), *Staphylococcus*. spp. (n = 43) and *S. felis* (n = 1). Seven isolates [*S. pseudintermedius* (n = 6) and *S. aureus* (n = 1)] were not included in subsequent analyses due to missing information. Therefore, this study focuses only on the 334 samples that were positive for *S. pseudintermedius* (n = 278) or *S. aureus* (n = 56) and that did not have missing information. Twenty-five different types of specimens tested positive for *Staphylococcus* spp. with the skin contributing the most samples (34.4%, 115/334), followed by ear canal (29.9%, 100/334) while the rest of the 23 different specimen types making up the remaining 35.6% (119/334).

Over 50% of the *S. aureus* isolates were resistant to ampicillin (66.1%), penicillin (64.3%), lincospectin (64.3%), and clindamycin (51.8%). Similarly, over 50% of the *S. pseudintermedius* isolates were resistance to ampicillin (57.9%) and penicillin (54.3%) (Fig. 1). In addition, significant differences were observed in the proportion of *S. pseudintermedius* and *S. aureus* resistance to lincospectin (p = 0.0006) and clindamycin (p = 0.0055) (Fig. 1). In both instances, the proportion of *S. aureus* isolates were significantly higher than those of *S. pseudintermedius* isolates. These results show that the level of resistance among *Staphylococcus* isolates from dogs presented at the teaching hospital was very high, and also showed that *S. aureus* tended to exhibit higher resistance levels to certain antimicrobials compared to *S. pseudintermedius*.

Temporal patterns in resistance patterns of *S. aureus* and *S. pseudintermedius*

The proportions of *S. aureus* isolates resistant to the different antimicrobials is shown in Table 1. Cochran-Armitage trend test showed that the proportion of *S. aureus* isolates that were resistant to doxycycline (p = 0.0412) or tylosin (p = 0.0083) significantly decreased from 37.5% in 2007 to 0.0% in 2012, while the proportion resistant to kanamycin significantly (p = 0.0167) decreased from 26.7% in 2008 to 0.0% in 2012. Similarly, a significant (p = 0.0317) decrease (37.5 to 0%) in the proportion of *S. aureus* isolates resistant to amoxicillin/clavulanic acid was observed between 2007 and 2011. However,

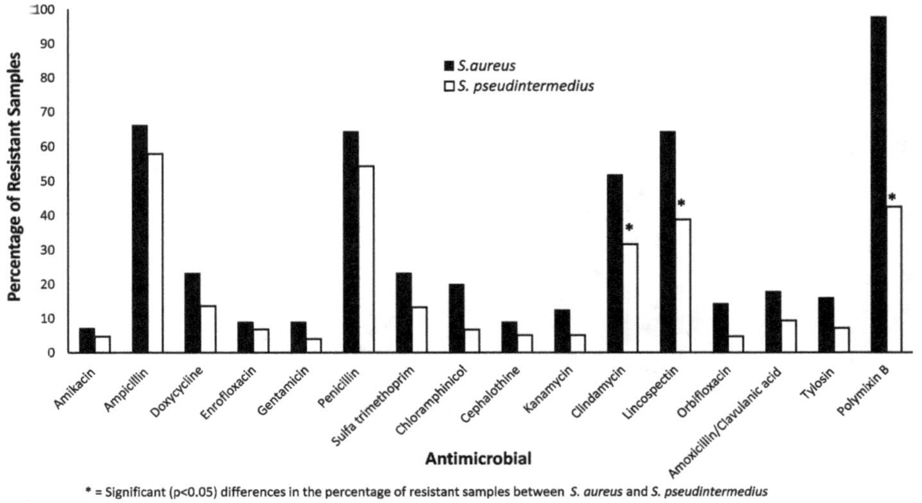

Fig. 1 Proportions of *S. aureus* and *S. pseudintermedius* samples resistant to each of the 15 antimicrobials tested at the University of Pretoria bacteriology laboratory, 2007 and 2012

increasing levels of resistance among *S. aureus* isolates to amoxicillin/clavulanic acid emerged by the end of 2012. A significant (p = 0.0052) increase in the level of resistance to enrofloxacin among *S. aureus* isolates was also observed between 2007 and 2012 (Fig. 2).

The distributions of resistance among *S. pseudintermedius* isolates to the different antimicrobials is shown in Table 2. Significant increases in the proportions of resistant isolates to trimethoprim-sulphamethoxazole (p = 0.0040), clindamycin (p = 0.0221) and orbifloxacin (p = 0.0418) were observed among *S. pseudintermedius* isolates between 2007 and 2012 (Fig. 3, Table 2). Among *S. pseudintermedius* isolates, the proportion that were resistant to clindamycin increased until 2011 (59%) but subsequently decreased to 28% in 2012, while, the proportion of isolates that were resistant to orbifloxacin increased from 0 to 11% by 2012. Similarly, we observed an increase in the proportion of isolates resistant to

Table 1 Trends in antimicrobial resistance of *S. aureus* from samples tested at the University of Pretoria bacteriology laboratory, 2007–2012

Group	Antimicrobials	Resistance to antimicrobial agents by year						[a]*P*-values of CAT Test
		2007	2008	2009	2010	2011	2012	
β-lactams	Penicillin	75.0 (6/8)	80.0 (12/15)	63.6 (7/11)	50.0 (5/10)	50.0 (3/6)	50.0 (3/6)	0.089
	Ampicillin	75.0 (6/8)	80.0 (12/15)	63.6 (7/11)	60.0 (6/10)	50.0 (3/6)	50.0 (3/6)	0.124
	Cephalothin	25.0 (2/8)	6.7 (1/15)	9.1 (1/11)	10.0 (1/10)	0.0 (0/6)	0.0 (0/6)	0.181
Aminoglycosides	Amikacin	0.0 (0/8)	20.0 (3/15)	9.1 (1/11)	0.0 (0/10)	0.0 (0/6)	0.0 (0/6)	0.258
	Gentamicin	12.5 (1/8)	20.0 (3/15)	9.1 (1/11)	0.0 (0/10)	0.0 (0/6)	0.0 (0/6)	0.098
	Kanamycin	25.0 (2/8)	26.7 (4/15)	9.1 (1/11)	0.0 (0/10)	0.0 (0/6)	0.0 (0/6)	0.017
Tetracyclines	Doxycycline	37.5 (3/8)	26.7 (4/15)	36.4 (4/11)	20.0 (2/10)	0.0 (0/6)	0.0 (0/6)	0.041
Fluoroquinolones	Enrofloxacin	0.0 (0/8)	6.7 (1/15)	0.0 (0/11)	0.0 (0/10)	16.7 (1/6)	50.0 (3/6)	0.005
	Orbifloxacin	12.5 (1/8)	20.0 (3/15)	9.1 (1/11)	0.0 (0/10)	16.7 (1/6)	33.3 (2/6)	0.718
Potentiated-sulfas	Co-trimoxazole[b]	37.5 (3/8)	33.3 (5/15)	27.3 (3/11)	10.0 (1/10)	0.0 (0/6)	16.7 (1/6)	0.067
Amphenicols	Chloramphenicol	33.3 (1/3)	20.0 (3/15)	9.1 (1/11)	10.0 (1/10)	40.0 (2/5)	33.3 (2/6)	0.552
Macrolides	Tylosin	37.5 (3/8)	33.3 (5/15)	0.0 (0/11)	10.0 (1/10)	0.0 (0/6)	0.0 (0/6)	0.008
Aminoglycoside-lincosamides	Lincospectin[c]	37.5 (3/8)	80.0 (12/15)	54.6 (6/11)	70.0 (7/10)	50.0 (3/6)	83.3 (5/6)	0.478
Lincosamides	Clindamycin	50.0 (4/8)	60.0 (9/15)	45.5 (5/11)	60.0 (6/10)	50.0 (3/6)	33.3 (2/6)	0.552
Others	Amoxicillin/clavulanic acid	37.5 (3/8)	33.3 (5/15)	9.1 (1/11)	0.0 (0/10)	0.0 (0/6)	16.7 (1/6)	0.032

[a]*P*-values of CAT Test= *P*-value of Cochran-Armitage trend test
[b]Co-trimoxazole = Trimethoprim-sulphamethoxazole
[c]Lincospectin = Espectinomycine-lincomycine

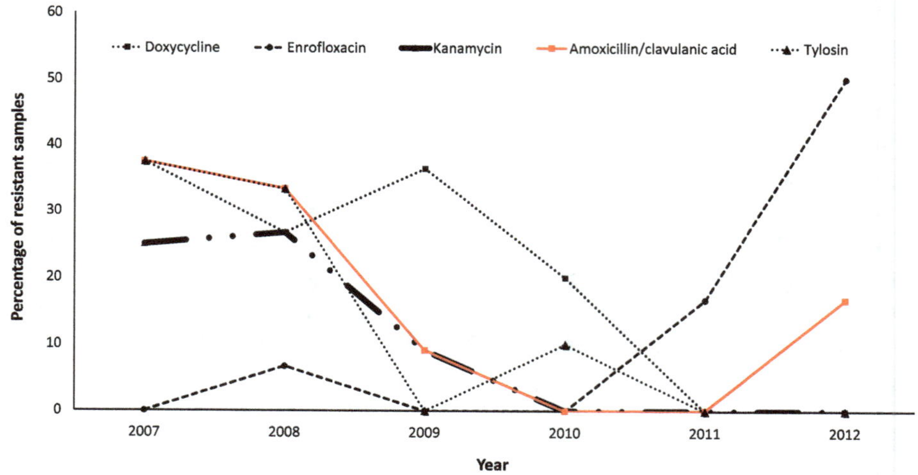

Fig. 2 Antimicrobial agents showing significant temporal trends in resistance based on the Cochran-Armitage trend tests among the *S. aureus* isolates from canine samples tested at the University of Pretoria bacteriology laboratory, 2007–2012

trimethoprim-sulphamethoxazole from 2.5% in 2007 to 22% in 2012 among *S. pseudintermedius* isolates.

Proportions of AMR or MDR among isolates of *S. aureus* and *S. pseudintermedius*

Of the 334 isolates, 80.5% (269/334) exhibited antimicrobial resistance (AMR) to at least one drug, while 28.7% (96/334) were multidrug resistant resistant (MDR). AMR was significantly (p = 0.0003) more common among *S. aureus* (98.2%, 55/56) than *S. pseudintermedius* (76.98%, 214/278). Similarly, MDR was also significantly (p = 0.0105) more frequent among *S. aureus* (42.9%, 24/56) than *S. pseudintermedius* (25.9%, 72/278).

No significant temporal trends were observed in the proportion of AMR *S. aureus* (p = 0.1580) or *S. pseudintermedius* (p = 0.7312) between 2007 and 2012 (Fig. 4). However, the proportion of AMR samples was significantly (p = 0.0003) higher among *S. aureus* than S.

Table 2 Trends in antimicrobial susceptibility of *S. pseudintermedius* to antimicrobial agents from samples tested at the University of Pretoria academic veterinary laboratory, 2007–2012

Group	Antimicrobial	Resistance to antimicrobial agents by year						[a]*P*-value of CAT Test
		2007	2008	2009	2010	2011	2012	
β-lactams	Penicillin	37.5 (15/40)	58.6 (34/58)	50.0 (30/60)	51.2 (22/43)	73.2 (30/41)	55.6 (16/36)	0.052
	Ampicillin	50.0 (20/40)	56.9 (33/58)	53.3 (32/60)	55.8 (24/43)	73.2 (30/41)	61.1 (22/36)	0.104
	Cephalothin	7.5 (3/40)	5.2 (3/58)	5.0 (3/60)	2.3 (1/43)	7.3 (3/41)	2.8 (1/36)	0.555
Aminoglycosides	Amikacin	0.0 (0/40)	13.8 (8/58)	3.3 (2/60)	0.0 (0/43)	4.9 (2/41)	2.8 (1/36)	0.382
	Gentamicin	0.0 (0/40)	10.3 (6/53)	3.3 (2/60)	0.0 (0/43)	2.4 (1/41)	5.6 (2/36)	0.777
	Kanamycin	2.5 (1/40)	3.5 (2/58)	8.3 (5/60)	4.7 (2/43)	4.9 (2/41)	5.6 (2/36)	0.612
Tetracyclines	Doxycycline	12.5 (5/40)	22.4 (13/58)	15.0 (9/60)	2.3 (1/43)	17.1 (7/41)	8.3 (3/36)	0.213
Fluoroquinolones	Enrofloxacin	5.0 (2/40)	5.2 (3/58)	6.7 (4/60)	4.7 (2/43)	4.9 (2/41)	16.7 (6/36)	0.122
	Orbifloxacin	0.0 (0/40)	3.5 (2/58)	6.7 (4/60)	0.0 (0/43)	7.3 (3/41)	11.1 (4/36)	0.042
Potentiated sulfas	Co-trimoxazole[b]	2.5 (1/40)	5.2 (3/58)	20.0 (3/60)	14.0 (2/41)	17.1 (7/41)	22.2 (8/36)	0.004
Amphenicols	Chloramphenicol	4.8 (1/21)	7.0 (4/57)	5.0 (3/60)	4.9 (2/41)	12.8 (5/36)	5.6 (2/36)	0.626
Macrolides	Tylosin	7.5 (3/40)	6.9 (4/58)	6.7 (4/60)	7.0 (3/43)	9.8 (4/41)	5.6 (2/36)	1
Aminoglycoside-lincosamides	Lincospectin[c]	22.5 (9/40)	48.3 (28/58)	26.7 (16/60)	39.5 (17/43)	58.5 (24/41)	38.9 (14/36)	0.066
Lincosamides	Clindamycin	22.5 (9/40)	25.9 (15/58)	26.7 (16/60)	32.6 (14/43)	58.5 (24/41)	27.8 (10/36)	0.022
Others	Amoxicillin/clavulanic acid	22.5 (9/40)	6.9 (4/58)	5.0 (3/60)	2.3 (1/43)	17.1 (7/41)	5.6 (2/36)	0.225

[a]*P*-value of CAT Test = *P*-value of Cochran-Armitage trend test
[b]Co-trimoxazole = Trimethoprim-sulphamethoxazole
[c]Lincospectin = Espectinomycine-lincomycine

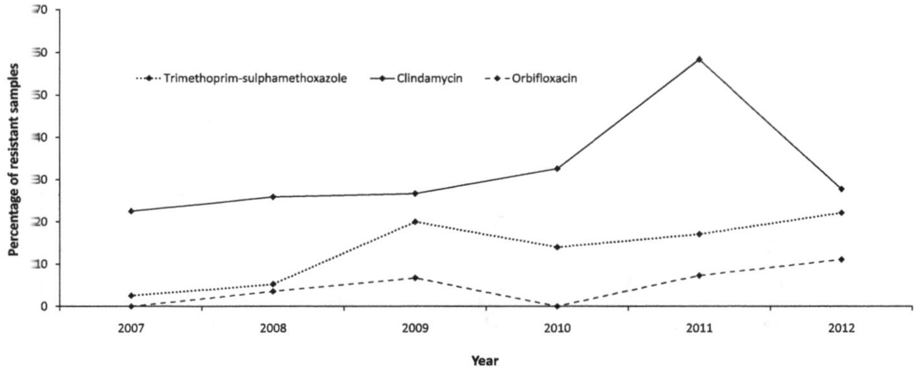

Fig. 3 Antimicrobial agents showing significant temporal trends in resistance based on the Cochran-Armitage trend tests among the *S. pseudintermedius* isolates from canine samples tested at the University of Pretoria bacteriology laboratory, 2007–2012

pseudintermedius. For example, between 2007 and 2012 the proportion of AMR *S. aureus* ranged from 87.5 to 100% compared to 68% to 84% among S. *pseudintermedius* isolates.

MDR *S. aureus* were more common than MDR *S. pseudintermedius* during the period 2007 to 2012 with the exception of 2011. In 2011, 39% of *S. pseudintermedius* were MDR compared to 33% of *S. aureus* isolates. While, between 2007–2010 and 2012 the proportion of MDR *S. aureus* ranged from 53 to 30% compared to 16% to 39% among *S. pseudintermedius* isolates. No significant temporal trends were observed in the proportions of MDR S. *aureus* (p = 0.8212) or MDR *S. pseudintermedius* (p = 0.0932) (Fig. 5).

Predictors of AMR or MDR *Staphylococcus* spp.

None of the variables investigated in this study had significant association with the log odds of either AMR or MDR.

Discussion

Antimicrobial resistance in veterinary medicine and especially in companion animals is of increasing public health concern [2, 19]. This problem is exacerbated by the fact that the relationship between companion animals and their owners have been implicated in the cross-transmission and spread of antimicrobial resistant organisms [20–22]. Since South Africa lacks continuous assessment and reporting of veterinary related staphylococcal infections and antimicrobial resistance, the results of this study contribute significantly to improving our understanding of the trends in antimicrobial resistance among *S. aureus* and *S. pseudintermedius* clinical cases of dogs.

Antimicrobial resistance patterns

In the present study, we observed high proportions of *S. aureus* and *S. pseudintermedius* isolates resistant to β-lactam antibiotics (ampicillin and penicillin). This is consistent with previous studies that have reported

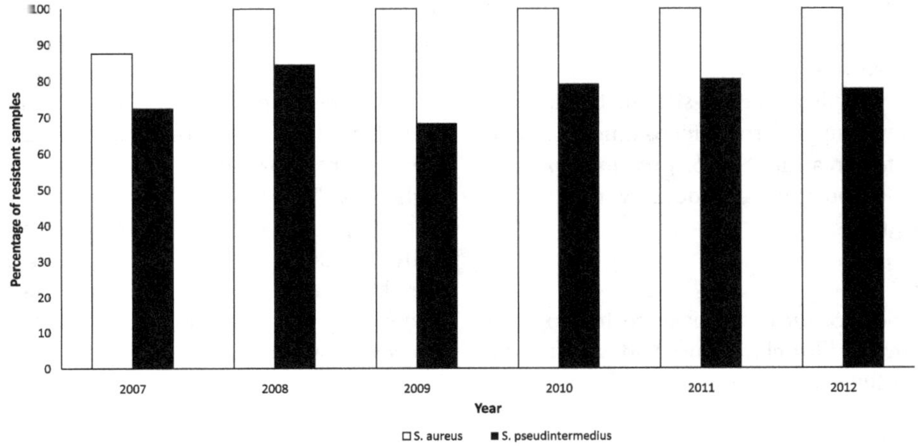

Fig. 4 Proportions of *S. aureus* and *S. pseudintermedius* isolates resistant to at least one antibiotic from samples tested at the University of Pretoria bacteriology laboratory, 2007–2012

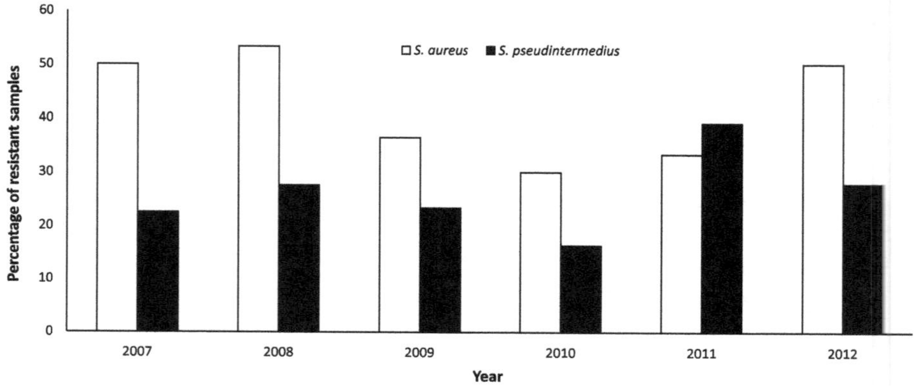

Fig. 5 Proportions of multidrug resistant *S. aureus* and *S. pseudintermedius* isolates from samples tested at the University of Pretoria veterinary bacteriology laboratory, 2007–2012

significantly higher levels of resistance of *Staphylococcus* species to β-lactam antibiotics compared to other classes of antimicrobials [23, 24]. This may be associated with the expression of intrinsic low-affinity to penicillin-binding proteins (PBPs) among *Staphylococcus* species [25] or the excessive use of β-lactam antibiotics in the treatment of *S. aureus* and *S. pseudintermedius* infections [3]. High levels of resistance to β-lactam antibiotics observed in this study will undoubtedly affect treatment and management of *Staphylococcus* spp. infections.

A significantly higher proportion of *S. aureus* than *S. pseudintermedius* isolates exhibited resistance to lincosamides (lincospectin and clindamycin). The reasons for this difference are unclear but these findings are consistent with reports of high levels of lincosamide resistance among *S. aureus* and *S. pseudintermedius* in the United States [26]. These findings suggest that lincosamides should not be used as alternative drugs in the treatment of staphylococcal infections in this population of dogs [27]. Of concern is the fact that lincosamides, such as clindamycin, have been generally known to be effective against Methicillin-Resistant *Staphylococcus aureus* (MRSA) and multidrug resistant staphylococci [28]. However, we observed that up to 59% of the *S. pseudintermedius* positive samples were resistant to lincosamides. This seems to suggest that lincosamides should not be considered for treatment of *S. pseudintermedius* infections in this population of dogs without first performing antibiograms.

Temporal patterns

Over the study period, *S. aureus* resistance to doxycycline, kanamycin, amoxicillin/clavulanic acid and tylosin decreased significantly while resistance to fluoroquinolones among *S. aureus* and *S. pseudintermedius* positive samples significantly increased. A study conducted over a 14-year period in Canada by Prescott et al. [3] reported no significant temporal changes in *S. aureus* resistance to fluoroquinolones. Similar to findings by Pellerin et al. [5] in France among *S. pseudintermedius* isolates tested between 1987 and 1996, we observed an increasing trend in resistance to trimethoprim-sulphamethoxazole among *S. pseudintermedius*. The observed decrease or increase in antimicrobial resistance in the current study may be due to changes in usage patterns as suggested by other authors [3, 26]. Moreover, a causal link between trimethoprim-sulphamethoxazole usage and trimethoprim-sulphametho xazole resistance in patients with urinary tract infections (UTI) has been established [29]. It has also been suggested that rapid introduction of fluoroquinolone and Trimethoprim-sulphamethoxazole drugs into companion veterinary medicine practice may also be a contributing factor to increased prevalence of resistance [30]. The authors of the present study think that this might be the case in this study. However, further investigations of the antimicrobial prescription practices among clinicians at the veterinary hospital is needed to better understand this.

Hauschild and Wójcik [4] reported 88% resistance to at least one antimicrobial drug among canine *Staphylococcus* isolates in Poland, whereas, Lilenbaum et al. [31] in Canada, reported 90.9% resistance among *Staphylococcus* spp. In our study, 80.5% of the *Staphylococcus* spp. isolates exhibited resistance to at least one antimicrobial drug. With regards to multi-drug resistance, the percentage MDR isolates in the current study was higher (28.7%) than the 24.5% reported by Gandolfi-Decristophoris et al. [32] in Switzerland and lower than the 34% as reported by Schmidt et al. [33] in the UK. The reasons for the high MDR among *Staphylococcus* spp. isolates in this study is unclear. However, we hypothesise that this may be an early indication of changes in the usage patterns among veterinarians caring for animals whose samples were included in the study. In view of this, more research needs to be done to provide a much clearer picture of the situation.

Distribution and predictors of AMR or MDR

Almost 100% of the *S. aureus* positive samples were resistant to at least one antimicrobial agent compared to only 77% of *S. pseudintermedius* positive samples. Although resistance to at least one antimicrobial agent was lower among *S. pseudintermedius,* it was much higher than 5.2% reported as by Vanni et al. [34] in Italy and 2–40% as reported by Blunt et al. [35] in South Africa. Our findings are consistent with reports of higher levels of MDR among *S. aureus* (ranging from 51% to 67%) compared to *S. pseudintermedius* (ranging from 5% to 14%) in the UK [36] and Canada [6]. On the contrary, Jung-Ho Youn et al. [37] reported no MDR in S. *aureus* compared to 10.4% MDR among *S. pseudintermedius* in Zambia. The results of this study suggest that MDR is more common in *S. aureus* isolates than *S. pseudintermedius* from dogs presented at the veterinary academic hospital in South Africa.

Study limitations

Hoekstra and Paulton [6] reported that the site of isolation is a risk factor of resistance. Unfortunately, we could not assess this in the current study due to the large number of categories (site types) and the small sample sizes associated with each category (site type). Some of the categories in some of the sub-analyses performed had low sample sizes and high variances hence lower precision. Previous exposure to antimicrobial agents has been associated with increased risk of development of antimicrobial resistance [20]. Unfortunately, due to the retrospective nature of the current study, the history of antibiotic use was not available. Therefore, we could not investigate the association between previous antibiotic use and antimicrobial resistance patterns. Furthermore, the study focused on canine clinical cases that were submitted to the bacteriology laboratory for diagnosis. Often such cases would include animals that have not responded well to previous treatments. Therefore, it is possible that a large population of dogs that responded to empirical treatments were not included in this study. Some sub-analyses were not possible due to relatively low sample sizes associated with some categories of some variables such as specimen type. Additionally, the time when culture and sensitivity test was done in relation to the time after hospital admission of the dogs was not available making it impossible to identify nosocomial from community acquired infections. Moreover, the geographic area covered by the study was limited to Gauteng Province which is not representative of South Africa as a whole nor is it representative of other veterinary hospitals in South Africa. These limitations, notwithstanding, the findings from this study provide useful information to guide future studies to better understand antimicrobial resistance in dogs.

Conclusion

Antibiotic resistance among *Staphylococcus* spp. from dogs presented to the veterinary academic hospital was high and continued to increase for enrofloxacin, trimethoprim-sulphamethoxazole, clindamycin and orbifloxacin during the 7-year study period. Of concern are the increasing levels of resistance to fluoroquinolones and sulphonamides among *S. pseudintermedius.* This calls for urgent action to address the problem. The actions may include development of antimicrobial stewardship program for veterinary and para-veterinary personnel to be offered by the university as part of continuing education. Furthermore, training of veterinary students should have a strong emphasis on antimicrobial stewardship. Lastly, the need for *Staphylococcus* species characterization and request for antibiogram as part of the protocol for diagnosis and treatment of *Staphylococcus* spp. infections should be emphasized and encouraged.

Abbreviations

AKC: American Kennel Club; AMR: Antimicrobial resistance; CAT: Cochran-Armitage trend; CI: Confidence interval; DNase: Deoxyribonuclease; MDR: Multidrug resistant resistance; MRSA: Methicillin-Resistant *Staphylococcus aureus*; OR: Odds ratio; PBPs: Penicillin-binding proteins; SAS: Statistical Analysis System; UTI: Urinary tract infection

Acknowledgements

The authors would like to thank the Department of Tropical Diseases and Companion Animal Clinical Studies for providing access to the records used in this study. We are also grateful to Ms. S Nxumalo and Mr. W Mbethe for helping with data entry and validation.

Funding

Not applicable.

Authors' contributions

DNQ was involved in study design and data management and performed all statistical analyses and interpretation as well as preparation of the manuscript draft. AO was involved in study design, data analysis and interpretation as well as extensive editing of the manuscript. JWO was involved in study design and editing of the manuscript. FS was involved in interpretation of results of the manuscript. All authors have read and approved the final manuscript.

Competing interests

The authors declare that they have no competing interests.

Consent for publication

The study does not involve human subjects and therefore no consent was required. However, the lab that supplied the study data provided consent for study results to be published.

Author details
[1]Section of Veterinary Public Health, Department of Paraclinical Sciences, Faculty of Veterinary Science, University of Pretoria, Pretoria, South Africa. [2]Department of Agriculture and Animal Health, College of Agriculture and Environmental Sciences, University of South Africa, Johannesburg, South Africa. [3]Ross University School of Veterinary Medicine, Basseterre, Saint Kitts and Nevis. [4]Biomedical and Diagnostic Sciences, College of Veterinary Medicine, University of Tennessee, Knoxville, USA.

References

1. Kim J, Song W, Kim H, Cho HC, Lee KM, Choi M, Kim E. Association between the methicillin resistance of clinical isolates of Staphylococcus aureus, their staphylococcal cassette chromosome mec (SCCmec) subtype classification, and their toxin gene profiles. Diagn Microbiol Infect Dis. 2006;56(3):289–95.
2. Werckenthin C, Cardoso M, Martel J-L, Schwarz S. Antimicrobial resistance in staphylococci from animals with particular reference to bovine Staphylococcus aureus, porcine Staphylococcus hyicus, and canine Staphylococcus intermedius. Vet Res. 2001;32(3–4):341–62.
3. Prescott JF, Hanna WJB, Reid-Smith R, Drost K. Antimicrobial drug use and resistance in dogs. Can Vet J. 2002;43(2):107–16.
4. Hauschild T, Wójcik A. Species distribution and properties of staphylococci from canine dermatitis. Res Vet Sci. 2007;82(1):1–6.
5. Pellerin JL, Bourdeau P, Sebbag H, Person JM. Epidemiosurveillance of antimicrobial compound resistance of Staphylococcus intermedius clinical isolates from canine pyodermas. Comp Immunol Microbiol Infect Dis. 1998;21(2):115–33.
6. Hoekstra KA, Paulton RJ. Clinical prevalence and antimicrobial susceptibility of Staphylococcus aureus and Staphylococcus intermedius in dogs. J Appl Microbiol. 2002;93:406–13.
7. Eagar H, Swan G, Van Vuuren M. A survey of antimicrobial usage in animals in South Africa with specific reference to food animals. J S Afr Vet Assoc. 2012;83(1):15–23.
8. Kudakwashe CJ. A survey of antimicrobial usage patterns by veterinarians treating dogs and cats in South Africa. Pretoria: University of Pretoria; 2014.
9. Moodley A, Damborg P, Nielsen SS. Antimicrobial resistance in methicillin susceptible and methicillin resistant Staphylococcus pseudintermedius of canine origin: Literature review from 1980 to 2013. Vet Microbiol. 2014;171(3–4):337–41.
10. Quinn PJ, Carter ME, Markey B, Carter GR. Clinical Veterinary Microbiology. 1st ed. England: Wolfe; 1994.
11. Clinical Laboratory Standards Institute. Performance standards for antimicrobial disk and dilution susceptibility tests for bacteria isolated from animals; Approved Standard – Fourth Edition. CLSI document VET01-A; 2013.
12. Clinical Institute Laboratory Standards. Performance Standards for Antimicrobial Susceptibility Testing. Seventeenth Informational Supplement. CLSI Document M100-S17. Wayne: Clinical and Laboratory Standards Institute; 2007.
13. Clinical Institute Laboratory Standards. Performance Standards for Antimicrobial Susceptibility Testing: Twenty-first Informational Supplement M100-S21. Wayne: Clinical and Laboratory Standards Institute; 2011.
14. Clinical Institute Laboratory Standards. Performance Standards for Antimicrobial Susceptibility Testing: Twentieth Informational Supplement M100-S20. Wayne: Clinical and Laboratory Standards Institute; 2010.
15. Clinical Institute Laboratory Standards. Clinical and Laboratory Standards Institute. Performance Standards for Antimicrobial Susceptibility Testing: Twenty-second Informational Supplement M100-S22. Wayne: Clinical and Laboratory Standards Institute; 2012.
16. Clinical Institute Laboratory Standards. Performance standards for antimicrobial susceptibility testing, 18th ed. CLSI/NCCLS M100-S18. Wayne: Clinical and Laboratory Standards Institute; 2008.
17. Clinical Institute Laboratory Standards. Performance Standards for Antimicrobial Susceptebility Testing: Nineteenth Informational Supplement M100-S19. Wayne: Clinical and Laboratory Standards Insitute; 2009.
18. Clinical Laboratory Standards Insitute. Performance Standards for Antimicrobial Susceptebility Testing: Twenty-second Informational Supplement M100-S25. Wayne: Clinical Laboratory Standards Institute; 2015.
19. Normand EH, Gibson NR, Reid SWJ, Carmichael S, Taylor DJ. Antimicrobial-resistance trends in bacterial isolates from companion-animal community practice in the UK. Prev Vet Med. 2000;46(4):267–78.
20. van den Bogaard AE, Stobberingh EE. Epidemiology of resistance to antibiotics: Links between animals and humans. Int J Antimicrob Agents. 2000;14(4):327–35.
21. Lloyd DH. Reservoirs of antimicrobial resistance in pet animals. Clin Infect Dis. 2007;45(Suppl 2):S148–52.
22. Guardabassi L, Schwarz S, Lloyd DH. Pet animals as reservoirs of antimicrobial-resistant bacteria. J Antimicrob Chemother. 2004;54(2):321–32.
23. Malik S, Peng H, Barton MD. Antibiotic resistance in staphylococci associated with cats and dogs. J Appl Microbiol. 2005;99(6):1283–93.
24. Boost MV, O'Donoghue MM, James A. Prevalence of Staphylococcus aureus carriage among dogs and their owners. Epidemiol Infect. 2008;136(7):953–64.
25. Rice LB. Mechanisms of Resistance and Clinical Relevance of Resistance to Î²-Lactams, Glycopeptides, and Fluoroquinolones. Mayo Clin Proc. 2012;87(2):198–208.
26. Gold RM, Lawhon SD. Incidence of Inducible Clindamycin Resistance in Staphylococcus pseudintermedius from Dogs. J Clin Microbiol. 2013;51(12):4196–9.
27. Guardabassi L, Houser GA, Frank LA, Papich MG. Guidelines for antimicrobial use in dogs and cats. In: Guardabassi L, Jensen LB, Kruse H, editors. Guide to Antimicrobial Use in Animals. Oxford: Blackwell Publishing, Ltd; 2008. p. 183–206.
28. Frank LA, Loeffler A. Meticillin-resistant Staphylococcus pseudintermedius: clinical challenge and treatment options. Vet Dermatol. 2012;23(4):283–91.
29. Metlay JP, Strom BL, Asch DA. Prior antimicrobial drug exposure: a risk factor for trimethoprim-sulfamethoxazole-resistant urinary tract infections. J Antimicrob Chemother. 2003;51(4):963–70.
30. Walker RD, Thornsberry C. Decrease in antibiotic susceptibility or increase in resistance? J Antimicrob Chemother. 1998;41(1):1–4.
31. Lilenbaum W, Veras M, Blum E, Souza GN. Antimicrobial susceptibility of staphylococci isolated from otitis externa in dogs. Lett Appl Microbiol. 2000;31(1):42–5.
32. Gandolfi-Decristophoris P, Regula G, Petrini O, Zinsstag J, Schelling E. Prevalence and risk factors for carriage of multi-drug resistant Staphylococci in healthy cats and dogs. J Vet Sci. 2013;14(4):449–56.
33. Schmidt VM, Williams NJ, Pinchbeck G, Corless CE, Shaw S, McEwan N, Dawson S, Nuttall T. Antimicrobial resistance and characterisation of staphylococci isolated from healthy Labrador retrievers in the United Kingdom. BMC Vet Res. 2014;10(1):1–14.
34. Vanni M, Tognetti R, Pretti C, Crema F, Soldani G, Meucci V, Intorre L. Antimicrobial susceptibility of Staphylococcus intermedius and Staphylococcus schleiferi isolated from dogs. Res Vet Sci. 2009;87(2):192–5.
35. Blunt C, van Vuuren M, Picard J. Antimicrobial susceptibility profiles of Staphylococcus intermedius isolates from clinical cases of canine pyoderma in South Africa. J S Afr Vet Assoc. 2013;84(1):1–6.
36. Wedley AL, Dawson S, Maddox TW, Coyne KP, Pinchbeck GL, Clegg P, Jamrozy D, Fielder MD, Donovan D, Nuttall T, Williams NJ. Carriage of Staphylococcus species in the veterinary visiting dog population in mainland UK: Molecular characterisation of resistance and virulence. Vet Microbiol. 2014;170(1–2):81–8.
37. Youn J, Park YH, Hang'ombe B, Sugimoto C. Prevalence and characterization of Staphylococcus aureus and Staphylococcus pseudintermedius isolated from companion animals and environment in the veterinary teaching hospital in Zambia, Africa. Comp Immunol Microbiol Infect Dis. 2014;37(2):123–30.

4

Impact of growth matrix on pharmacodynamics of antimicrobial drugs for pig pneumonia pathogens

Lucy Dorey* and Peter Lees

Abstract

Background: The most widely used measure of potency of antimicrobial drugs is Minimum Inhibitory Concentration (MIC). MIC is usually determined under standardised conditions in broths formulated to optimise bacterial growth on a species-by-species basis. This ensures comparability of data between laboratories. However, differences in values of MIC may arise between broths of differing chemical composition and for some drug classes major differences occur between broths and biological fluids such as serum and inflammatory exudate. Such differences must be taken into account, when breakpoint PK/PD indices are derived and used to predict dosages for clinical use. There is therefore interest in comparing MIC values in several broths and, in particular, in comparing broth values with those generated in serum. For the pig pneumonia pathogens, *Actinobacillus pleuropneumoniae* and *Pasteurella multocida*, MICs were determined for three drugs, florfenicol, oxytetracycline and marbofloxacin, in five broths [Mueller Hinton Broth (MHB), cation-adjusted Mueller Hinton Broth (CAMHB), Columbia Broth supplemented with NAD (CB), Brain Heart Infusion Broth (BHI) and Tryptic Soy Broth (TSB)] and in pig serum.

Results: For each drug, similar MIC values were obtained in all broths, with one exception, marbofloxacin having similar MICs for three broths and 4–5-fold higher MICs for two broths. In contrast, for both organisms, quantitative differences between broth and pig serum MICs were obtained after correction of MICs for drug binding to serum protein (fu serum MIC). Potency was greater (fu serum MIC lower) in serum than in broths for marbofloxacin and florfenicol for both organisms. For oxytetracycline fu serum:broth MIC ratios were 6.30:1 (*P. multocida*) and 0.35:1 (*A. pleuropneumoniae*), so that potency of this drug was reduced for the former species and increased for the latter species. The chemical composition of pig serum and broths was compared; major matrix differences in 14 constituents did not account for MIC differences. Bacterial growth rates were compared in broths and pig serum in the absence of drugs; it was concluded that broth/serum MIC differences might be due to differing growth rates in some but not all instances.

Conclusions: For all organisms and all drugs investigated in this study, it is suggested that broth MICs should be adjusted by an appropriate scaling factor when used to determine pharmacokinetic/pharmacodynamic breakpoints for dosage prediction.

Keywords: Minimum inhibitory concentration, Florfenicol, Oxytetracycline, Marbofloxacin, *A. Pleuropneumoniae*, *P. Multocida*

* Correspondence: ldorey@rvc.ac.uk
The Royal Veterinary College, Hawkshead Campus, Herts, AL97TA, Hatfield, UK

Background

Dosage regimens of antimicrobial drugs should be optimized first to achieve clinical and bacteriological cure and second to provide minimal opportunities for the selection of resistant organisms. The successful outcome of therapy depends on both the pharmacokinetic (PK) profile, which determines the drug concentration-time course at the site of infection and the pharmacodynamic (PD) profile that is drug effect on the pathogen [1–4]. Hence, a rational approach to dose prediction, for subsequent confirmation or adaptation in disease models and clinical trials, is dependent on PK/PD integration and modelling methods. These establish PK/PD breakpoints for pre-determined levels of kill [2–6].

Minimum Inhibitory Concentration (MIC) is the primary PD parameter used to determine potency; it is the lowest drug concentration that inhibits visible bacterial growth after 16–24 h incubation. Standardised methodologies for MIC determination are described in European Committee on Antimicrobial Susceptibility Testing (EUCAST) and Clinical and Laboratory Standards Institute (CLSI) [7] guidelines [VET01-A4 (formerly M31-A3)]. These ensure reproducibility between individual analysts, between laboratories and across both geographical regions and time [5, 8]. CLSI and EUCAST methods require the use of broths formulated to standardises the growth of bacteria of each bacterial species. Thus, the almost universal use of internationally recognised guidelines, methods and standards for MIC determination is highly beneficial. However, when the objective of potency determination is prediction of dosage for clinical efficacy based on PK/PD breakpoints, conditions should be representative of in vivo pathological circumstances. Zeitlinger et al. [9] commented that "bacteria with appropriate and well-defined growth in the selected medium should be employed" and "in order to be able to extrapolate data from various models to in vivo situations, models should always attempt to mimic physiological conditions as closely as possible".

Whilst serum is not identical to extravascular infection site fluids, it is likely to be closer to the biophase than broths in chemical composition and indeed in respect of immunological components also [9, 10]. A comparison of broth MICs with potency determined in biological fluids is therefore relevant to PK/PD breakpoint estimation, when the aim is optimal dose prediction for clinical use. For some drugs and pathogens, calculation of a scaling factor to bridge between broth and serum MICs may be warranted [4, 6, 10].

A second consideration, in relation to dose prediction, is that CLSI and EUCAST guidelines have limitations regarding accuracy for individual isolates, because they require use of two-fold dilutions, giving potential for approaching 100% error. For most purposes, this is wholly acceptable, and indeed is necessary, when large numbers of isolates are examined to establish MIC distributions. When plotted on a histogram, using a log-base 2 distribution, they are log-normal. These histograms facilitate the identification of wild-type distributions. Standardisation of methodology thereby enables determination of epidemiological cut-offs (ECOFF) by EUCAST and wild type cut-offs (CO_{WT}) by CLSI. However, modification of the two-fold dilution approach may be appropriate, when MICs are correlated with PK data for establishing PK/PD breakpoints. Based on methods previously described [11, 12] five overlapping sets of doubling dilutions were used in this study to decrease inaccuracy from up to 100% to no more than 20% for a small number of individual isolates. Hence, the quantitative determination potency with improved accuracy and in biological fluids may be appropriate for some drug classes and some microorganisms, when calculating PK/PD indices [6, 10, 12–16].

It is the hypothesis of this investigation that MICs determined in pig serum (potentially reflecting more closely concentrations required to achieve clinical efficacy than those determined in artificial broths) might differ from MICs determined in broths. The aims were to: (1) compare MICs measured in five broths with MICs determined in pig serum, using five sets of overlapping two-fold dilutions for three drugs, florfenicol, marbofloxacin and oxytetracycline, used in the treatment of pig pneumonia caused by the pathogens, *Actinobacillus pleuropneumoniae* and *Pasteurella multocida*; (2) determine whether any broth/serum MIC differences were attributable solely to drug binding to serum protein; (3) compare chemical compositions of CLSI recommended broths and pig serum; (4) determine rates of growth *A. pleuropneumoniae* and *P. multocida* in broths and pig serum in the absence of drugs. Aims 3 and 4 were included to investigate whether chemical composition differences and/or bacterial growth rate differences between broth and serum might account for matrix MIC differences over and above those attributable binding of the drugs to serum protein.

Methods

Selection of bacterial isolates for MIC studies

Don Whitley Scientific (Shipley, West Yorkshire, UK) supplied 20 isolates of *P. multocida* and three American Type Culture Collection (ATCC) reference strains to validate MIC tests; *A. pleuropneumoniae* ATCC 27090, *Enterococcus faecalis* ATCC 29212 and *Escherichia coli* ATCC 25922. Eight isolates of *A. pleuropneumoniae* were supplied by A. Rycroft (Royal Veterinary College, Hatfield, Herts, UK). All *P. multocida* and *A. pleuropneumoniae* isolates were obtained from European Union (EU) field cases of pig pneumonia, specifically the UK and France.

The quality control organisms were incorporated in each MIC test. Organisms were stored at -80 °C.

From the organisms supplied, three isolates of each species were selected, based on three criteria: (1) exhibiting logarithmic growth in all broths (see below) and pig serum; (2) sensitivity to florfenicol, marbofloxacin and oxytetracycline in disk diffusion assays (data not shown); and (3) the highest and lowest CLSI defined broth MICs and one isolate of intermediate MIC, determined using two-fold dilutions (data not shown).

Culture media and bacterial counts

For *A. pleuropneumoniae* Chocolate Mueller Hinton Agar (CMHA) was used to grow the organism on a solid medium. Mueller Hinton Agar (MHA), supplemented with 5% defibrinated sheep blood, was used to grow *P. multocida*. Columbia broth (CB) supplemented with 2 μg/mL nicotinamide adenine dinucleotide (NAD) was used as the principal liquid broth for *A. pleuropneumoniae* MIC determination. CLSI guidelines require use of Veterinary Fastidious Medium (VFM) for the liquid culture of *A. pleuropneumoniae*. However, for isolates used in this study, MIC end-points were more readily and reliably established using CB than with VFM. In the latter broth, there was difficulty defining MIC end-points, because the high density of red blood cells caused them to settle at the base of the well obscuring the result of MIC. The CLSI recommended broth for *P. multocida* is Cation Adjusted Mueller Hinton broth (CAMHB), and this was the principal liquid broth used in this study for this organism.

Both organisms were incubated in a static incubator at 37 °C for 18–24 h. For comparative purposes, MICs were determined for both organisms in five broths, CB, CAMHB, Mueller Hinton broth (MHB), Brain Heart Infusion broth (BHIB), Tryptic soy broth (TSB), and pig serum (Invitrogen Gibco Porcine Serum, Origin: New Zealand, ThermoFisher Scientific, UK).

Bacterial counts were determined by serial dilution and spot plate counts. Culture dilutions were carried out in phosphate buffered saline. Three 10 μL drops of the appropriate dilutions were dropped onto the agar surface and allowed to dry. After 24 h incubation, the mean colony forming unit (CFU) count for each 10 μL was determined and multiplied by 100 and then multiplied by the dilution factor to give the original CFU/mL count.

Minimum inhibitory concentrations in six growth matrices

MICs of florfenicol, marbofloxacin and oxytetracycline were determined by microdilution in 96-well plates for three isolates each of *A. pleuropneumoniae* and *P. multocida*, using CLSI guidelines, except that: (1) five sets of overlapping two-fold serial dilutions were used to reduce inaccuracy for individual isolates to no greater than 20%; (2) determinations were made in five broths, MHB, CAMHB, CB, BHIB, TSB and pig serum; (3) the bacterial culture was grown to 0.5 McFarland Standard and this was diluted ten-fold to obtain the intended starting inoculum of 1–2 × 10^7 CFU/mL. This starting inoculum count is higher than the CLSI recommendation of 5 × 10^5 CFU/mL, the higher inoculum count being selected deliberately to be equivalent clinically to a medium to heavy in vivo microbial challenge.

Drug solutions, media and culture were added sequentially to the wells of 96-well plates, with a total volume of 200 μL. These were sealed and incubated statically at 37 °C for 24 h. Spot plate counts were prepared immediately after plate inoculation. ATCC isolates were used in all assays at the CLSI recommended strength of 5 × 10^5 CFU/mL. A positive control well contained medium and pathogen only and a negative control well contained medium and drug only. Blank controls contained medium alone.

MICs were determined in triplicate for each isolate of each species and each drug. In previous studies in this laboratory, binding to pig serum protein had been determined for each drug over the therapeutic concentration range and shown to be independent of concentration [17–19]. Percentage binding was 49, 65 and 71 for marbofloxacin, florfenicol and oxytetracycline, respectively. As serum protein bound drug is microbiologically inactive, MICs for serum were reported first, as uncorrected, experimental values and second, as values corrected for free drug (that is unbound) concentration, termed the fu serum MIC.

Chemical composition of growth matrices

For analysis of 14 chemical constituents, three batches of each broth were prepared in 10 mL quantities, according to manufacturer's instructions and three batches each of pig and calf serum were obtained commercially (ThermoFisher Scientific, Paisley, UK). Calf serum was included to compare the composition of pig serum with another farm animal species. Samples were analysed for total protein, albumin, globulin, sodium, potassium, calcium, magnesium, chloride, inorganic phosphorus, urea, creatinine, glucose, iron and Unsaturated Iron Binding Capacity (UIBC) (ILAB 600 Instrumentation Laboratory Ltd., Cheshire UK; Nova Biomedical CCX and Phox, Cheshire UK).

Bacterial growth in broth and serum

Twenty isolates each of *P. multocida* and *A. pleuropneumoniae* (Don Whitley Scientific (Shipley, West Yorkshire, UK) supplied 20 isolates of both organisms for the purpose of determining growth in media), from clinical cases of pig pneumonia, were used to investigate bacterial growth in the absence of antimicrobial drugs. Growth rates were determined in pig serum and the CLSI recommended broths,

VFM for *A. pleuropneumoniae* and CAMHB for *P. multocida*.

Three mL of serum, CAMHB or VFM were aseptically added to the wells of a 96-well plate. Two control wells containing medium alone ensured the absence of contamination. Six independent colonies were removed from a fresh agar plate aseptically and mixed into the medium within the wells. The well plates were placed in a static incubator at 37 °C for 24 h. At times of 0, 6 and 24 h viable counts were determined. Bacterial growth was monitored in triplicate for each of 20 isolates of each species.

Results

Minimum inhibitory concentration

Tables 1, 2 and 3 present MIC data for each drug as geometric means and standard deviation for pig serum, MHB, CAMHB, CB, BHIB and TSB.

Marbofloxacin

P. multocida MICs were similar for three broths, MHB, CAMHB and TSB (range = 0.05–0.07 µg/mL). MICs were 4–5-fold higher for CB and BHIB (0.25–0.27 µg/mL). Serum MIC was 0.09 µg/mL and, corrected for protein binding, fu serum MIC was 0.04 µg/mL. The mean MIC ratio fu serum:CAMHB was 0.63:1.

For *A. pleuropneumoniae* broth MICs were similar (range = 0.91 µg/mL for CAMHB to 1.37 µg/mL for TSB). Serum MIC was 0.69 µg/mL and fu serum MIC was 0.35 µg/mL; mean MIC ratio fu serum:CB was 0.35:1.

Florfenicol

For *P. multocida* MICs in all broths were similar; range = 0.47 µg/mL for MHB to 0.55 µg/mL for CAMHB. Serum MIC was 0.30 µg/mL and fu serum MIC was 0.10 µg/mL. The mean MIC ratio fu serum:CAMHB was 0.19:1.

Table 1 *P. multocida* (PM) and *A. pleuropneumoniae* (APP) Minimum Inhibitory Concentrations for marbofloxacin; mean and standard deviation (SD) in pig serum and five broths[a]

	PM (*n* = 3)		APP (*n* = 3)	
Matrix	Mean	SD	Mean	SD
Serum	0.09	0.52	0.69	0.23
fu Serum	0.04	0.27	0.35	0.12
MHB	0.06	0.01	0.93	0.17
CAMHB	0.07	0.05	0.91	0.13
CB	0.25	0.14	1.00	0.00
BHIB	0.27	0.18	1.14	0.25
TSB	0.05	0.01	1.37	0.22

[a]Cation Adjusted Mueller Hinton Broth (CAMHB), Mueller Hinton Broth (MHB), Columbia Broth supplemented with NAD (CB), Brain Heart Infusion broth (BHI) and Tryptic Soy broth (TSB)

Table 2 *P. multocida* (PM) and *A. pleuropneumoniae* (APP) Minimum Inhibitory Concentrations for florfenicol; mean and standard deviation (SD) in pig serum and five broths[a]

	PM (*n* = 3)		APP (*n* = 3)	
Matrix	Mean	SD	Mean	SD
Serum	0.30	0.13	0.47	0.18
fu Serum	0.10	0.05	0.16	0.06
MHB	0.47	0.03	0.36	0.02
CAMHB	0.55	1.19	0.36	0.04
CB	0.50	0.00	0.43	0.03
BHI	0.50	0.00	0.45	0.05
TSB	0.49	0.02	0.44	0.04

[a]Cation-adjusted Mueller Hinton Broth (CAMHB), Mueller Hinton Broth (MHB),, Columbia Broth supplemented with NAD (CB), Brain Heart Infusion broth (BHI) and Tryptic Soy broth (TSB)

For *A. pleuropneumoniae* broth MICs ranged from 0.36 µg/mL for both MHB and CAMHB to 0.45 µg/mL for BHIB. Serum MIC was 0.47 µg/mL and fu serum MIC was 0.16 µg/mL, so that mean MIC ratio fu serum:CB was 0.38:1.

Oxytetracycline

For *P. multocida* broth MICs were similar, ranging from 0.28 µg/mL (MHB) to 0.38 µg/mL (TSB). Serum MIC was 6.20 µg/mL and fu serum MIC was 1.80 µg/mL. The mean MIC ratio fu serum:CAMHB was 6.30:1.

Broth MICs for *A. pleuropneumoniae* ranged from 2.34 µg/mL (CAMHB) to 3.22 µg/mL (TSB). Serum MIC and fu serum MIC were 3.47 and 1.01 µg/mL, respectively, so that the mean MIC ratio fu serum:CB was 0.35:1.

Chemical composition of broths and serum

Table 4 presents comparative data on the chemical composition of six broths and pig serum for 14 constituents. In addition, for comparison with the latter, the composition

Table 3 *P. multocida* (PM) and *A. pleuropneumoniae* (APP) Minimum Inhibitory Concentrations for oxytetracycline; mean and standard deviation (SD) in pig serum and five broths[a]

	PM (*n* = 3)		APP (*n* = 3)	
Matrix	Mean	SD	Mean	SD
Serum	6.20	2.06	3.47	2.38
fu Serum	1.80	0.60	1.01	0.69
MHB	0.28	0.04	2.56	0.29
CAMHB	0.29	0.04	2.34	0.24
CB	0.30	0.04	2.92	0.28
BHI	0.34	0.05	3.06	0.21
TSB	0.38	0.03	3.22	0.42

[a]Cation-adjusted Mueller Hinton Broth (CAMHB), Mueller Hinton Broth (MHB),, Columbia Broth supplemented with NAD (CB), Brain Heart Infusion broth (BHI) and Tryptic Soy broth (TSB)

Table 4 Chemical composition of broths[a] and pig and calf sera: mean and standard deviation (SD) (n = 3 batches)[a]

Matrix	Total protein (g/L)	Albumin (g/L)	Globulin (g/L)	Sodium (mmol/L)	Potassium (mmol/L)	Calcium (mmol/L)	Magnesium (mmol/L)	Chloride (mmol/L)	Inorganic phosphorus (mmol/L)	Urea (mmol/L)	Creatinine (μmol/L)	Glucose (mmol/L)	Iron (μmol/L)	Unsaturated Iron Binding Capacity (μmol/L)
Porcine serum	79.3	40.3	39.0	153	7.13	2.59	0.98	115	2.82	4.67	139	5.47	19.1	78.00
SD	2.20	0.17	2.03	4.4	0.06	0.14	0.09	8.96	0.61	3.35	5.5	0.84	0.15	0.36
Bovine serum	74.3	38.1	37.1	148	7.07	2.55	1.00	108	3.28	5.23	149	4.43	22.2	71.00
SD	3.65	2.11	1.31	15.4	1.04	0.55	0.17	7.55	0.98	0.60	9.9	0.29	0.61	0.43
MHB	3.23	0.00	3.23	125	2.49	0.13	0.23	99.23	2.55	0.93	61.3	2.57	9.47	-6.90
SD	0.12	0.00	0.12	0.2	0.01	0.02	0.00	0.32	0.03	0.06	2.31	0.06	0.15	0.44
CAMHB	4.10	0.07	4.03	127	2.87	5.21	4.20	117	2.96	2.97	83.3	2.57	9.53	-7.20
SD	0.44	0.06	0.46	11.5	0.21	2.14	1.68	5.29	0.34	0.64	2.08	0.25	0.17	1.24
CB	12.6	0.10	12.5	130	14.58	0.22	1.41	112	4.99	2.90	217	12.90	63.9	-56.50
SD	0.20	0.00	0.20	0.1	0.01	0.01	0.02	0.26	0.02	0.10	2.31	0.00	0.62	1.74
BHI	9.67	0.10	9.57	168	10.01	0.13	0.25	123	6.86	5.97	418	10.20	7.50	-3.17
SD	0.21	0.00	0.21	0.2	0.01	0.01	0.01	0.56	0.07	0.06	3.61	0.20	0.10	1.11
TSB	9.07	0.10	9.00	118	9.56	0.05	0.18	79.33	4.85	2.17	260	11.77	6.86	-2.20
SD	0.06	0.06	0.10	0.1	0.01	0.02	0.00	0.06	0.02	0.06	1.53	0.15	0.25	1.74
VFM	11.4	0.87	10.5	132	38.73	0.33	1.16	104	14.31	4.87	198	3.40	25.9	-3.00
SD	0.26	0.12	0.15	3.5	0.31	0.03	0.10	4.04	0.44	0.72	9.07	0.10	0.52	1.31

[a]Mueller Hinton Broth (MHB), Cation Adjusted Mueller Hinton Broth (CAMHB),, Veterinary Fastidious Medium (VFM), Columbia Broth supplemented with NAD (CB), Brain Heart Infusion broth (BHIB), Tryptic Soy broth (TSB) and Veterinary Fastidious Medium (VFM)

of serum for another farm animal species, the calf, was determined (Fig. 1). The data were derived for the mean of three batch samples of each fluid.

Protein, albumin and globulin

For the six broths, total protein concentration was low in MHB and CAMHB (3.23 and 4.10 g/L, respectively) but higher and similar for the four other broths (range 9.07–12.6 g/L). Serum total protein concentrations were higher, 79.3 g/L (pig) and 74.3 g/L (calf). For all broths, the principal protein constituent was globulin (range 3.23 to 12.5 g/L) whilst albumin concentrations were uniformly low, ranging from 0.00 to 0.87 g/L, for MHB and VFM, respectively. Albumin serum concentrations were much higher; 40.2 g/L (pig) and 38.1 g/L (calf). Expressed as serum:broth albumin concentration ratios, these ranged from greater than 400:1 for CAMHB to 46:1 for VFM.

Electrolytes

There were moderate differences in sodium concentration between the growth matrices; the lowest concentration was 118 mmol/L (TSB) and the highest was 168 mmol/L (BHI) and serum concentrations were intermediate, 153 and 148 mmol/L, for pig and calf, respectively. Similarly, serum chloride ion concentrations for pig and calf were intermediate (115 and 108 mmol/L, respectively) between the lowest, 79 mmol/L for TSB, and highest broth concentration of 123 mmol/L for BHI. MHB had the lowest potassium concentration (2.49 mmol/L) whereas the highest concentration was 39 mmol/L for VFM. Serum potassium concentrations were intermediate, 7.13 and 7.07 mmol/L for pig and calf, respectively.

With the exception of CAMHB, the concentration of calcium was much lower in broths, ranging from 0.05 to 0.33 mmol/L, in comparison with serum, 2.59 and 2.55 mmol/L for pig and calf, respectively. For CAMHB the calcium concentration was 5.21 mmol/L. Concentrations of magnesium were lower in three broths (0.23 mmol/L MHB, 0.25 mmol/L BHI and 0.18 mmol/L TSB) than in serum of pig and calf, 0.98 and 1.00 mmol/L, respectively, whereas concentrations in CAMHB, CB and VFM were higher, 4.20, 1.41 and 1.16, respectively.

Inorganic phosphorus, urea, creatinine and glucose

Broth inorganic phosphorus concentrations ranged from 2.55 mmol/L (MHB) to 14.3 mmol/L (VFM) and serum concentrations were similar to MHB, 2.82 and 3.28 mmol/L for pig and calf, respectively. Broth urea concentrations ranged from 0.93 mmol/L (MHB) to 5.97 mmol/L (BHI) and concentrations in serum were slightly less than the highest broth value, 4.67 and 5.23 mmol/L, pig and calf,

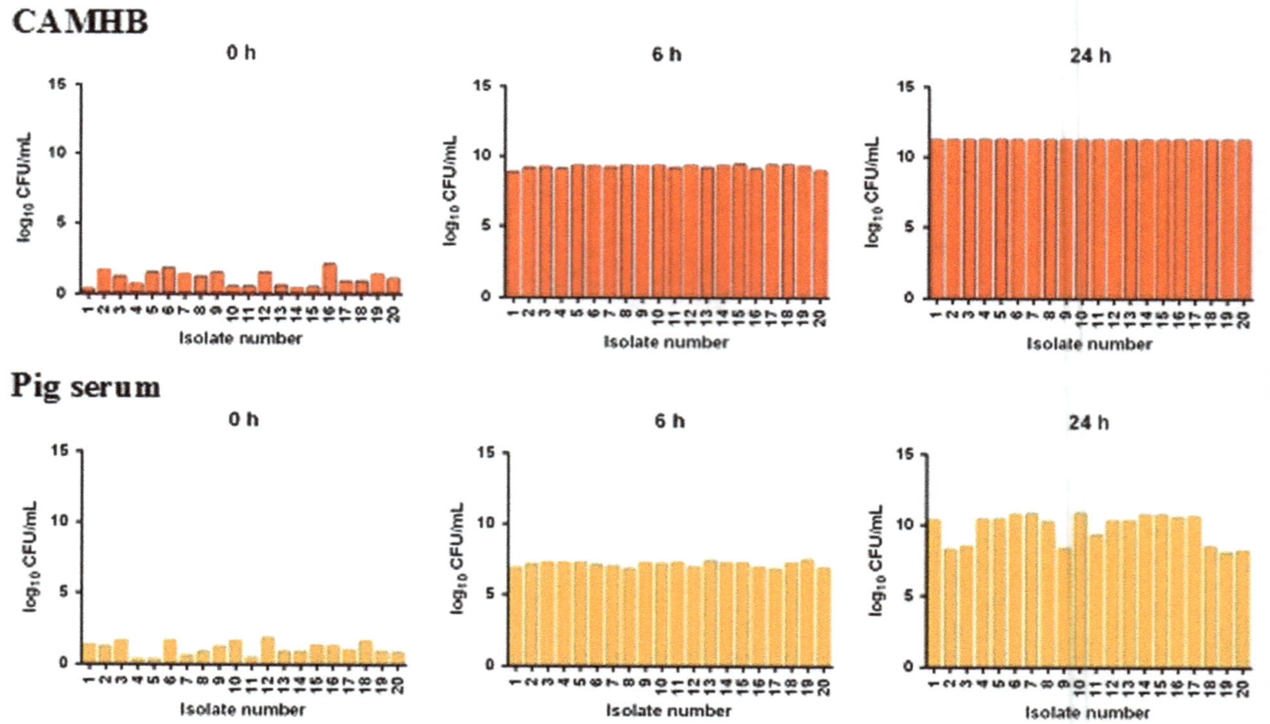

Fig. 1 Pie chart comparing the concentrations of constituents in eight matrices: Porcine serum, bovine serum, cation-adjusted Mueller Hinton Broth (CAMHB), Mueller Hinton Broth (MHB), Columbia broth supplemented with NAD (CB), Veterinary Fastidious Medium (VFM), Trypic Soy broth (TSB) and Brain Heart Infusion broth (BHI). Highlighted with a star is one of the more notably important components, total protein

respectively. In broths, creatinine concentration was lowest in MHB (61 μmol/L) and highest in BHI (418 μmol/L) and serum concentrations were intermediate (139 and 149 μmol/L, for pig and calf). Broth glucose concentrations ranged from 1.56 mmol/L (MHB and CAMHB) to 12.9 mmol/L (CB) whilst serum concentrations were intermediate, 5.47 mmol/L (pig) and 4.43 mmol/L (calf).

Iron and unsaturated iron binding capacity

Iron broth concentrations varied almost 10-fold, from 6.86 μmol/L (TSB) to 63.9 μmol/L (CB) and serum concentrations were intermediate, 19.1 μmol/L (pig) and 22.2 μmol/L (calf). Unsaturated iron binding capacity also varied widely (data not shown).

Bacterial growth in absence of antimicrobial drugs

Figures 2 and 3 illustrate bacterial growth rates of *P. multocida* and *A. pleuropneumoniae*, respectively. There were no apparent inter-isolate differences in *P. multocida* growth rates in CAMHB at 6 and 24 h. For all isolates at 6 h, bacterial counts had increased to 6-7x10^{9}CFU/mL in broth and at 24 h counts exceeded 10^{10} CFU/mL for all isolates. In serum, there was again minimal inter-isolate difference in growth of *P. multocida* at 6 h but the count, 5-6x10^{7}CFU/mL, was lower at this time than in CAMHB by some 2 × 10^2 CFU/mL. After 24 h, there was further increase in growth but there were some inter-isolate differences in count, which ranged from 8-10 × 10^{10} CFU/mL, and the serum count was somewhat lower than the 24 h count in CAMHB at this time.

For *A. pleuropneumoniae*, bacterial growth was much slower initially (at 6 h) in both media than for *P. multocida*. At 6 h the mean CFU/mL count for 20 isolates was 5.37 × 10^5 in broth and in in serum it was significantly lower, 1.36x10^{2}CFU/mL. In contrast with *P. multocida* there was clear inter-isolate variability in growth rate at 6 h. However, by 24 h considerable growth had occurred and counts were of a similar order in both media, approaching or exceeding slightly 10log$_{10}$ CFU/mL.

Discussion

For some drug classes, MICs measured in broths using internationally standardised procedures (for example, those of CLSI and EUCAST) may not differ significantly from potency estimated in biological fluids. The absence of growth matrix differences implies no significant impact on PK/PD breakpoint estimation, as a basis for dose determination, provided that the protein bound serum drug concentration is corrected for [4, 16, 20]. However, broth/biological fluid differences in potency do occur for other drug classes, even after correction for drug binding

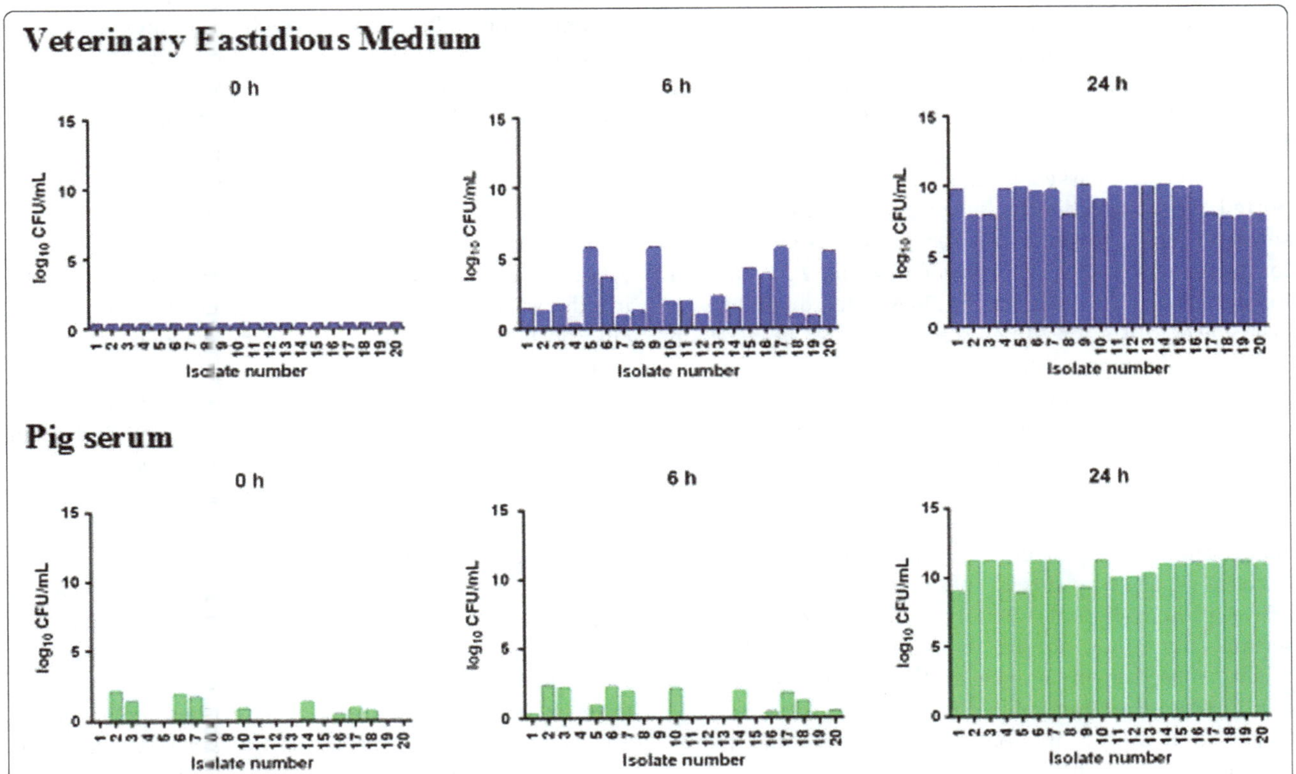

Fig. 2 In vitro growth of *P. multocida* (*n* = 20 isolates) at time points 0, 6 and 24 h in CAMHB and pig serum (*n* = 20). Growth quantified in log$_{10}$ CFU/mL (ordinate); each bar represents mean of triplicate analyses

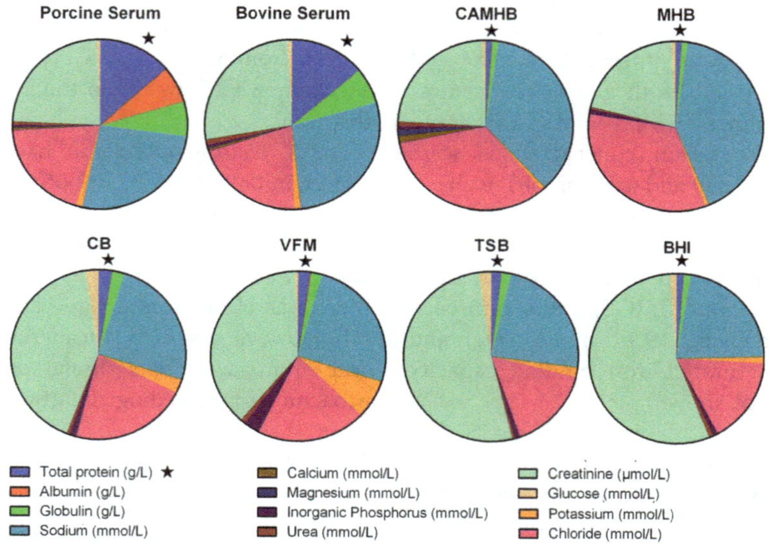

Fig. 3 In vitro growth of *A. pleuropneumoniae* (n = 20 isolates) at time points 0, 6 and 24 h in VFM and pig serum. Growth quantified in $\log_{10}$ CFU/mL (ordinate); each bar represents mean of triplicate analyses

to proteins in biological fluids. For example, Honeyman et al. [21] compared potencies of several tetracyclines in broth and a 50% broth: 50% serum mixture. They established marked differences in MIC for the two growth matrices. Moreover, MICs differed and had to be determined on a matrix-by-matrix, species-by-species, compound-by-compound basis. Likewise, Brentnall et al. [10, 14] reported for oxytetracycline, after correction for serum protein binding, for a calf isolate of *Mannheimia haemolytica*, a MIC in serum 6 times *greater* than the broth MIC. In marked contrast, Toutain et al. [6] reported, after correction for serum protein binding, MICs some 80-fold *smaller* in calf serum compared to broth for tulathromycin for *M. haemolytica* and *P. multocida* isolates from calves. Similar findings, with quantitatively even lower MICs for *Mycoplasma mycoides mycoides* in calf serum compared to broth, were reported for the macrolides, tulathromycin and gamithromycin by Mitchell et al. [22–24]. Thus, whilst correction for serum protein binding is always necessary, it is not always sufficient to account for potency differences between matrices.

These published data suggest: first, that serum MIC values should be considered on both a drug-by-drug and bacterial species-by-species basis to allow for the inactive protein bound fraction; and second, corrected serum values may not be the same as, and therefore might be used in preference to, the broth MIC for PK/PD breakpoint estimation.

Only free drug is microbiologically active and therefore protein binding is a major factor, and unfortunately sometimes the only factor, considered in seeking to explain growth medium differences in antimicrobial drug potency [2, 3, 9, 16, 20, 25–27]. The magnitude of drug binding to serum protein can vary with methodology [16] and, moreover, for single drugs, intra-species differences have been reported. In addition, it is necessary to consider possible differences in protein binding in serum obtained from different sources, differing animal breeds, ages and indeed between healthy and diseased animals. Such variations must be borne in mind in considering the present findings, for which protein binding was determined for pig serum from a single source in healthy animals. In fact, for all three drugs investigated, the degree of binding was independent of total concentration over therapeutic ranges [17–19].

For both organisms investigated in this study, correcting the serum MIC for protein binding for marbofloxacin, florfenicol and oxytetracycline yielded fu serum MICs differing from broth MICs in most instances. Fu serum:broth MIC ratios were: marbofloxacin 0.63:1 (*P. multocida*) and 0.35:1 (*A. pleuropneumoniae*); florfenicol 0.19:1 (*P. multocida*) and 0.38:1 (*A. pleuropneumoniae*); oxytetracycline 6.30:1 (*P. multocida*) and 0.35:1 (*A. pleuropneumoniae*). Thus, for marbofloxacin and florfenicol there were small to moderate trends for both pathogens of increased (1.6- to 5.2-fold) potency in serum compared to broth. Likewise, for oxytetracycline and *A. pleuropneumoniae* the greater potency in serum was 2.8-fold, whereas for *P. multocida* potency was 6.3-fold lower in serum. Consequently, correction of serum MIC for protein binding is, as stated, *necessary but not sufficient* for determination of potency differences between the two matrices for these two bacterial species and these three drugs. The consistent finding of differences, which were nevertheless unpredictable in direction (increased or reduced potency) and magnitude indicates the possibility of similar differences for human pathogens also more frequently than is commonly recognised.

Possibly the most important difference in chemical composition between all broths and serum was in albumin concentration, which was much higher in serum. Correction for drug binding to serum albumin revealed broth/serum potency differences for all drugs. It is therefore necessary to consider whether other differences, as well as albumin content, in chemical composition might explain the protein binding corrected potency differences. The chemical analyses indicated wide differences in composition of five broths for electrolytes, iron and organic compounds. Possibly surprisingly, these frequently large inter-broth differences resulted in, at most, very minor differences in MICs, with one exception, namely marbofloxacin, and for *P. multocida* only. However, even for this drug and species, MICs were similar for two broths and different but again similar for other three broths. In contrast, the broth and corrected serum MICs differed, despite the finding that chemical composition of pig serum for every analyte was within the lower and upper ranges for the five broths. Therefore, chemical composition indicated no readily apparent explanation for the broth/serum MIC differences.

In addition to the chemical differences between broths and serum, for circulating blood there are other differences e.g. the presence of white and red cells as well as a wide range of immunological components in blood. Future studies should therefore be directed towards evaluating which of these might interact with drugs, and how, to modulate drug potency. One factor, pH, is known to influence the rate and extent of growth of microorganisms [28, 29]. An effect of pH on weakly basic drugs such as macrolides and triamilides is well recognised [6].

Zeitlinger et al. [26] compared growth curves of *Staphylococcus aureus* and *Pseudomonas aeruginosa* in MHB and serum. Slower logarithmic growth was obtained for both species in serum compared to broth, and this might be expected to provide more rapid kill in serum, as a consequence of a smaller microbial challenge [5, 30]. Indeed, Illambas et al. [31, 29] reported significant effects of inoculum count (high, medium and low) on MIC for marbofloxacin and florfenicol and the calf pneumonia pathogens, *M. haemolytica* and *P. multocida*, while Dorey et al. [17–19] reported similar dependency of MIC on inoculum strength for the three drugs and the two pig pathogens investigated in this study.

In the present study, bacterial growth was initially greater in broths than serum for both *P. multocida* and *A. pleuropneumoniae*. This difference persisted for *P. multocida* at 24 h, whereas for *A. pleuropneumoniae* logarithmic growth was similar for the two media at this time. Slower growth, resulting potentially in lesser challenge to bacterial kill, therefore might explain, at least in part, the greater potency in serum compared to broth in five of six instances. The one notable exception, however, was the 6-fold reduction in potency of oxytetracycline in serum compared to broth for *P. multocida*. This finding indicates that some serum factor, presently unknown, operates to reduce potency of this drug for this species, whilst conversely potency was increased in serum for *A. pleuropneumoniae*.

The differences in MIC between serum and broth reported in this study do not provide a rationale for abandoning broths by diagnostic laboratories reporting MIC distributions of wild type organisms. This would be impractical and unnecessary. Rather, the present data suggest that, for marbofloxacin, florfenicol and oxytetracycline and the two bacterial species studied, it will be appropriate and possible to apply a scaling factor, to bridge between MICs in broths and pig serum when calculating PK/PD breakpoints.

Conclusion

For three commonly used drugs, florfenicol, oxytetracycline and marbofloxacin, and two pathogenic species of bacteria causing pig pneumonia, *A. pleuropneumoniae* and *P. multocida*, differences between serum and broth MICs were obtained, after correction was made for binding to serum protein. In contrast, major differences were not obtained when MICs were determined in five broths, marked differences in chemical composition between the broths notwithstanding. In the absence of drugs, the rate of logarithmic growth of *A. pleuropneumoniae* and *P. multocida* was slower in pig serum than in broth. It is suggested that, in using MIC data as a pharmacodynamic parameter to determine PK/PD breakpoints, the use of a scaling factor to bridge between broth and biological fluids may be required more commonly than currently recognised.

Highlights

- For florfenicol, oxytetracycline and marbofloxacin and the pig pathogens, A. pleuropneumoniae and P. multocida, there were no major differences in MICs measured in five broths, widely differing in chemical composition.
- Significant differences between serum and broth MICs were obtained, after correction for binding to serum protein, indicating that such correction is necessary but that it does not alone account for potency differences.
- With one exception potency was greater in serum than broths.
- In using MIC data to predict dosages for clinical use, the use of a scaling factor to bridge between broth and biological fluids may be required.

Abbreviations

ATCC: American Type Culture Collection; BHI: Brain Heart Infusion Broth; CAMHB: cation-adjusted Mueller Hinton Broth; CB: Columbia Broth; CLSI: Clinical and Laboratory Standards Institute; EUCAST: Committee on Antimicrobial Susceptibility Testing; MHB: Mueller Hinton Broth; MIC: Minimum inhibitory concentration; NAD: Nicotinamide Adenine Dinucleotide; PD: Pharmacodynamics; PK: Pharmacokinetics; TSB: Tryptic Soy Broth; VFM: Veterinary Fastidious Medium

Acknowledgements

Lucy Dorey was a BBSRC CASE AWARD Scholar. A. Pridmore, Don Whitley Scientific, and A. Rycroft, Royal Veterinary College, supplied bacterial isolates.

Funding

This project was funded by a BBSRC and Norbrook Laboratories Ltd. CASE Award; grant number BB/101649X1.

Authors' contributions

LD and PL were responsible for the study design and co-ordination, data analysis and both were involved in writing the manuscript. LD conducted the experiments. Both authors approved the final manuscript.

Authors' information

Address: Comparative Biological Sciences, Royal Veterinary College, London University, United Kingdom.

Competing interests

The authors declare that they have no competing interests.

Consent for publication

Not applicable.

References

1. Toutain PL, Lees P. Integration and modelling of pharmacokinetic and pharmacodynamic data to optimize dosage regimens in veterinary medicine. J Vet Pharmacol Ther. 2004;27(6):467-7.
2. Nielsen EI, Cars O, Friberg LE. Pharmacokinetic/pharmacodynamic (PK/PD) indices of antibiotic predicted by a semimechanistic PK/PD model: a step toward model-based dose optimization. Antimicrob Agents Chemother. 2011;55(10):4619–30.
3. Nielsen EI, Friberg LE. Pharmacokinetic-Pharmacodynamic modeling of antibacterial drugs. Pharmacol Rev. 2013;65(3):1053–90.
4. Lees P, Pelligand L, Illambas J, Potter T, Lacroix M, Rycroft A, et al. Pharmacokinetic/pharmacodynamic integration and modelling of amoxicillin for the calf pathogens Mannheimia haemolytica and Pasteurella multocida. J Vet Pharmacol Ther. 2015;38(5):457–70.
5. Martinez MN, Papich MG, Drusano GL. Dosing regimen matters: the importance of early intervention and rapid attainment of the pharmacokinetic/pharmacodynamic target. Antimicrob Agents Chemother. 2012;56(6):2795–805.
6. Toutain PL, Potter T, Pelligand L, Lacroix M, Illambas J, et al. Standard PK/PD concepts can be applied to determine a dosage regimen for a macrolide: the case of tulathromycin in the calf. J Vet Pharmacol Ther 2016; doi: 10.1111/jvp.12333, in press.
7. CLSI. Performance Standards for Antimicrobial Disk and Dilution Susceptibility Tests for Bacteria Isolated from Animals: Approved Standard - Fourth Edition. CLSI document VET01-A4 (formerly M31-A3, 2008) Supplementary information VET01-S, 2015. ISBN 1–56238–877-0 [print]; ISBN 1–56238–878-9 [electronic]. Clinical and Laboratory Standards Institute, 950 West Valley Road, Suite 2500, Wayne, Pennsylvania 19087 USA, 2013.
8. Papich MG. Pharmacokinetic-Pharmacodynamic (PK-PD) modelling and the rational selection of dosage regimes for the prudent use of antimicrobial drugs. Vet Micro. 2014;171(3):480 6.
9. Zeitlinger MA, Derendorf H, Mouton JW, Cars O, Craig WA, et al. Protein Binding: Do We Ever Learn? Antimicrob Agents Chemother. 2011;55(7): 3067–74.
10. Brentnall C, Cheng Z, McKellar QA, Lees P. Pharmacodynamics of oxytetracycline administered alone and in combination with carprofen in calves. Vet Rec. 2012;171(11):273–7.
11. Aliabadi FS, Lees P. Pharmacokinetics and pharmacodynamics of danofloxacin in serum and tissue fluids of goats following intravenous and intramuscular administration. Amer J Vet Res. 2001;62(12):1979–89.
12. Sidhu P, Landoni MF, Aliabadi FS, Lees P. Pharmacokinetic and pharmacodynamic modelling of marbofloxacin administered alone and in combination with tolfenamic acid in goats. Vet J. 2010;184(2):219–29.
13. Aliabadi FS, Lees P. Pharmacokinetics and pharmacokinetic/pharmacodynamic integration of marbofloxacin in calf serum, exudate and transudate. J Vet Pharmacol Ther. 2002;25(3):161–74.
14. Brentnall C, Cheng Z, McKellar QA, Lees P. Pharmacokinetic-pharmacodynamic integration and modelling of oxytetracycline administered alone and in combination with carprofen in calves. Res Vet Sci. 2013;94(3):687–94.
15. Nightingale CH, Murakawa T. Microbiology and pharmacokinetics. In Microbiology and pharmacokinetics Eds Nightingale, C.H., Murakawa, T. Ambrose, P.G. Marcel Dekker, A.G. New York: Marcel Dekker, Inc.; 2002. pp. 23–39.
16. Barbour AM, Schmidt S, Zhuang L. Application of pharmacokinetic/pharmacodynamic modelling and simulation for the prediction of target attainment of ceftobiprole against meticillin-resistant *Staphylococcus aureus* using minimum inhibitory concentration and time–kill curve based approaches. Int J Antimicrob A. 2014;43(1):60–7.
17. Dorey L, Hobson S, Lees P. What is the true in vitro potency of oxytetracycline for the pig pneumonia pathogens A. pleuropneumoniae and P. multocida ? J Vet Pharmacol Ther. 2016. doi:10.1111/jvp.12386.
18. Dorey L, Hobson S, Lees P. Activity of florfenicol for the porcine pneumonia pathogens Actinobacillus pleuropneumoniae and Pasteurella multocida using standardised versus non-standardised methodology. Vet J. 2016; doi:10.1016/j.tvjl.2016.11.004.
19. Dorey L, Hobson S, Lees P. Potency of marbofloxacin for pig pneumonia pathogens Actinobacillus pleuropneumoniae and Pasteurella multocida: comparison of growth media. Res Vet Sci. 2016; doi:10.1016/j.rvsc.2016.11.001.
20. Gonzalez D, Schmidt S, Derendorf H. Importance of relating efficacy measures to unbound drug concentrations for anti-infective Agents. Clin Microbiol Rev. 2013;26(2):274–88.
21. Honeyman L, Ismail M, Nelson ML, Bhatia B, Bowser TE, Chen J, et al. Structure-activity relationship of the aminomethylcyclines and the discovery of omadacycline. Antimicrob Agents Chemother. 2015;59:7044–53.
22. Mitchell JD, McKellar QA, McKeever DJ. Pharmacodynamics of antimicrobials against Mycoplasma mycoides mycoides small colony, the causative agent of contagious bovine pleuropneumonia: PLoS One 2012; v. 7, p. e44158.
23. Mitchell JD, Goh S, McKellar QA, DJ MK. In vitro pharmacodynamics of gamithromycin against Mycoplasma mycoides subspecies mycoides small Colony. Vet J. 2013;197(3):806–11.
24. Mitchell JD, McKellar QA, McKeever DJ. Evaluation of antimicrobial activity against Mycoplasma mycoides subsp. mycoides small Colony using an in vitro dynamic dilution pharmacokinetic/pharmacodynamic model. J Med Microbiol. 2013;62(1):56–61.
25. Wise R. The clinical relevance of protein binding and tissue concentrations in antimicrobial therapy. Clin Pharmacokinet. 1986;11(6):470–82.
26. Zeitlinger MA, Sauermann R, Traunmüller F, Georgopoulos A, Müller M, Joukhadar C. Impact of plasma protein binding on antimicrobial activity using time-killing curves. J Antimicrob Chemother. 2004;54(5): 876–80.
27. Zeitlinger M, Sauermann R, Fille M, Hausdorfer J, Leitner I, Müller M. Plasma protein binding of fluoroquinolones affects antimicrobial activity. J Antimicrob Chemother. 2008;61(3):561–7.
28. Russell JB, Dombrowski DB. Effect of pH on the efficiency of growth by pure cultures of rumen bacteria in continuous culture. Appl Environ Microbiol. 1980;39(3):604–10.
29. Illambas J, Potter T, Sidhu P, Rycroft AN, Cheng Z et al. Pharmacodynamics of florfenicol for calf pneumonia pathogens. Vet Rec. 2013;172(13):340–6.
30. Drusano GL. What are the properties that make an antibiotic acceptable for therapy of community acquired pneumonia? J Antimicrob Chemother. 2011;66(suppl 3):iii61–iii67. doi:10.1093/jac/dkr100 PMID: 21482571

5

A novel composite formulation of palmitoylethanolamide and quercetin decreases inflammation and relieves pain in inflammatory and osteoarthritic pain models

Domenico Britti[1], Rosalia Crupi[2], Daniela Impellizzeri[2], Enrico Gugliandolo[2], Roberta Fusco[2], Carlo Schievano[3], Valeria Maria Morittu[1], Maurizio Evangelista[4], Rosanna Di Paola[2] and Salvatore Cuzzocrea[2,5*]

Abstract

Background: Osteoarthritis (OA) is a common progressive joint disease in dogs and cats. The goal of OA treatment is to reduce inflammation, minimize pain, and maintain joint function. Currently, non-steroidal anti-inflammatory drugs (e.g., meloxicam) are the cornerstone of treatment for OA pain, but side effects with long-term use pose important challenges to veterinary practitioners when dealing with OA pain. Palmitoylethanolamide (PEA) is a naturally-occurring fatty acid amide, locally produced on demand by tissues in response to stress. PEA endogenous levels change during inflammatory and painful conditions, including OA, i.e., they are typically increased during acute conditions and decreased in chronic inflammation. Systemic treatment with PEA has anti-inflammatory and pain-relieving effects in several disorders, yet data are lacking in OA. Here we tested a new composite, i.e., PEA co-ultramicronized with the natural antioxidant quercetin (PEA-Q), administered orally in two different rat models of inflammatory and OA pain, namely carrageenan paw oedema and sodium monoiodoacetate (MIA)-induced OA. Oral treatment with meloxicam was used as benchmark.

Results: PEA-Q decreased inflammatory and hyperalgesic responses induced by carrageenan injection, as shown by: (i) paw oedema reduction, (ii) decreased severity in histological inflammatory score, (iii) reduced activity of myeloperoxidase, i.e., a marker of inflammatory cell infiltration, and (iv) decreased thermal hyperalgesia. Overall PEA-Q showed superior effects compared to meloxicam. In MIA-treated animals, PEA-Q exerted the following effects: (i) reduced mechanical allodynia and improved locomotor function, (ii) protected cartilage against MIA-induced histological damage, and (iii) counteracted the increased serum concentration of tumor necrosis factor alpha, interleukin 1 beta, metalloproteases 1, 3, 9 and nerve growth factor. The magnitude of these effects was comparable to, or even greater than, those of meloxicam.

(Continued on next page)

* Correspondence: salvator@unime.it
[2]Department of Chemical, Biological, Pharmaceutical and Environmental Sciences, University of Messina, Viale Ferdinando Stagno D'Alcontres 31-, I-98166 Messina, Italy
[5]Manchester Biomedical Research Centre, Manchester Royal Infirmary, School of Medicine, University of Manchester, Manchester, UK
Full list of author information is available at the end of the article

(Continued from previous page)

Conclusion: The present findings shed new light on some of the inflammatory and nociceptive pathways and mediators targeted by PEA-Q and confirm its anti-inflammatory and pain-relieving effects in rodent OA pain models. The translatability of these observations to canine and feline OA pain is currently under investigation.

Keywords: Osteoarthritis, Disease models, Pain, Inflammation, Drug combinations, Palmitoylethanolamide, Quercetin, Co-ultra micronization, N-acylethanolamines

Background

Osteoarthritis (OA) represents one of the most frequently occurring painful conditions in both humans and small animals [1]. In dogs, it affects approximately 20% of those over the age of 1 year [2]. OA is also very common in elderly domesticated cats, its prevalence being greater than 50% [3]. Clinical signs (i.e., lameness, stiffness, behavioral and lifestyle changes) are largely related to persistent and chronic pain [1–3], i.e. a mixed phenomenon involving both inflammatory and neuropathic mechanisms at the peripheral (joint) and central (spinal and supraspinal) levels [4]. Currently, the most frequently used analgesics for canine and feline OA are non-steroidal anti-inflammatory drugs (NSAIDs) [4]. Despite their widespread use, the main drawbacks of NSAIDs relate to both poor efficacy against the neuropathic component of OA pain [5] and unwanted side effects, especially with long-term use [6]. Thus, research is now focused on the identification of more effective and safe analgesic tools, as part of an ideal multimodal management of pain in veterinary OA patients [4, 7].

Given the aetiological and clinical heterogeneity of canine and feline OA, several animal models have been employed to investigate the multifaceted mechanisms of OA pain and to evaluate the analgesic efficacy of different compounds [8, 9]. Experimental OA pain models that provide ease of induction and reproducibility without the need for surgery are favored [9]. Of these, subplantar carrageenan (CAR) injection is recognized as a model of acute and highly reproducible inflammatory pain [10, 11], the main signs of inflammation - oedema, hyperalgesia, and erythema – developing immediately following subcutaneous injection. Neutrophils readily migrate to sites of CAR-induced inflammation and generate pro-inflammatory mediators, such as bradykinin, histamine, and reactive oxygen and nitrogen species, with consequent sensitization of local nociceptors and inflammatory pain development [11]. Recently, the intra-articular injection of sodium monoiodoacetate (MIA) has been suggested to be more predictive of OA pain drug efficacy than other models [8, 9]. MIA inhibits a key glycolytic enzyme, leading to chondrocyte cell death and bone lesions [9]. Pain-related characteristics in the MIA model are considered to originate from an inflammatory pain state induced by the local increase of inflammatory cytokines, followed by gradual initiation of neuronal cell injury and nerve sensitization, culminating in neuropathic pain [9, 12].

Palmitoylethanolamide (PEA) is a naturally-occurring N-acylethanolamine and a congener of the endocannabinoid anandamide [13]. First discovered in the 1950s as the active anti-inflammatory component of some food sources (recently reviewed in [14]), PEA has emerged as a disease-modifying agent in conditions eliciting both inflammatory and neuropathic pain, both in experimental (e.g. intraplantar injection of formalin, chronic constriction injury, viscerovisceral hyperalgesia) and naturally occurring conditions (eg. diabetic neuropathy, low back pain and pelvic pain in human patients) [13–15]. Moreover, PEA is currently considered a negative regulator of tissue inflammation [14, 16]. However, its effect on joint disease-related pain remains to be fully investigated. Available data are mainly limited to changes in endogenous levels of PEA, with an increase being reported in the spinal cord of MIA-treated rats [17] and a marked decrease in the synovial fluid of human patients with OA or rheumatoid arthritis [18]. These findings posit that PEA metabolism is deregulated during joint disorders and that exogenous supply of PEA may be beneficial in such conditions [19].

Oxidative stress is considered to be an important etiologic factor in OA [20], and the antioxidant quercetin has been used with success as an adjunct in human and experimental arthritic diseases [21, 22]. New formulations of PEA have recently been introduced in the Italian and international health market, both in the human and veterinary fields [14]. These mainly comprise micronized or ultramicronized formulations of PEA (i.e., micron- or submicron-sized particles with better solubility), that show superior activity compared to naïve PEA [23]. In some formulations, PEA is micronized (or ultramicronized) together with natural polyphenols, showing a synergistic effect and the ability to target also the oxidative stress cascade [14]. The newest of these formulations is a co-ultramicronized composite of PEA with quercetin (PEA-Q).

Based on the above considerations, the present study aimed to investigate the anti-inflammatory and pain-relieving effects of PEA-Q. Two sets of experiments were carried out. In the first (preliminary study) the CAR-induced inflammatory rat pain model was used.

The encouraging results thus obtained led us to then test PEA-Q in the MIA-induced rat OA pain model. In both sets of experiments pain thresholds were evaluated and inflammatory/nociceptive markers measured. In all these studies meloxicam was used as a representative NSAID commonly prescribed in Europe for treating chronic OA pain in dogs and cats.

Methods

Animals

This study was performed on Sprague–Dawley male rats (200–230 g, 7 weeks old, Envigo RMS Srl, S. Pietro al Natisone, Udine, Italy). Ten rats were used for each treatment group (see below). Food and water were available ad libitum. The University of Messina Review Board for the care and use of animals authorized the study. Animal care was in accordance with Italian regulations on protection of animals used for experimental and other scientific purposes (D.M.116192) as well as with EEC regulations (C.J. of E.C. L 358/1 12/18/1986).

Reagents

Co-ultramicronized PEA-Q was kindly provided by Epitech group SpA (Saccolongo, Italy). PEA-Q is the result of the joint ultramicronization - by jet-milling technology - of a mixture made of PEA and quercetin in a 5:1 ratio by mass. All other compounds were obtained from Sigma-Aldrich, Milan, Italy. All chemicals were of the highest commercial grade available. All stock solutions were prepared in non-pyrogenic saline (0.9% NaCl, Baxter International, Rome, Italy).

Experimental models

CAR-induced inflammation

Rats were anesthetized with 5.0% isoflurane in 100% O_2 (Baxter International, Rome, Italy) and received a subplantar injection of CAR (0.1 ml/rat of a 1% suspension in saline) (Sigma–Aldrich, Milan, Italy) as previously reported [11]. Injections were performed using a 27-gauge needle inserted into the pad region of the glabrous skin on the underside of the right hind paw. At 6 h following CAR injection, rats were sacrificed by anaesthetic (isoflurane) overdose.

All analyses conducted in CAR-injected rats (see details below) were performed in a blinded manner.

MIA induction model

OA was induced by intra-articular injection of MIA in the right knee joint as previously described [24]. On day 0, rats were anesthetized with 5.0% isoflurane in 100% O_2. A volume of 25 μl saline +3 mg of MIA was injected into the knee joint through the right intrapatellar ligament. The left knee received an equal volume of saline. MIA was prepared in sterile conditions and injected using a 50 μl Hamilton syringe with a 27 gauge needle that was inserted into the joint for about 2–3 mm. On day 21 post-MIA injection, rats were sacrificed by anaesthetic overdose and perfused with 4% paraformaldehyde. All analyses conducted in MIA-injected rats (see details below) were performed in a blinded manner.

Experimental design

Treatment groups

The experiment was divided in two steps. First, we conducted a preliminary study to evaluate the effect of PEA-Q on inflammation and pain-related events (i.e., thermal hyperalgesia) in the CAR-induced paw oedema model. Rats were arbitrarily allocated to the following treatment groups, each compound being administered orally 30 min before CAR injection:

(i) CAR + vehicle (saline): rats were subjected to CAR-induced paw oedema, as described above (N = 10);
(ii) CAR + quercetin: same as the CAR + vehicle group plus 3.3 mg/kg quercetin dissolved in carboxymethylcellulose (1.5% *w*/*v* in saline) (N = 10);
(iii) CAR + PEA-Q (10): same as the CAR + vehicle group plus 10 mg/kg PEA-Q dissolved in carboxymethylcellulose (1.5% *w*/*v* in saline) (N = 10);
(iv) CAR + PEA-Q (20): same as the CAR + vehicle group plus 20 mg/kg PEA-Q dissolved in carboxymethylcellulose (1.5% *w*/*v* in saline) (N = 10);
(v) CAR + meloxicam: same as the CAR + vehicle group plus 0.2 mg/kg meloxicam dissolved in saline (N = 10).
(vi) sham group: same surgical procedure as the CAR group, except that saline was administered instead of CAR (N = 10).

Doses were chosen based on a dose-response studied carried out in our lab and on existing literature data. The dose of quercetin used is equivalent to 20 mg/kg PEA-Q. Based on preliminary results, we evaluated the anti-inflammatory and analgesic effects of PEA-Q in an experimental model of MIA-induced OA pain (definitive study). Rats were randomly divided into the following treatment groups, each compound being administered orally three times per week for 21 days, starting the third day after MIA injection:

(i) MIA + vehicle (saline): rats were subjected to induction of OA pain as described above (N = 10).

(ii) MIA + PEA-Q (10): same as the MIA + vehicle group plus 10 mg/kg PEA-Q dissolved in carboxymethylcellulose (1.5% *w/v* in saline) (*N* = 10);
(iii) MIA + PEA-Q (20): same as the MIA + vehicle group plus 20 mg/kg PEA-Q dissolved in carboxymethylcellulose (1.5% *w/v* in saline) (*N* = 10);
(iv) MIA + meloxicam: same as the MIA + vehicle group plus 0.2 mg/kg meloxicam dissolved in carboxymethylcellulose (1.5% *w/v* in saline) (*N* = 10);
(v) sham-operated group: rats received an intra-articular injection of saline (25 μl) instead of MIA (*N* = 10).

Quercetin was not tested in this set of experiments, given the lack of effect observed in the previous set. Doses were chosen based on a dose-response study carried out in our lab and on existing literature data. The timing of oral administration was based on a previous study [25].

The effect of PEA alone was not investigated, since oral administration of micronized and ultramicronized PEA had been shown to reduce inflammation and pain in several experimental models, the effective dose being 10 mg/kg [13, 14], thus higher than the dose equivalent to 10 mg/kg PEA-Q used here. Moreover, oral administration of naïve PEA (non-micronized) did not exert any significant effect against inflammation and hyperalgesia up to 10 mg/kg [23].

Assessment of CAR-induced paw oedema

Oedma was assessed by directly measuring changes in paw volume using a plethysmometer (Ugo Basile, Varese, Italy), as previously described [11]. Paw volume was measured immediately prior to CAR injection and thereafter at hourly intervals for 6 h. Oedema was expressed as the increase in paw volume (ml) after CAR injection relative to pre-injection value. Six hours after CAR injection, percentage inhibition (protection) against oedema formation was calculated as follows and taken as an index of anti-inflammatory activity:

Percentage inhibition of inflammation = [(Vc-Vt)/Vc] × 100, where;

Vc = mean paw oedema volume in the control group at 6 h;

Vt = mean paw oedema volume in the drug-treated group at 6 h.

Pain-related behavioral analysis in the CAR model

The hyperalgesic response to heat was measured at different time points (0, 30 min, 1, 2, 3, 4 and 5 h) based on the method described by Hargreaves et al. [26] using Plantar Test 7371 (Ugo Basile, Italy). Briefly, animals were allowed to move freely within an open-topped transparent plastic chamber. After an acclimation period, a mobile infrared (I.R.) radiant heating source (IR 60) was placed under the glass floor and focused onto the hind paw. When the animal felt pain and withdrew its paw, the I.R. source switched off and the reaction time counter stopped. The withdrawal latency to the nearest 0.1 s was then automatically determined and recorded. A cutoff time of 20 s was set, i.e., if the rat failed to respond by 20 s the test was stopped in order to prevent tissue damage in non-responsive animals. Each point represents the delta change (sec) in withdrawal latency (withdrawal latency of contralateral minus withdrawal latency of injected paw) at each time point. Results are expressed as paw withdrawal latency changes (sec).

Percentage anti-hyperalgesic activity 5 h after CAR injection was calculated as follows.

Percentage anti-hyperalgesic activity = [(Vt-Vc)/Vt] × 100 where:

Vc = mean paw withdrawal latency in the control group at 5 h;

Vt = mean paw withdrawal latency in the drug-treated group at 5 h.

Histological analysis following CAR injection

Six hours after intraplantar CAR injection, animals were terminally anesthetized and paw biopsies collected. Histological analysis of haematoxylin and eosin-stained paw tissue was performed as previously described [23]. The degree of paw damage was evaluated according to Bang and Coll. [27], on a six-point score: 0 = no inflammation, 1 = mild inflammation, 2 = mild/moderate inflammation, 3 = moderate inflammation, 4 = moderate/severe inflammation and 5 = severe inflammation. The photographs obtained (*n* = 5 photos from five slides for each sample) were collected from all animals in each experimental group. The histological coloration (5 slides for each same sample) was repeated three times on different days.

Myeloperoxidase (MPO) activity following CAR injection

MPO activity, an index of neutrophilic granulocyte infiltration, was evaluated as previously described [28]. Briefly, after animals were terminally anesthetized paw tissues were collected and homogenized in a solution containing 0.5% hexadecyltrimethylammoniumbromide dissolved in 10 mM potassium phosphate buffer (pH 7) and centrifuged for 30 min at 20000 *g* (4 °C). The supernatant was allowed to react with a solution of tetramethylbenzidine (1.6 mM) and 0.1 mM H_2O_2. The rate of change in absorbance was measured spectrophotometrically at 650 nm. MPO activity was measured as the quantity of enzyme degrading 1 mM of peroxide min^{-1} at 37 °C, and expressed in units per gram of wet tissue weight.

Assessment of MIA-induced mechanical allodynia

Mechanical allodynia was evaluated using a dynamic plantar Von Frey hair aesthesiometer on day 0 and 3, 7, 14 and 21 days post-injection (Ugo Basile, Comerio, Italy). Rats were located on a metal mesh surface in a chamber in a room with controlled temperature (21-22° C) and were allowed to adapt for 15 min before testing began. The touch stimulator part was positioned under the rat. When the aesthesiometer was activated, a plastic monofilament touched the paw in the metatarsal region. The filament exercised a gradually increasing force on the plantar surface, starting below the threshold of detection and increasing until the stimulus became painful and the rat removed its paw. The force required to produce a paw withdrawal reflex was recorded automatically and measured in grams. A maximum force of 50 g and a ramp speed of 20 s were used for all the aesthesiometry tests. Paw withdrawal latency (PWL) and paw withdrawal threshold (PWT) were calculated.

Motor function analysis (walking track analysis) following MIA injection

Motor functional recovery of the rear limb was evaluated by walking track analysis, a reliable and easily quantifiable noninvasive method based on gait analysis by means of specific footprint parameters [29]. In brief, rats were previously trained to walk down a track with a dark end, covered with strips of white paper. Tracks were obtained by wetting the rat's hind feet with water soluble black ink. Walking track analysis was performed in all animal groups before MIA injection (day 0) and 3, 7, 14 and 21 days post-injection. From the footprints, several measurements are taken between different anatomic landmarks (e.g., width and length of the footprint) and then incorporated in a mathematical formula, allowing the calculation of the functionality index of the sciatic nerve (SFI), with values close to 0 indicating normal function, and values tending to −100 indicating total impairment [29].

Histological analysis of MIA-injected rats

On day 21 post-MIA injection, rats were sacrificed and perfused with 4% paraformaldehyde. The MIA- and vehicle-injected tibiofemoral joints were dissected and post-fixed in neutral buffered formalin (containing 4% formaldehyde), decalcified in EDTA and processed as previously described. After decalcification, the specimens were embedded in paraffin. Mid-coronal tissue sections (5 μm) were stained for evaluation; all histomorphometric analyses were performed by an observer blinded to the treatment group. Sections were stained with haematoxylin and eosin and observed by light microscopy (Dialux 22 Leitz; Leica Microsystems SpA, Milan, Italy). Histopathological analysis of the cartilage was assessed by the modified Mankin score [30]. Briefly, the score assessed: (i) structure, (ii) cellular abnormalities, and (iii) matrix staining of cartilage sections and ranged from 0 (= normal histology) to 12 (= complete disorganization and hypocellularity). The photographs obtained (n = 5 photos from five slides for each sample) were collected from all animals in each experimental group. The histological coloration (5 slides for each same sample) was repeated three times on different days.

Serum concentration of inflammatory, nociceptive and matrix degradation markers following MIA injection

The concentration of tumor necrosis factor alpha (TNF-α), interleukin-1beta (IL-1β), nerve growth factor (NGF), and matrix metalloproteinase-1-3-9 (MMP-1, MMP-3, MMP-9) were measured in serum using commercial colorimetric ELISA kits (TNF-α, IL-1β, NGF: Thermo Fisher Scientific, DBA s.r.l. Milan Italy; MMP-1 MMP-3 MMP-9: Cusabio, DBA s.r.l. Milan Italy).

Data analysis

Data are expressed as mean ± standard error of the mean (SEM) of N observations, N representing the number of animals analyzed, with the exception of the ordinal level variable (i.e., histological score), for which median and range were used. In experiments involving histology, the figures are representative of at least three experiments performed on different days. The response over time was analyzed using a generalized linear mixed model (GLMM) for repeated measures, followed by Tukey-Kramer *post-hoc* analysis. One time evaluations with continuous level data were analyzed using ANOVA followed by Bonferroni-Holm post hoc analysis. Kruskal-Wallis test followed by Dunn's test for *post-hoc* comparisons with Bonferroni-Holm p correction was used for the histological score, due the ordinal level nature of the variable (i.e., 0 to 5 point scale). Data were analyzed using SAS v9.2 (SAS Institute, Cary, NC, USA). The significance threshold was set at 0.05. Exact p values are reported, unless less than 1 out of 10,000 (reported as $p < 0.0001$), 0.0001 being the lower limit for the statistical program.

Results

Preliminary study

A. Effect of PEA-Q on the time-course of CAR-induced paw oedema

Intraplantar injection of CAR in rats led to a significant time-dependent increase in paw volume, reaching a peak after 3 h ($p < 0.0001$) (Fig. 1a). Oral treatment with PEA-Q at 10 mg/kg significantly reduced paw volume at 3, 4, 5 and 6 h after injection ($p = 0.0007$, $p = 0.0005$, $p = 0.0250$ and $p = 0.0029$ respectively). The same results were observed for 20 mg/kg ($p < 0.0001$ at all time points) (Fig. 1a). Overall the effect of both doses of

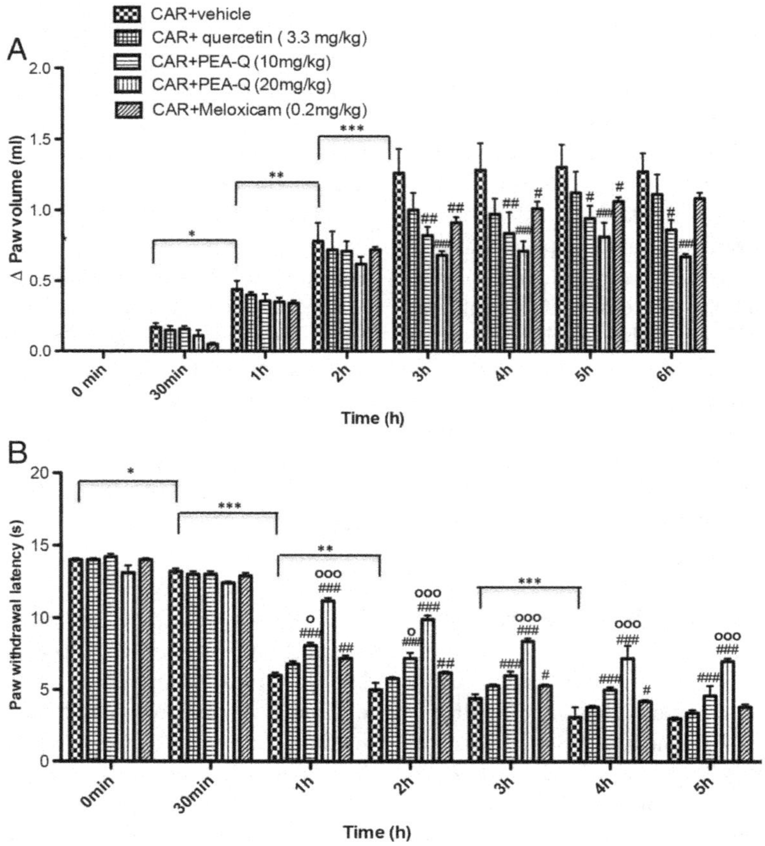

Fig. 1 Effects of PEA-Q on CAR-induced paw oedema and heat hyperalgesia. Paw oedema and hyperalgesia were measured at the time points indicated. Oral treatment with PEA-Q (10 and 20 mg/kg) produced a significant improvement in paw volume that, unlike meloxicam, lasted up to the latest time point (**a**). In addition, PEA-Q was more effective in decreasing the hyperalgesia compared meloxicam (**b**). See Methods for further details. Values are means ± SEM of 10 animals for each group. *$p < 0.05$, **$p < 0.001$ and ***$p < 0.0001$ vs previous time point. #$p < 0.05$, ##$p < 0.001$, ###$p < 0.0001$ vs CAR + vehicle. $^{\circ}p < 0.05$ and $^{\circ\circ\circ}p < 0.0001$ vs CAR + meloxicam. The exact p values are reported in the text

PEA-Q was longer compared to meloxicam, whose effect was no more statistically significant at 6 h. No significant difference was observed at any time points between the two doses of PEA-Q or between either dose of PEA-Q and meloxicam. Quercetin did not achieve a significant reduction at any of these time points (Fig. 1a). The percentage of anti-inflammatory activity of the tested compounds (quercetin, 10 and 20 mg/kg PEA-Q, and meloxicam) was, respectively, 10%, 30%, 45% and 12% (Fig. 2a).

B. Effect of PEA-Q on the time-course of CAR-induced thermal hyperalgesia

Intraplantar injection of CAR led to a statistically significant time-dependent development of thermal hyperalgesia, latency being increasingly decreased at 30 min, 1 h, 2 h and 4 h after injection (p = 0.0209, $p < 0.0001$, p = 0.0004, $p < 0.0001$ respectively) (Fig. 1b). Oral treatment with PEA-Q (10 and 20 mg/kg) was efficacious in decreasing the hyperalgesic response from the first to the fifth hour after injection ($p < 0.0001$ for both doses and all time points) (Fig. 1b). Moreover, the higher dose of PEA-Q resulted to be superior to the lower ($p < 0.0001$ at all time points). Similarly to paw oedema, the effect of meloxicam was shorter, statistical significance being lost at the fifth hour. Limited to the first and the second hour post-injection, the anti-hyperalgesic effect exerted by 10 mg/kg PEA-Q was significantly higher than that of meloxicam (p = 0.0309 and p = 0.0230 respectively). Superiority of 20 mg/kg PEA-Q over meloxicam was maintained at all time points ($p < 0.0001$). Quercetin was unable to change withdrawal latency (Fig. 1b). The percentage of anti-hyperalgesic activity of the tested compounds ranged from 12% (quercetin) to 57% (20 mg/kg PEA-Q) (Fig. 2b).

C. Effect of PEA-Q on CAR-induced histological damage

Sham rats exhibited no histological damage (Fig. 3a and inset a1). In contrast, CAR paw injection led to a marked infiltration of inflammatory cells (Fig. 3b and inset b1). Clear improvements were seen in paw tissues

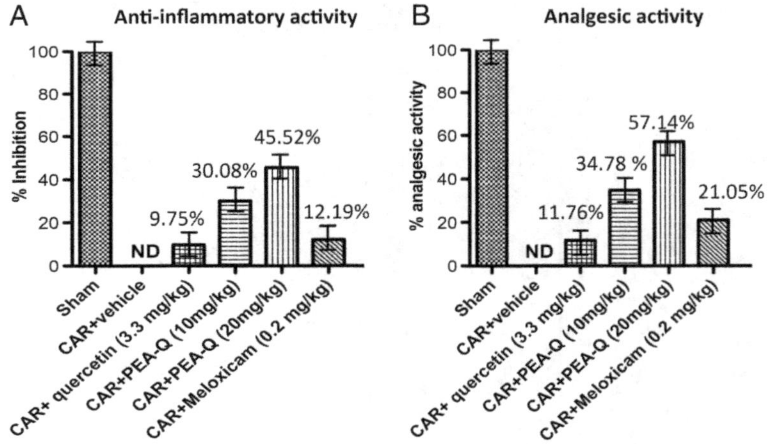

Fig. 2 Effects of PEA-Q on CAR-induced inflammation and analgesic activity. Percentages of anti-inflammatory (**a**) and analgesic activity (**b**) for the tested compounds as measured, respectively, at 6 h and 5 h post-CAR injection. See Methods for further details

of rats treated with PEA-Q at both doses (Fig. 3 d, d1; e, e1), while little effect was observed in the quercetin- and meloxicam-treated groups (Fig. 3c, c1, and Fig. 3f, f1). Histological score in the vehicle group (median 4, range 4–5) was significantly improved by PEA-Q both at 10 mg/kg (median 2, range 2–3) and 20 mg/kg dose (median 1, range 1–2) ($p < 0.0001$ for both doses). Quercetin (median 4, range 3–4) and meloxicam (median 3, range 3–4) did not significantly change the severity of the histological score compared to vehicle (Fig. 3g).

D. Effect of PEA-Q on CAR-induced increase in MPO activity

The development of histological damage was associated with a statistically significant increase in MPO activity ($p < 0.0001$), a marker of neutrophilic infiltration (Fig. 3h). Treatment with PEA-Q ($p < 0.0001$, both doses) and meloxicam ($p = 0.0014$), but not quercetin, significantly reduced MPO activity compared to vehicle (Fig. 3h). PEA-Q at the higher dose showed a statistically significant higher effect compared to meloxicam ($p = 0.0051$).

Definitive study

A. Effect of PEA-Q on pain and motor function deficits following MIA induction

Because pain is the hallmark of MIA-induced OA, mechanical allodynia in MIA-injected rats was assessed. In the von Frey hair assessment test, PWT (Fig. 4a) and PWL (Fig. 4b) were significantly decreased in the MIA + vehicle group compared to sham animals ($p < 0.0001$ for both variables at any time point). Treatment with PEA-Q at both doses ($p < 0.0001$ at any time point and either dose) and meloxicam ($p = 0.0103$ day 3 and $p < 0.0001$ at the following time points) significantly prolonged PWT compared to the MIA + vehicle group at different time points (Fig. 4a).

Similar findings were obtained on PWL ($p < 0.0001$ at all time points for any treatment), with the only difference that the effect of the lower dose of PEA-Q became significant at the seventh day ($p < 0.0001$ at 7, 14 and 21 days post-injection, Fig. 4b). The sham group showed no evident time-dependent changes (Fig. 4a, b). PEA-Q at 20 mg/kg dose resulted to exert a superior effect on both PWT and PWL compared to the lower dose and to meloxicam ($p < 0.0001$ for both variables and both comparisons, at any time point) (Fig. 4a, b). Furthermore, rats treated with PEA-Q at 20 mg/kg exhibited nociceptive behaviors that were not statistically different from the sham group up to day 14 and 21 for PWT and PWL respectively. In addition, motor function at different time points was assessed by walking track analysis. The sham group showed normal motor activity, with SFI approximating 0. In the MIA + vehicle group, SFI values were significantly lower than in sham animals, locomotor function being increasingly impaired at 3, 7, 14 and 21 days (Fig. 4c) ($p < 0.0001$ at all time points). Treatment with both PEA-Q and meloxicam significantly improved locomotor function at both 14 and 21 days ($p < 0.0001$ for each treatment and either time points) with no statistically significant differences being observed among treatments (Fig. 4c).

B. Effect of PEA-Q on MIA-induced histopathological changes

Histological examination of haematoxylin/eosin-stained knee sections 21 days after intra-articular injection of MIA showed a reduction in blood cells, irregularities in the surface layer, and multi-layering in transition and radial zones of the cartilage compared to sham (Fig. 5a, b see Mankin score F) ($p < 0.0001$). Treatment with PEA-Q at both doses reduced the histological cartilage changes induced by MIA injection (Fig. 5c,d see Mankin score F) ($p < 0.0001$ for either doses), the higher dose showing superior effect compared to the lower dose

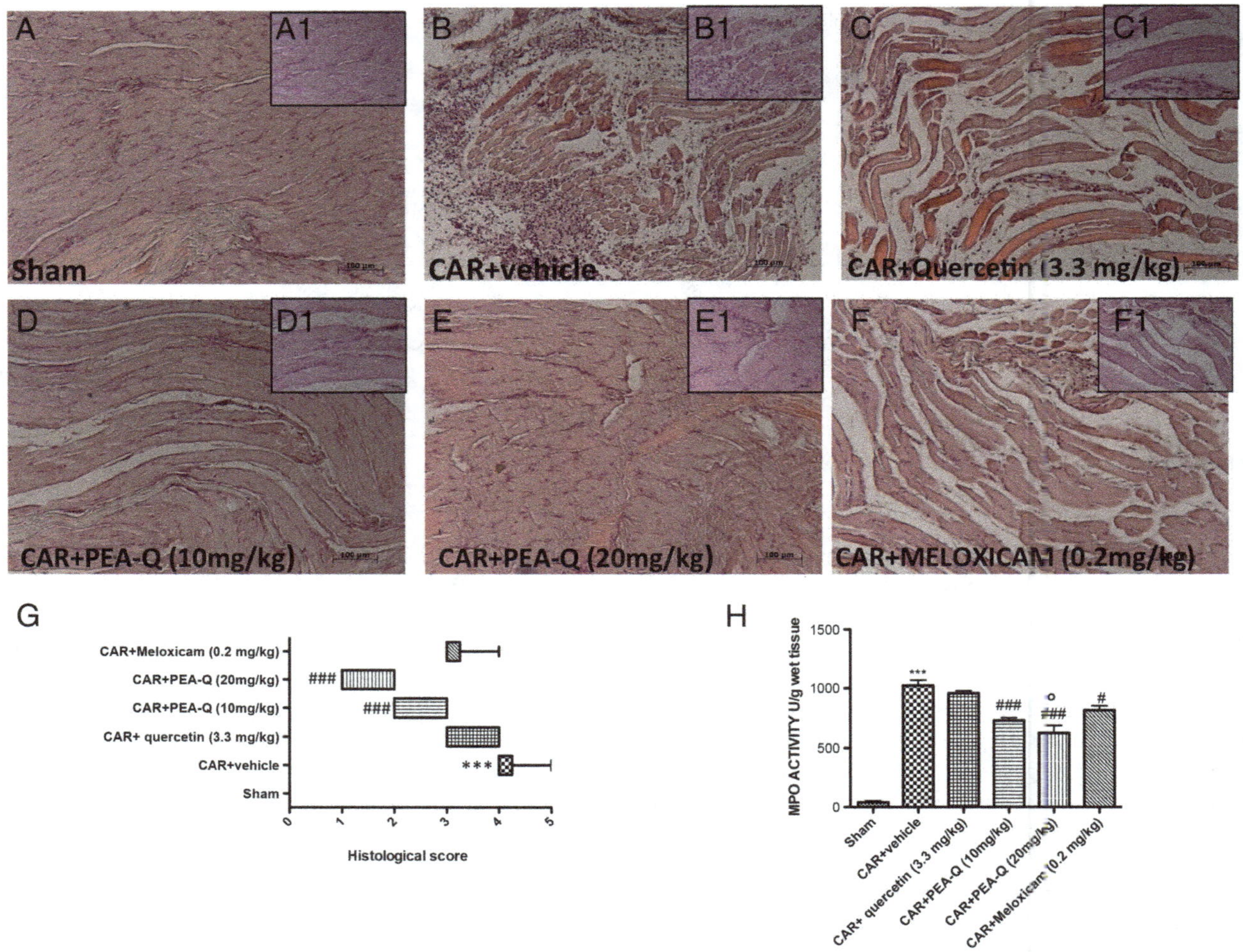

Fig. 3 Effects of PEA-Q on CAR-induced histological damage and neutrophil infiltration. Histological evaluation was performed by haematoxylin and eosin staining. Panels **a-a1**, sham; panels B-B1, CAR-injected; Panels **c-c1**, quercetin treatment; Panels **d**, **d1** and **e**, **e1**, PEA-Q treatment; Panels **f**, **f1** meloxicam treatment. Figures are representative of all animals in each group. Panel **g**, histological score for the various treatment groups. Distribution of data is represented by box plot analysis. Panel **h**, MPO activity. Values are means ± SEM of 10 animals for each group. $^{***}p < 0.0001$ vs sham. $^{\#}p < 0.05$ and $^{\#\#\#}p < 0.0001$ vs CAR + vehicle. $^{\circ}p < 0.05$ vs CAR + meloxicam. The exact p values are reported in the text

(p = 0.0058) and meloxicam (p = 0.0113, Fig. 5e see Mankin score F).

C. Effects of PEA-Q on plasma concentration of inflammatory, nociceptive and matrix degradation markers

A significant increase in serum concentration of the pro-inflammatory cytokines TNF-α (p = 0.0047, Fig. 6a) and IL-1β (p = 0.0007, Fig. 6b) and a similar increase in the level of the nerve sensitizer NGF ($p < 0.0001$, Fig. 6c) were observed in the MIA + vehicle group compared to sham animals. Treatment with PEA-Q significantly counteracted such increases at both 10 mg/kg (TNF-α, p = 0.0003; IL-1β, p = 0.0029; NGF, p = 0.0226) and 20 mg/kg dose (TNF-α, $p < 0.0001$; IL-1β, p = 0.0001; NGF, p = 0.0002). Similar findings were observed for meloxicam (TNF-α, $p < 0.0001$; IL-1β, $p < 0.0001$; NGF, p = 0.0017). Limited to TNF-α concentration, PEA-Q at the higher dose sowed a superior effect compared to the lower dose (p = 0.0070) and to meloxicam (p = 0.0443).

In addition, MIA + vehicle rats showed a markedly higher expression of the matrix degradation enzymes MMP-1 (Fig. 6d), MMP-3 (Fig. 6e), and MMP-9 (Fig. 6f) compared to the sham group ($p < 0.0001$ for all the three). PEA-Q significantly decreased MMP concentration compared to the vehicle-treated group, both at the 10 mg/kg dose (MMP-1, p = 0.0120; MMP-3, p = 0.0032; MMP-9, p = 0.0142) and at the 20 mg/kg one (MMP-1, p = 0.0002; MMP-3, $p < 0.0001$; MMP-9, p = 0.0003), similar to that observed with meloxicam (MMP-1, p = 0.0019; MMP-3, p = 0.0011; MMP-9,

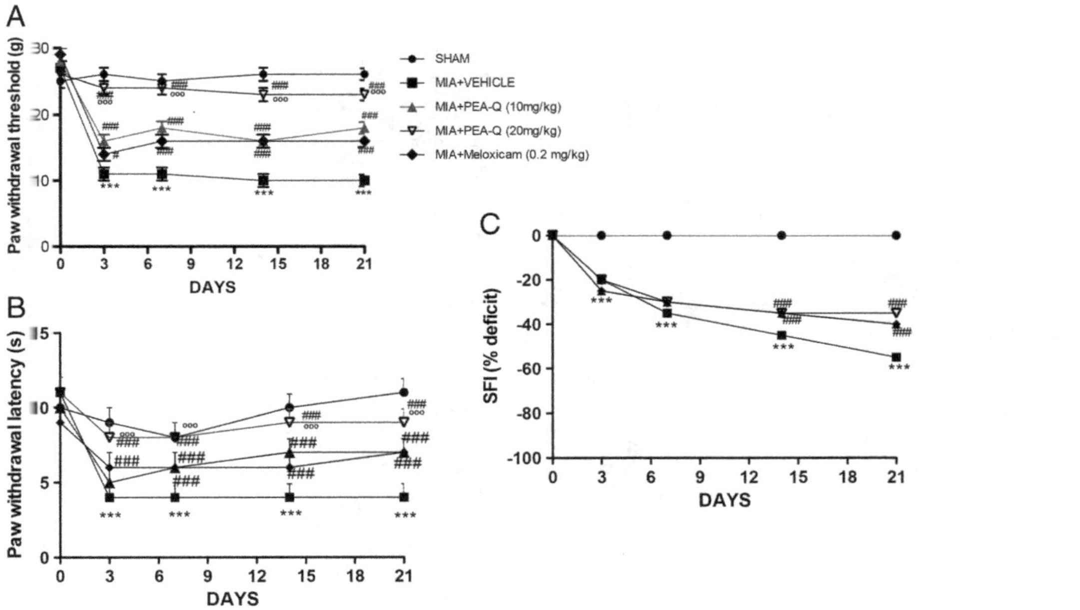

Fig. 4 Effects of PEA-Q on MIA-induced OA pain and motor function. Paw withdrawal threshold **a**, paw withdrawal latency **b** and motor function **c** as recorded for each treatment group before and after 3, 7, 14 and 21 days from the intra-articular injection of MIA. Data are means ± SEM of 10 rats for each group. ***$p < 0.0001$ versus sham. $^{\#}p < 0.05$ and $^{\#\#\#}p < 0.0001$ vs MIA + vehicle. $^{\circ\circ\circ}p < 0.0001$ vs MIA + PEA-Q (10 mg/kg) and MIA + meloxicam. The exact p values are reported in the text

$p = 0.0044$) (Fig. 6c–f). No statistically significant difference was observed between different PEA-Q doses or between either dose of PEA-Q and meloxicam.

Discussion

Here we show for the first time that a new co-ultramicronized composite, made of the anandamide congener PEA and the natural polyphenol quercetin (PEA-Q), exerts beneficial effects in both inflammatory and mixed persistent OA pain in rats. Although the anti-inflammatory and anti-hyperalgesic activities of PEA have been clearly demonstrated in several inflammatory and neuropathic pain models [13–15, 31], reports on joint disease-related pain states are scarce, with no study having yet been performed with PEA-Q. Conceivably, PEA-Q could dissociate into its single components (PEA and quercetin) after oral administration, although there is evidence supporting the synergistic effect of PEA and polyphenols [32]. OA pain is, without doubt, complex in its cellular/molecular mechanisms. As such, designing therapeutics that provide optimal efficacy may call for the use of models that allow one to evaluate distinct features of the disease in the context of the agent being evaluated. Indeed, we used both the CAR paw oedema and MIA-induced OA models, since previous studies gave information about the potential effect of the two components of PEA-Q on both inflammatory and neuropathic pain.

Intraperitoneal administration of ultramicronized PEA, alone or co-micronized with the polyphenol luteolin, is able to restore normal pain sensitivity and decrease inflammation in a rat model of rheumatoid arthritis [32]. In human patients, a two-week oral treatment with micronized PEA showed superior activity compared to the NSAID ibuprofen in decreasing temporomandibular joint inflammatory pain and improving joint function (better mandibular range of motion) [33]. Further, pharmacological inhibition of PEA degradation (which elevates tissue PEA levels), results in anti-hyperalgesic effects in arthritic pain models [34–36]. The pain relieving activity observed for PEA-Q is in line with these earlier findings, although direct comparisons are difficult due to different models and PEA formulations employed.

Quercetin has been reported to exert pain-relieving effects in different pain models [37] and, in particular, is able to reduce: (i) CAR-induced mechanical hyperalgesia [37], (ii) chemotherapy-induced neuropathic pain [38], (iii) diabetic neuropathic pain [37], and (iv) muscle mechanical hyperalgesia [39]. We were unable to confirm these observations, since quercetin did not show any significant effect on paw oedema or thermal sensitivity in the CAR-induced inflammatory pain model. This apparent lack of effect could result from differences in dosage used: we tested quercetin at 3.3 mg/kg (equivalent to 20 mg/kg PEA-Q), while the dosage used in the above-mentioned studies was approximately 100 mg/kg. Further synergistic studies will be

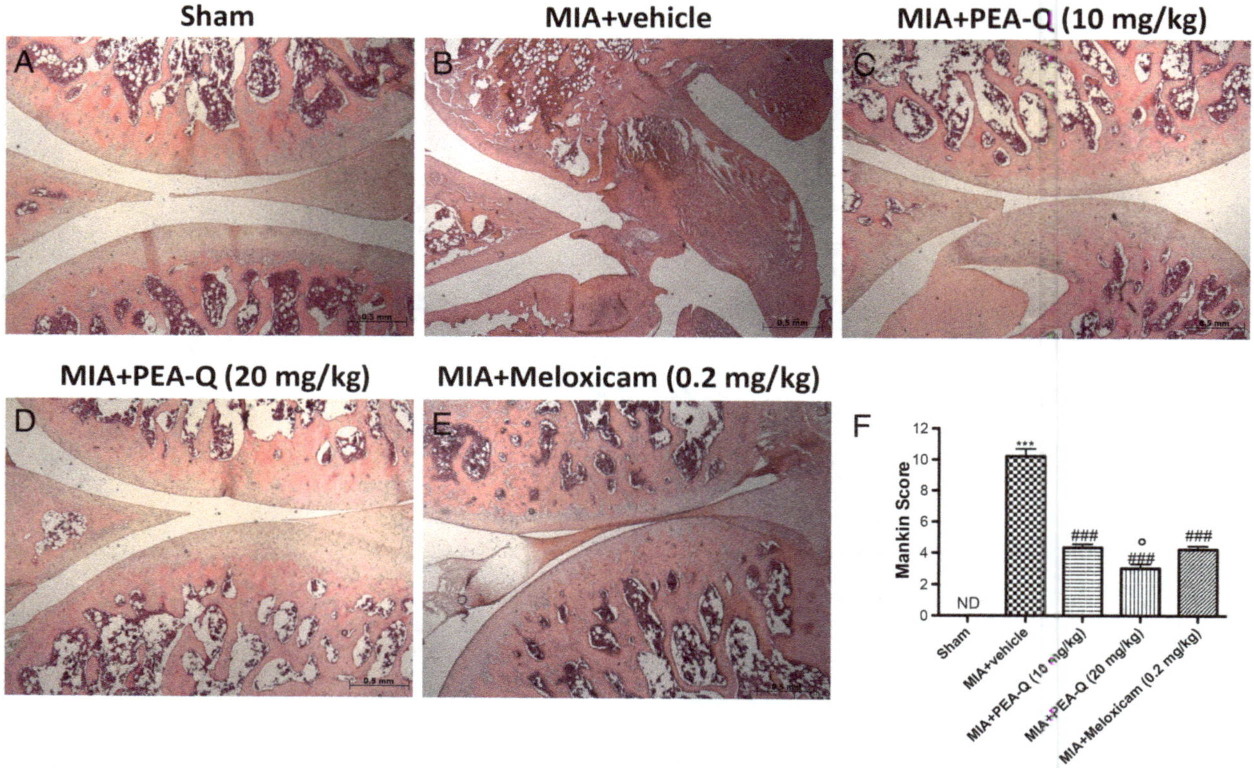

Fig. 5 Effects of PEA-Q on MIA-induced histological features of OA knee tissue. Histological evaluation was performed by haematoxylin and eosin staining. Panel (**a**), sham; panel (**b**), MIA–injected; Panels (**c**) and (**d**), PEA-Q treatment; Panels **d** and (**e**), meloxicam treatment. Figures are representative of all animals in each group. Panel (**f**), Mankin score for the various treatment groups. Values are means ± SEM of 10 animals for each group. $^{***}p < 0.0001$ vs sham. $^{###}p < 0.0001$ vs MIA + vehicle. $^{\circ}p < 0.05$ vs MIA + PEA-Q (10 mg/kg) and MIA + meloxicam

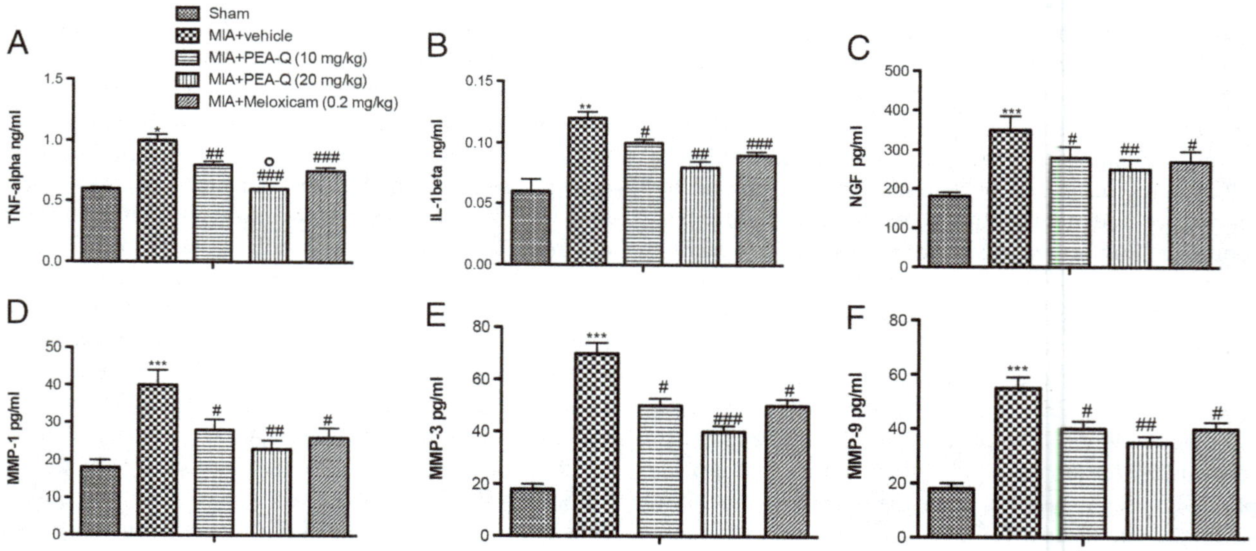

Fig. 6 Effects of PEA-Q on MIA-induced plasma cytokines, metalloproteinases and NGF in OA rats. Increased TNF-α (**a**) IL-1β (**b**), NGF (**c**) and MMP1 (**d**), MMP-3 (**e**), MMP-9 (**f**) plasma concentrations were detected in the MIA + vehicle group compared to sham animals. PEA-Q treatment significantly reduced the plasma concentration of all measured parameters, with effects being comparable to the meloxicam group. Values are means ± SEM of 10 animals for each group. $^{*}p < 0.05$, $^{**}p < 0.001$ and $^{***}p < 0.0001$ vs sham. $^{\#}p < 0.05$, $^{\#\#}p < 0.001$ and $^{\#\#\#}p < 0.0001$ vs MIA + vehicle. $^{\circ}p < 0.05$ vs MIA + PEA-Q (10 mg/kg) and MIA + meloxicam. The exact *p values* are reported in the text

needed to better characterize the contribution of quercetin to the activity of PEA-Q.

It was somewhat surprising that meloxicam exerted an anti-allodynic effect in the MIA model (significant improvement of PWL and PWT). NSAIDs are usually considered to be ineffective on allodynia, as recently shown in naturally-occurring OA in cats subjected to punctuate tactile allodynia quantification [40]. Again, differences in dosages used in the former study and ours, as well as species differences and nature of the disease (spontaneous versus chemically-induced OA) could be responsible for the apparent discrepancy. Although allodynia might not be the main target of meloxicam, its ability to improve functional parameters and pain scores in dogs with joint pain has been repeatedly demonstrated [41, 42]. Our findings on improved mechanical sensitivity and motor function following meloxicam are in line with the above-cited studies. PEA-Q also significantly improved locomotor function, as measured by walking track analysis. Interestingly, this analysis combines gait with the temporal and spatial relationship of one footprint to another during walking [29]. MIA injection is known to cause dropping of the foot to the ground, resulting in visible footprint changes [29]. One can envisage that these changes are associated with enhanced nociception and "antalgic gait". That is to say, OA animals minimize contact with the floor during walking. This could well correlate with the situation of OA dogs, in which walking likely causes enhanced nociception in the affected limb(s) leading to lameness. The decrease of walking alterations observed in our study might thus be clinically relevant and can be considered a measure of the motor functional recovery exerted by PEA-Q, as well as meloxicam.

The ability to decrease not only pain and locomotor deficits, but also inflammation is a further point in favor of the therapeutic use of PEA-Q in animals affected with OA. Inflammation and related soluble mediators are involved in: (i) the generation of acute pain, (ii) the vicious cycle of pain maintenance and chronicity, and (iii) the predominance of catabolic processes over anabolic ones, ultimately resulting in tissue degradation and damage at the cartilage and bone levels [7]. PEA-Q significantly reduced inflammatory paw oedema, and is in accordance with data obtained in the same model using either PEA [23, 43, 44], or PEA co-ultramicronized with various polyphenols [45]. Interestingly, PEA-Q showed a longer anti-inflammatory effect compared to meloxicam, whose effect lost significance at an earlier time point.

Neither meloxicam nor quercetin achieved statistical significance in decreasing histological signs of inflammation, while oral treatment with PEA-Q resulted in a clear reduction in histological inflammatory score. The effect was paralleled by a significant reduction in MPO activity (the most abundant pro-inflammatory enzyme of neutrophilic granulocytes) in PEA-Q treated rats, which proved to be superior to meloxicam in reducing neutrophil infiltration in paw tissues. These results are in agreement with previous studies, showing that PEA decreased inflammatory cell infiltration in different inflammatory models [23, 46, 47]. Notably, the increase of pro-inflammatory, nociceptive and proteolytic markers analyzed was significantly counteracted by PEA-Q to the same extent (and even better concerning TNF-α) as with meloxicam. Interestingly, cytokines (e.g., IL-1β, TNF-α) and MMPs are considered to play a crucial role in chondrocyte cell death and matrix degeneration [7, 48] and NGF is currently viewed as a key regulator of nociceptive and neuropathic pain [49]. Given that (i) the concentration of NGF in canine synovial fluid is significantly increased in chronically lame dogs [50], and (ii) feline OA-associated pain improves under treatment with a anti-NGF antibody [51], the ability of PEA-Q to reduce NGF levels during experimentally-induced OA holds promise for a disease-modifying effect against pain in canine and feline OA patients.

PEA-Q counteracted histological OA changes caused by MIA injection in the tibiofemoral joint and significantly decreased the severity of cartilage degeneration, the effect being superior to meloxicam. To the best of our knowledge no study has investigated the effect of either PEA or quercetin on histological joint damage, and so it is difficult to compare our data with previous findings. The only available data in this regard involves the effectiveness of intra-articular injected meloxicam, which decreased joint histologic score in MIA rats - albeit without reaching statistical significance [52].

Although complete extrapolation of efficacy from the pre-clinical models used here to veterinary patients would be unadvised, the present findings shed new light on some of the inflammatory and nociceptive pathways and molecules targeted by PEA-Q. In the present study, the use of two different models and assessment of the effect at different levels (behavioural, tissue, and molecular) to a large extent address the most relevant questions. Moreover, the pain-relieving effect of PEA-Q not only on CAR-inflammation but also on MIA-related pain supports its use in OA pain states, where inflammatory and neuropathic mechanisms frequently coexist. Studies on the effects of PEA-Q on pain and locomotion in lame dogs are in progress.

Conclusions

PEA-Q is a novel co-ultramicronized formulation of PEA and quercetin whose effects were investigated in two pre-clinical models of OA pain in rats. Oral administration of PEA-Q decreased pain sensitivity, improved locomotor function, reduced inflammatory signs and mediators and lowered histological damage score. Although the underlying mechanism(s) of the observed effects are beyond the scope of our study, the particular cellular targets of PEA (e.g., mast cells and microglia) [19], redundancy of its receptors (direct and direct agonism on nuclear and membrane cannabinoid receptors) [14] and oxidative stress addressed by quercetin [22, 37] comprise targets that could be different from standard pharmacological tools (i.e., NSAIDs). Importantly, toxicological studies show that micronized and ultramicronized PEA is safe, the LD50 being greater than 2000 mg/kg [53]. Individually or in association with different antioxidant polyphenols, micronized and ultramicronized PEA has a long track record of use in human and veterinary patients, with good-to-excellent tolerability [14]. Moreover, prolonged use of PEA is not associated with the development of tolerance [43, 54]. There is an unmet need in veterinary medicine for the development of new agents to treat OA-associated pain which target alternative mechanisms distinct from currently approved drugs. The collective observations presented here propose that PEA-Q shows promise for multimodal pain management in canine and feline OA.

Acknowledgements
The authors would like to thank Mrs. Maria Antonietta Medici for excellent technical assistance, Mr. Francesco Soraci for secretarial and administrative assistance and Miss Valentina Malvagni for editorial assistance with the manuscript.

Funding
The authors received no specific funding for this work.

Authors' contributions
DB conceived of the study and drafted the manuscript. RF, EG, RC and DI carried out the experiments and revised the manuscript. VMM and CS performed the statistical analysis. RDP, ME and SC designed the study and critically revised the manuscript. All authors read and approved the final manuscript.

Consent for publication
Not applicable

Competing interests
Dr. Salvatore Cuzzocrea is co-inventor on patent WO2013121449 A8 (Epitech Group SpA) which deals with compositions and methods for the modulation of amidases capable of hydrolysing N-acylethanolamines useable in the therapy of inflammatory diseases. Moreover, Dr. Cuzzocrea is also a co-inventor with Epitech group on the following patents: (1). EP2821083; (2). EP 2985037 A1; (3). 102,015,000,067,344. No other authors have competing interests.

Author details
[1]Department of Health Sciences V. le Europa, Campus S. Venuta, Germaneto, 88100 Catanzaro, Italy. [2]Department of Chemical, Biological, Pharmaceutical and Environmental Sciences, University of Messina, Viale Ferdinando Stagno D'Alcontres 31-, I-98166 Messina, Italy. [3]Innovative Statistical Research SRL, Prato Della Valle 24, I-35123 Padova, Italy. [4]Institute of Anaesthesiology and Reanimation, Catholic University of Sacred Heart, Rome, Italy. [5]Manchester Biomedical Research Centre, Manchester Royal Infirmary, School of Medicine, University of Manchester, Manchester, UK.

References
1. Malek S, Sample SJ, Schwartz Z, Nemke B, Jacobson PB, Cozzi EM, Schaefer SL, Bleedorn JA, Holzman G, Muir P. Effect of analgesic therapy on clinical outcome measures in a randomized controlled trial using client-owned dogs with hip osteoarthritis. BMC Vet Res. 2012;8:185.
2. Johnston SA. Osteoarthritis. Joint anatomy, physiology, and pathobiology. Vet Clin North Am Small Anim Pract. 1997;27(4):699–723.
3. Bennett D, Zainal Ariffin SM, Johnston P. Osteoarthritis in the cat: 1. How common is it and how easy to recognise? J Feline Med Surg. 2012;14(1):65–75.
4. Epstein M, Rodan I, Griffenhagen G, Kadrlik J, Petty M, Robertson S, et al. 2015 AAHA/AAFP pain management guidelines for dogs and cats. J Am Anim Hosp Assoc. 2015;51(2):67–84.
5. Moore SA. Managing neuropathic pain in dogs. Front Vet Sci. 2016;3:12.
6. Monteiro-Steagall BP, Steagall PV, Lascelles BD. Systematic review of nonsteroidal anti-inflammatory drug-induced adverse effects in dogs. J Vet Intern Med. 2013;27(5):1011–9.
7. Fox SM. Painful decisions for senior pets. Vet Clin North Am Small Anim Pract. 2012;42(4):727–48.
8. D'Souza WN, Ng GY, Youngblood BD, Tsuji W, Lehto SG. A review of current animal models of osteoarthritis pain. Curr Pharm Biotechnol. 2011;12:1596–612.
9. Kuyinu EL, Narayanan G, Nair LS, Laurencin CT. Animal models of osteoarthritis: classification, update, and measurement of outcomes. J Orthop Surg Res. 2016;11:19.
10. De Vito V, Salvadori M, Poapolathep A, Owen H, Rychshanova R, Giorgi M. Pharmacokinetic/pharmacodynamic evaluation of grapiprant in a carrageenan-induced inflammatory pain model in the rabbit. J Vet Pharmacol Ther. 2016; doi:10.1111/jvp.12380. [Epub ahead of print]
11. Morris CJ. Carrageenan-induced paw edema in the rat and mouse. Methods Mol Biol. 2003;225:115–21.
12. Orita S, Ishikawa T, Miyagi M, Ochiai N, Inoue G, Eguchi Y, et al. Pain-related sensory innervation in monoiodoacetate-induced osteoarthritis in rat knees that gradually develops neuronal injury in addition to inflammatory pain. BMC Musculoskelet Disord. 2011;12(1):134.
13. Re G, Barbero R, Miolo A, Di Marzo V. Palmitoylethanolamide, endocannabinoids and related cannabimimetic compounds in protection against tissue inflammation and pain: potential use in companion animals. Vet J. 2007;173(1):23–32.
14. Petrosino S, Di Marzo V. The pharmacology of palmitoylethanolamide and the therapeutic efficacy of some of its new formulations. Br J Pharmacol. 2017;174(11):1349–65.
15. Skaper SD, Facci L, Fusco M, della Valle MF, Zusso M, Costa B, et al. Palmitoylethanolamide, a naturally-occurring disease modifying agent in neuropathic pain. Inflammopharmacology. 2014;22(2):79–94.
16. Solorzano C, Zhu C, Battista N, Astarita G, Lodola A, Rivara S, et al. Selective N-acylethanolamine-hydrolyzing acid amidase inhibition reveals a key role for endogenous palmitoylethanolamide in inflammation. Proc Natl Acad Sci U S A. 2009;106(49):20966–71.
17. Sagar DR, Staniaszek LE, Okine BN, Woodhams S, Norris LM, Pearson RG, et al. Tonic modulation of spinal hyperexcitability by the endocannabinoid receptor system in a model of osteoarthritic pain. Arthritis Rheum. 2010; 62(12):3666–76.
18. Richardson D, Pearson RG, Kurian N, Latif ML, Garle MJ, Barrett DA, et al. Characterisation of the cannabinoid receptor system in synovial tissue and fluid in patients with osteoarthritis and rheumatoid arthritis. Arthritis Res Ther. 2008;10(2):R43.
19. Fusco M, Skaper SD, Coaccioli S, Paladini A, Varrassi G. Degenerative joint diseases and neuroinflammation. Pain Pract. 2017;17(4):522–32.
20. Vo N, Niedernhofer LJ, Nasto LA, Jacobs L, Robbins PD, Kang J, et al. An overview of underlying causes and animal models for the study of age-related degenerative disorders of the spine and synovial joints. J Orthop Res. 2013;31(6):831–7.
21. Kanzaki N, Saito K, Maeda A, Kitagawa Y, Kiso Y, Watanabe K, et al. Effect of a dietary supplement containing glucosamine hydrochloride, chondroitin sulfate and quercetin glycosides on symptomatic knee osteoarthritis: a

randomized, double-blind placebo-controlled study. J Sci Food Agric. 2012; 92(4):862–9.
22. Gardi C, Bauerova K, Stringa B, Kuncirova V, Slovak L, Ponist S, et al. Quercetin reduced inflammation and increased antioxidant defense in rat adjuvant arthritis. Arch Biochem Biophys. 2015;583:150–7.
23. Impellizzeri D, Bruschetta G, Cordaro M, Crupi R, Siracusa R, Esposito E, et al. Micronized/ultramicronized palmitoylethanolamide displays superior oral efficacy compared to nonmicronized palmitoylethanolamide in a rat model of inflammatory pain. J Neuroinflammation. 2014;11(1):136.
24. Vonsy JL, Ghandehari J, Dickenson AH. Differential analgesic effects of morphine and gabapentin on behavioural measures of pain and disability in a model of osteoarthritis pain in rats. Eur J Pain. 2009;13(8): 786–93.
25. Woo YJ, Joo YB, Jung YO, Ju JH, Cho ML, Oh HJ, et al. Grape seed proanthocyanidin extract ameliorates monosodium iodoacetate-induced osteoarthritis. Exp Mol Med. 2011;43(10):561–70.
26. Hargreaves K, Dubner R, Brown F, Flores C, Joris J. A new and sensitive method for measuring thermal nociception in cutaneous hyperalgesia. Pain. 1988;32(1):77–88.
27. Bang JS, Oh DH, Choi HM, Sur BJ, Lim SJ, Kim JY, et al. Anti-inflammatory and antiarthritic effects of piperine in human interleukin 1beta-stimulated fibroblast-like synoviocytes and in rat arthritis models. Arthritis Res Ther. 2009;11(2):R49.
28. Cuzzocrea S, Mazzon E, Esposito E, Muià C, Abdelrahman M, Di Paola R, et al. Glycogen synthase kinase-3beta inhibition attenuates the development of ischaemia/reperfusion injury of the gut. Intensive Care Med. 2007;33(5): 880–93.
29. Sarikcioglu L, Demirel BM, Utuk A. Walking track analysis: an assessment method for functional recovery after sciatic nerve injury in the rat. Folia Morphol (Warsz). 2009;68(1):1–7.
30. Xu Y, Liu Q, Liu ZL, Lim L, Chen WH, Lin N. Treatment with SiMiaoFang, an anti-arthritis chinese herbal formula, inhibits cartilage matrix degradation in osteoarthritis rat model. Rejuvenation Res. 2013;16(5):364–76.
31. Esposito E, Cuzzocrea S. Palmitoylethanolamide is a new possible pharmacological treatment for the inflammation associated with trauma. Mini Rev Med Chem. 2013;13(2):237–55.
32. Impellizzeri D, Esposito E, Di Paola R, Ahmad A, Campolo M, Peli A, et al. Palmitoylethanolamide and luteolin ameliorate development of arthritis caused by injection of collagen type II in mice. Arthritis Res Ther. 2013;15(6):R192.
33. Marini I, Bartolucci ML, Bortolotti F, Gatto MR, Bonetti GA. Palmitoylethanolamide versus a nonsteroidal anti-inflammatory drug in the treatment of temporomandibular joint inflammatory pain. J Orofac Pain. 2012;26(2):99–104.
34. Ahn K, Smith SE, Liimatta MB, Beidler D, Sadagopan N, Dudley DT, et al. Mechanistic and pharmacological characterization of PF-04457845: a highly potent and selective fatty acid amide hydrolase inhibitor that reduces inflammatory and noninflammatory pain. J Pharmacol Exp Ther. 2011;338(1): 114–24.
35. Lowin T, Apitz M, Anders S, Straub RH. Anti-inflammatory effects of N-acylethanolamines in rheumatoid arthritis synovial cells are mediated by TRPV1 and TRPA1 in a COX-2 dependent manner. Arthritis Res Ther. 2015; 17(1):321.
36. Bonezzi F, Sasso O, Pontis S, Realini N, Romeo E, Ponzano S, et al. An important role for N-acylethanolamine acid amidase in the complete Freund's adjuvant rat model of arthritis. J Pharmacol Exp Ther. 2016;356(3):656–63.
37. Carullo G, Cappello AR, Frattaruolo L, Badolato M, Armentano B, Aiello F. Quercetin and derivatives: useful tools in inflammation and pain management. Future Med Chem. 2017;9(1):79–93.
38. Gao W, Zan Y, Wang ZJ, Hu XY, Huang F. Quercetin ameliorates paclitaxel-induced neuropathic pain by stabilizing mast cells, and subsequently blocking PKCe-dependent activation of TRPV1. Acta Pharmacol Sin. 2016;37(9):1166–77.
39. Borghi SM, Pinho-Ribeiro FA, Fattori V, Bussmann AJ, Vignoli JA, Camilios-Neto D, et al. Quercetin inhibits peripheral and spinal cord nociceptive mechanisms to reduce intense acute swimming-induced muscle pain in mice. PLoS One. 2016;11(9):e0162267.
40. Guillot M, Moreau M, Heit M, Martel-Pelletier J, Pelletier JP, Troncy E. Characterization of osteoarthritis in cats and meloxicam efficacy using objective chronic pain evaluation tools. Vet J. 2013;196(3):360–7.
41. Walton MB, Cowderoy E, Wustefeld-Janssens B, Lascelles D, Innes J. Mavacoxib and meloxicam for canine osteoarthritis: a randomised clinical comparator trial. Vet Rec. 2014;175(11):280.
42. Gruet P, Seewald W, King JN. Evaluation of subcutaneous and oral administration of robenacoxib and meloxicam for the treatment of acute pain and inflammation associated with orthopedic surgery in dogs. Am J Vet Res. 2011;72(2):184–93.
43. Wise LE, Cannavacciulo R, Cravatt BF, Marun BF, Lichtman AH. Evaluation of fatty acid amides in the carrageenan-induced paw edema model. Neuropharmacology. 2008;54(1):181–8.
44. Costa B, Conti S, Giagnoni G, Colleoni M. Therapeutic effect of the endogenous fatty acid amide, palmitoylethanolamide, in rat acute inflammation: inhibition of nitric oxide and cyclo-oxygenase systems. Br J Pharmacol. 2002;137(4):413–20.
45. Esposito E, Impellizzeri D, Bruschetta G, Cordaro M, Siracusa R, Gugliandolo E, et al. A new co-micronized composite containing palmitoylethanolamide and polydatin shows superior oral efficacy compared to their association in a rat paw model of carrageenan-induced inflammation. Eur J Pharmacol. 2016;782:107–18.
46. Impellizzeri D, Ahmad A, Bruschetta G, Di Paola R, Crupi R, Paterniti I, et al. The anti-inflammatory effects of palmitoylethanolamide (PEA) on endotoxin-induced uveitis in rats. Eur J Pharmacol. 2015;761:28–35.
47. Pessina F, Capasso R, Borrelli F, Aveta T, Buono L, Valacchi G, et al. Protective effect of palmitoylethanolamide, a naturally-occurring molecule, in a rat model of cystitis. J Urol. 2015;193(4):1401–8.
48. Wojdasiewicz P, Poniatowski LA, Szukiewicz D. The role of inflammatory and anti-inflammatory cytokines in the pathogenesis of osteoarthritis. Mediat Inflamm. 2014;2014:561459.
49. Mizumura K, Murase S. Role of nerve growth factor in pain. Handb Exp Pharmacol. 2015;227:57–77.
50. Isola M, Ferrari V, Miolo A, Stabile F, Bernardini D, Carnier P, et al. Nerve growth factor concentrations in the synovial fluid from healthy dogs and dogs with secondary osteoarthritis. Vet Comp Orthop Traumatol. 2011;24(4):279–84.
51. Gruen ME, Thomson AE, Griffith EH, Paradise H, Gearing DP, Lascelles BD. A feline-specific anti-nerve growth factor antibody improves mobility in cats with degenerative joint disease-associated pain: a pilot proof of concept study. J Vet Intern Med. 2016;30(4):1138–48.
52. TenBroek EM, Yunker L, Nies MF, Bendele AM. Randomized controlled studies on the efficacy of antiarthritic agents in inhibiting cartilage degeneration and pain associated with progression of osteoarthritis in the rat. Arthritis Res Ther. 2016;18:24.
53. Nestmann ER. Safety of micronized palmitoylethanolamide (microPEA): lack of toxicity and genotoxic potential. Food Sci Nutrition. 2016; doi:10.1002/fsn3.392.
54. Lo Verme J, Russo R, La Rana G, Fu J, Farthing J, Raso G, et al. Rapid broad-spectrum analgesia through activation of peroxisome proliferator-activated receptor-α. J Pharmacol Exp Ther. 2006;319(3):1051–61.

6

Effect of benazepril, robenacoxib and their combination on glomerular filtration rate in cats

Jonathan N. King[1*], Alessandro Panteri[2], Melanie Graille[2], Wolfgang Seewald[1], Gabriele Friton[1] and Cyril Desevaux[3]

Abstract

Background: Combined use of angiotensin-converting enzyme inhibitors and nonsteroidal anti-inflammatory drugs may induce acute kidney injury in humans, especially when combined with diuretics. The objective of this investigation was to evaluate the effects of benazepril, robenacoxib and their combination in healthy cats.

In each of two studies (study 1 followed by study 2), 32 healthy cats were randomised to one of four groups ($n = 4$ male and 4 female cats per group) in a parallel-group design. The groups received orally once daily for 7 days either placebo (control group), benazepril, robenacoxib or benazepril plus robenacoxib. In study 2, all groups received in addition 0.5 mg/kg furosemide twice daily by subcutaneous injection for 7 days.

Results: Benazepril, robenacoxib and their combination were well tolerated as evidenced from lack of clinical signs and no negative effects on body weight, feed consumption and clinical chemistry, haematology and urinalysis variables. The primary endpoint of the study was the glomerular filtration rate (GFR), which was estimated from the plasma clearance of iohexol. In the absence of furosemide, GFR was significantly higher in cats receiving the combination of benazepril plus robenacoxib compared to the other three groups, and was also significantly higher in females receiving only benazepril compared to the control.

Administration of furosemide induced diuresis, reduced GFR and activated the renin-aldosterone-angiotensin system, evidenced from increased plasma renin activity and plasma aldosterone concentrations. Compared to the control group in cats treated with furosemide, GFR was increased by benazepril (females only) but decreased by robenacoxib (males only). Benazepril, robenacoxib and their combination significantly inhibited the increase in plasma aldosterone induced by furosemide.

Conclusions: The combination of benazepril and robenacoxib was well tolerated and either increased or had a neutral effect on GFR in healthy cats without or with concomitant furosemide. The combination of benazepril and robenacoxib reduced plasma aldosterone concentrations increased by furosemide. It is recommended to test the efficacy and safety of the combined use of benazepril and robenacoxib in cats with clinical disease, notably proteinuric chronic kidney disease.

Keywords: ACE inhibitor, Benazepril, Cat, Glomerular filtration, NSAID, Robenacoxib, Safety

* Correspondence: jonathan.king@elanco.com
[1]Companion Animal Development, Elanco Animal Health, Basel, Switzerland
Full list of author information is available at the end of the article

Background

Angiotensin-converting enzyme (ACE) inhibitors (ACEIs) are used in the management of various diseases in cats, notably chronic kidney disease (CKD) [1]. Nonsteroidal anti-inflammatory drugs (NSAIDs) are used to treat fever, inflammation and pain. Administration of an ACEI and an NSAID to the same animal may be considered, for example, in cats suffering from both CKD and osteoarthritis. In addition, ACEIs and NSAIDs may have additive efficacy in certain cardiovascular diseases in which inflammation is present, notably proteinuric CKD [2]. Additive effects of ACEIs and NSAIDs in reducing proteinuria have been reported in humans [3].

Negative pharmacodynamic interactions between ACEIs and NSAIDs have been described in humans, however [4]. First, NSAIDs reduce the synthesis of vasodilatory prostaglandins and as a consequence may inhibit the systemic anti-hypertensive efficacy of ACEIs [5]. Second, as a result of reduction in vasodilatory prostaglandins, NSAIDs can constrict the renal afferent arteriole leading to reduced glomerular filtration rate (GFR) and in extreme cases acute kidney injury (AKI). The risk of AKI with NSAIDs is increased by dehydration or reduced blood pressure, for example with general anaesthesia or administration of an ACEI [6].

One of the principal mechanisms of action of ACEIs in slowing the progression of CKD in humans is reduction in glomerular capillary hypertension, mediated via selective dilation of the efferent arterioles in the kidney [1]. As a result of reduced glomerular capillary pressure, ACEIs may reduce GFR in patients with CKD. The benefit to risk ratio of ACEIs in human CKD is positive, however, provided that the reduction in GFR, usually evidenced by increased plasma creatinine concentrations, is not excessive [7]. The combination of vasoconstriction of the renal afferent arterioles by an NSAID and dilation of the efferent arterioles by an ACEI can however produce excessive reduction in GFR potentially leading to AKI [3]. The risk of AKI is further increased by concomitant use of diuretics which themselves reduce blood flow to the kidney via intravascular volume depletion. The danger of the combination of ACEIs, diuretics and NSAIDs in humans was described as a "triple whammy" [8, 9].

To our knowledge, no controlled studies have been reported on the combination of ACEIs and NSAIDs in cats. In contrast to humans, a benefit of ACEIs in slowing the progression of CKD has not been demonstrated in cats, although the ACEI benazepril has been shown to increase GFR while reducing glomerular hypertension in an experimental model of renal insufficiency [10] and to reduce proteinuria in clinical cases of CKD [11]. No significant effect of the NSAID robenacoxib on GFR was reported recently in healthy cats administered furosemide [12]. The effect of the combination of benazepril and robenacoxib on GFR in cats is not known.

The objective of this study was to evaluate the effect of benazepril, robenacoxib and their combination in healthy cats. Two studies were conducted, the first without and the second with concomitant administration of the diuretic furosemide. The primary endpoint was the GFR, which was estimated from the plasma clearance of iohexol.

Methods

Studies and approvals

Two studies (termed study 1 and study 2) were conducted using similar study designs, except that in addition in study 2 furosemide was administered and plasma renin activity (PRA) and plasma aldosterone concentration, urine variables including volume and specific gravity (USG), and water intake were measured. Both studies followed a randomised and parallel-group design comparing three treatment groups (benazepril, robenacoxib and their combination) to the control group (Table 1).

Studies 1 and 2 were performed respectively in compliance with the registered permit numbers 2011_11_FR and 2012_34E_FR approved by the Swiss cantonal animal welfare committee, and after approval of the protocol by the company Global Animal Welfare Unit. The studies were designed to use the fewest number of animals possible while being consistent with the objectives. The current state of scientific knowledge did not provide acceptable alternatives, *in vitro* or otherwise, to the use of live animals to accomplish the purpose of the studies. The cat is a target species for the test items. Study 2 was initiated only after positive tolerability results were obtained from study 1. All cats were returned to the site's animal facilities upon completion of the study.

This manuscript was prepared in compliance with the ARRIVE Guidelines Checklist for animal *in vivo* experiments [13].

Table 1 Treatment groups

Group	Treatment (mg/kg) once daily orally		Study 1	Study 2
A	None (placebo, control)	Cohort 1	4 f	2 m & 2 f
		Cohort 2	4 m	2 m & 2 f
B	Benazepril (0.5–1.0)	Cohort 1	4 f	2 m & 2 f
		Cohort 2	4 m	2 m & 2 f
C	Robenacoxib (1.0–2.4)	Cohort 1	4 f	2 m & 2 f
		Cohort 2	4 m	2 m & 2 f
D	Benazepril (0.5–1.0) + Robenacoxib (1.0–2.4)	Cohort 1	4 f	2 m & 2 f
		Cohort 2	4 m	2 m & 2 f

f female, *m* male

Study animals

A total of 48 unneutered European short-haired cats (26 males plus 22 non-pregnant and nulliparous females) were used, with 16 males and 16 females included in each of the two studies. All cats had been bred specifically for research purposes and were owned by the laboratory. A total of 6 males and 10 females were used in both studies, with a washout of 4 months. All cats were healthy and had not received an ACEI or NSAID for at least 2 months prior to each study.

Housing and management

The acclimatisation phase lasted approximately two weeks and started on day -14 (study 1, Table 2) or -15 (study 2, Table 3). During this phase, the cats were acclimatised to their housing and management and were confirmed to be healthy based on a physical examination, feed consumption and results of clinical chemistry, haematology and urinalyses.

The cats were housed in groups in a climate-controlled building with artificial light from 6.00 to 18.00. The animals were placed in individual cages for up to 5 h daily to record feed consumption, and in study 2 the cats were also placed individually into cages two times for 24 h to measure water consumption and urine volume, and to facilitate collection of urine samples.

Each cat was offered 40–70 g of dried pelleted feed (Purina® Pro Plan Adult, Switzerland) once a day at 12.00 (±1 h), approximately 4 h after dosing with the test items. On the days that blood samples were taken, cats were fed approximately 4 h after dosing with the test items and after the 4 h time point for iohexol determination. Drinking water was supplied *ad libitum*.

Randomisation and blinding

The cats were assigned at random to one of four groups A, B, C or D (4/gender/group, Table 1), while maintaining homogeneous distribution of body weight where possible. The randomisation was made by the statistician using SAS/STAT® procedure *plan* [14]. Due to the experimental workload, the cats in both studies were divided into two cohorts with the first day of dosing staggered by 1 day in study 1 and 7 days in study 2. In study 1, cohort 1 consisted of all females and cohort 2 all males. In study 2, each cohort consisted of 2 males and 2 females per group.

The study was not blinded. This was judged acceptable since the main endpoints, including the primary endpoint, were objective.

Test items and furosemide

Benazepril was dosed once daily orally at a minimum dose of 0.5 mg/kg (as the hydrochloride salt) with a range of 0.5–1.0 mg/kg (Fortekor® Flavour 2.5 or 5 mg tablets, Elanco Animal Health, Huningue, France). This is the dosage of benazepril registered for the reduction of proteinuria in cats with CKD in the EU [11].

Robenacoxib was dosed once daily orally at a minimum dose of 1.0 mg/kg with a range of 1.0–2.4 mg/kg (Onsior® 6 mg flavoured tablets, Elanco Animal Health, Huningue, France). This is the dosage of robenacoxib registered for the treatment of acute musculoskeletal disorders in cats in the EU [15].

The seven day treatment time for the test items was selected in order to reach steady state for benazeprilat (steady state plasma concentrations within 2–3 days [16]) and robenacoxib (terminal half-life 1–2 h in blood and ~24 h in peripheral sites of inflammation [17, 18]).

In study 2, furosemide was administered at a target dose of 0.5 ± 0.2 mg/kg twice daily (BID) by subcutaneous injection (Dimazon® Solution for injection, Merck Animal Health, Kenilworth, NJ, USA). Injection was chosen as the route of administration in order to minimise variability in absorption. The manufacturer's recommended dose of furosemide is 5 mg/kg followed by maintenance at 1-2 mg/kg every 6–8 h. However in a pilot study, furosemide doses of 1 or 2 mg/kg BID for 9 days to cats led to unacceptable reduction in feed intake and body weight. In a second pilot study, 0.5 furosemide mg/kg BID for 7 days produced a significant diuretic effect and compared to 1 mg/kg BID was better tolerated and produced numerically greater stimulation of the renin-angiotensin-aldosterone-system (RAAS), as assessed from PRA and aldosterone.

In order to avoid multiple administrations, benazepril and robenacoxib were dosed together in combinations of whole and part tablets in a single size 00 gelatin capsule. The control group received a placebo consisting of a single empty size 00 gelatin capsule. All treatments were administered at

Table 2 Schedule of study 1

Category	Cohort 1 study days		Cohort 2 study days	
	Pre-treatment	Post-treatment	Pre-treatment	Post-treatment
Administration of test items	0 to 6		1 to 7	
Haematology, coagulation, clinical chemistry	−14	2, 9	−14	3, 10
Body weight	−15, −8, −1	6	−15, −7, −1	7
Feed consumption	−15 to −8, −7 to −1	0 to 6, 7 to 10	−15 to −8, −7 to 0	1 to 7, 8 to 10
Iohexol concentration (0, 2, 3 & 4 h)	−8	6	−7	7

Table 3 Schedule of study 2

Category	Cohort 1 study days		Cohort 2 study days	
	Pre-treatment	Post-treatment	Pre-treatment	Post-treatment
Administration of test items and furosemide[a]	0 to 6		7 to 13	
Haematology, coagulation	−15	5	−15	12
Clinical chemistry	−15, −8	5	−15, −8	12
Urinalysis and water consumption	−14, −7[b]	6	−14, −7[b]	13
Body weight	−16, −13, −9, −6, −1	7	−16, −13, −9, −6, −1, 5	14
Feed consumption	−16 to −1	0 to 6	−16 to 6	7 to 14
Iohexol concentration	−8 (0, 2, 3 & 4 h)	6 (0, 2, 3 & 4 h)	−7 (0, 2, 3 & 4 h)	13 (0, 2, 3 & 4 h)
Plasma renin activity and aldosterone concentration	0[c] 6 (0 h)	6 (2, 6, 12 & 24 h)	7[c] 13 (0 h)	13 (2, 6, 12 & 24 h)

h hour
[a]Furosemide was administered subcutaneously twice daily on days 0 to 5 (cohort 1) or 7 to 12 (cohort 2) and then as a single dose on the morning of day 6 (cohort 1) or 13 (cohort 2)
[b]Urinalysis at day −7 only if no sample was taken at day −14
[c]For plasma renin activity and plasma aldosterone, the day 0/7 value not used in the analysis

8.00 ± 1 h (in study 2 furosemide was administered at 8.00 ± 1 h and 20.00 ± 2 h). After dosing, 2.5 mL of water was administered via a syringe to facilitate passage of the capsules into the stomach, and the cats were observed for several minutes to ensure that the capsules had been swallowed.

Doses were determined using the body weight measured on day -1, or day 5 for cohort 2 in study 2 (Table 3). Except for unplanned medical treatments, additional medications were prohibited during the studies.

Endpoints

The primary endpoint of the study was the GFR, which was estimated from the plasma clearance of iohexol (CLioh).

Secondary endpoints included general clinical monitoring (body weight, clinical examination, feed consumption, clinical chemistry, coagulation and haematology). In study 2, additional secondary endpoints were PRA and plasma aldosterone concentration, water intake, urine volume and USG, and fractional excretions of potassium and sodium.

Clinical monitoring

Cats were checked at least once daily. A detailed clinical examination was made once during the acclimatisation phase, and then again 96 h after the first dose of the test items and the day following the last dosing.

Cats were weighed in the morning before feeding at least three times in the baseline period and again at the end of the study (Tables 2 and 3). Daily feed consumption was determined as the difference between rations offered and remaining uneaten after approximately 4 h.

Blood samples for clinical pathology (standard haematology, coagulation and plasma clinical chemistry variables) were taken from a cephalic or jugular vein, after feed was removed for at least 12 h, once during the acclimatisation phase (for animal selection and as baseline), once during the treatment phase and in study 1 again after the end of treatment (Tables 2 and 3).

Glomerular filtration rate (GFR)

The GFR was estimated from the CLioh after intravenous (IV) administration of iohexol (Accupaque® 350, GE Healthcare Buchler GmbH & Co., Braunschweig, Germany). This was performed once during the acclimatisation phase prior to administration of the test item(s) (day -8 or -7) and again after the last treatment.

Cats had free access to water but feed was withheld for at least 12 h before IV administration of iohexol. A target dose of 90 mg of iodine/kg iohexol was administered via an IV catheter placed in a cephalic vein followed by flushing with physiological saline solution. Actual mean (range) doses administered were 90.0 (86.4.2–93.8) iodine/kg in study 1 and 88.9 (81.8–94.3) iodine/kg in study 2. Blood was sampled from a jugular or antebrachial vein (i.e. not a vein used for iohexol administration) in 1.2 mL heparin tubes before and 2, 3 and 4 h after administration of iohexol. Samples were stored on ice until centrifuged at approximately 3,000 g for 15 min at 4 °C. Once centrifuged, plasma was collected and stored at -20 °C before analysis.

Due to breakdown of equipment between studies, plasma iohexol concentrations were analysed using two different methods in studies 1 and 2. Both methods were validated in cat plasma in terms of selectivity, linearity, repeatability, reproducibility and stability according to the document "Guidance for Industry: Bioanalytical Method Validation" (U.S. Department of Health and Human Services et al., 2001, http://www.labcompliance.com/info/links/methods/guidelines.aspx).

In study 1, the endo- and exo-iohexol isomers were quantified separately. Analyses were performed on a high performance liquid chromatography system (Hewlett Packard 1100, Palo Alto, CA, USA) coupled with an ultraviolet detector (Hewlett Packard 1050). The method was linear over the calibration ranges 1 to 80 μg/mL and 2 to 320 μg/mL for endo- and exo-iohexol respectively. Intra-day and inter-day precisions were lower than 9 % for both isomers. The accuracy varied from 98 to 102 %. The lower limit of quantification (LLOQ) was 1 μg/mL with precision 8 % and accuracy 99 % for endo-iohexol, and 2 μg/mL with precision 10 % and accuracy 109 % for exo-iohexol.

In study 2, total plasma iohexol concentrations were measured using an ultra-high performance liquid chromatography system (Acquity UPLC, Waters, Milford, MA, USA) coupled with a triple quadrupole mass spectrometer (Xevo, Waters). The method was validated with a calibration curve ranging from 5 to 400 μg/mL. Intra-day and inter-day precisions were respectively lower than 11 and 12 %. The accuracy varied from 87 to 102 %. The LLOQ was 5 μg/mL with a precision of 7 % and an accuracy of 91 %.

The CLioh was calculated using the methods described by Laroute et al., [19]. In brief, it was first checked that the pre-administration concentrations of iohexol in plasma were below the LLOQ. Next, a log-linear regression of total iohexol concentration versus time was calculated using:

$$\text{log concentration} = \alpha + (\beta \times \text{time})$$

The area under the curve (AUC) is then:

$$\text{AUC} = \exp(\alpha)/(-\beta)$$

Clearance (CL) was calculated as:

$$\text{CL} = \text{dose}/\text{AUC}$$

The CL was calculated relative to body weight (BWT) and relative to body surface area (BSA), the latter being estimated by:

$$(\text{BSA}\ [\text{m}^2]) = 0.00101 \times (\text{BWT}\ [\text{g}])^{0.71}$$

Urine variables

In study 2, the cats were placed in cages with specialised litter trays for 24 h on days -14 or -7 and 6 or 13. Water consumption and urine volume were measured and urine samples collected.

The total volume of water consumed over 24 h was calculated from the difference in volume of water provided and remaining in bowls which were suspended above the floor. The volume was checked repeatedly during the day.

Urine was collected from litter trays by using Catrine Pearl Cat Litter® (Kruuse, Langeskov, Denmark).

Urine samples were stored at below -70 °C before analysis for creatinine, potassium and sodium concentrations and USG. The fractional excretions of potassium (FE_K) and sodium (FE_{Na}) were calculated according to the following formulae:

$$\text{K fractional excretion } (\%) = \frac{\text{Urine K x Plasma Creatinine}}{\text{Plasma K x Urine Creatinine}}$$

$$\text{Na fractional excretion } (\%) = \frac{\text{Urine Na x Plasma Creatinine}}{\text{Plasma Na x Urine Creatinine}}$$

Plasma renin activity (PRA) and aldosterone concentration

In study 2, pre-treatment and on the last day of dosing, approximately 1.2 mL of blood was collected in the morning before administration of furosemide and test items (pre-dose) and 2, 6, 12 and 24 h later (post-dose). Blood was collected into pre-cooled tubes containing K_3 EDTA and aprotinin (500 KIU/mL of blood) and kept on ice until centrifugation at approximately 3,000 g for 15 min at 4 °C. The plasma was collected and stored below -70 °C until analysis. Plasma angiotensin-1 concentrations were measured using an enzyme immuno-assay (Penisula Labs, San Carlos, CA, USA). The PRA was calculated by comparing the concentration of angiotensin-1 obtained after incubation of the samples at +4 °C (absence of renin activity) and +37 °C (presence of renin activity). The angiotensin-1 assay was validated, over the concentration range 30 to 700 pg/mL. Quality control samples at 60, 145 and 500 pg/mL were analysed in each run; the accuracy was within the defined acceptable range of 75–125 % for all 48 samples, with a mean (coefficient of variation (CV%)) accuracy of 96.7 (7.7 %).

Aldosterone was determined in plasma using a Symbiosis liquid chromatography-mass spectrometry system (online SPE, Spark Holland, Emmen, Netherlands). Concentrations of aldosterone are low in urine of cats and therefore plasma concentrations are more relevant clinically [20]. The assay was validated over the concentration range 0.05 to 2.0 ng/mL. Quality control samples at 0.12, 0.6 and 1.8 ng/mL were analysed in each run; the accuracy was within the defined acceptable range of 75–125 % for all 27 samples, with a mean (CV%) accuracy 96.6 (5.7 %).

Statistical analysis

The software SAS®, Version 9.2 or higher, was used for all analyses [14]. Data are presented as mean (± SD) or range. The experimental unit was results from each individual cat. Two tailed P values less than 0.05 were defined as significant with no correction for multiple analyses, in order not to inflate the type II error.

Variables that were analysed only once post-treatment, including GFR, were analysed using analysis of covariance (ANCOVA) with the pre-treatment value as covariate and sex, treatment, and "treatment by sex" interaction as effects (Tables 4 and 6). Various data transformations were attempted and the adequacy of each statistical model was assessed by evaluation of the normality of the residuals (Shapiro-Wilk test, SAS® procedure *univariate*). In all cases, no or a log transformation was selected.

Table 4 Results of statistical analyses for selected variables in study 1 analysed by ANCOVA

Variable	Transformation	*P* values in ANCOVA				*P* value for normality	*P* < 0.05 in post-hoc tests*
		Treatment	Sex	Treatment by sex	Baseline		
Iohexol clearance per BWT	None	0.0030*	0.0002*	**0.0017***	0.0003*	0.1957	A, B & C < D (all & f)
Iohexol clearance per BSA	None	0.0036*	0.0005*	**0.0013***	0.0005*	0.6001	A, B & C < D (all & f), A < B (f)
Body weight	None	0.1823	0.3007	**0.0303***	< 0.0001*	0.4012	B < A (m), A < C (f), D < C (all & f)

Only results of variables with a significant ($P < 0.1$) treatment or "treatment by sex" effect are shown. For sex, baseline, normality and post-hoc comparisons, $P < 0.05$ was defined as significant

BWT body weight, *BSA* body surface area, *f* female, *m* male

*Results were primarily interpreted from the effect with the *P* value shown in bold

Variables that were measured pre-treatment and multiple times post-treatment were analysed using repeated measures analysis of covariance (RMANCOVA) (Table 7). The pre-treatment value was the covariate and effects were sex, treatment, time and "treatment by sex" and "treatment by time" interactions.

In the event that the *P* value was less than 0.1 for treatment or the "treatment by sex" or "treatment by time" interactions, individual groups were compared by linear contrasts with $P < 0.05$ defined as significant.

SAS® procedure *mixed* was used for the (RM)ANCOVA analyses.

Results

Study 1

The 32 cats were aged 8 months to 7 years with bodyweight 2.5–6 kg at baseline. Groups were well matched at baseline. The mean (range) doses of the test items in mg/kg administered orally once daily alone and in combination were respectively 0.69 (0.51–0.88) and 0.70 (0.51–0.98) for benazepril hydrochloride and 1.67 (1.16–2.27) and 1.67 (1.23–2.36) for robenacoxib.

Clinical monitoring

All test items were well tolerated. One isolated event of bloody loose stools on day 7 was observed in one cat in group B (benazepril) but was not considered to be caused by the test item. No other clinical signs were reported.

There was no significant ($P > 0.1$) treatment effect or "treatment by time" or "treatment by sex" interactions for feed intake or for relevant haematology, coagulation or clinical chemistry variables (data not shown).

Certain variables showed significant ($P < 0.05$) changes from baseline. These included the red cell variables (cell count, haemoglobin and haematocrit) which decreased in all four groups. For coagulation variables, fibrinogen decreased in group B (benazepril) and the activated partial thromoplastin time increased in group B (benazepril) and group D (benazepril plus robenacoxib). For clinical chemistry variables, plasma albumin and calcium decreased and chloride increased in all four groups. There were also increases in plasma potassium (C and D) and sodium (A, B and D), and decreases in aspartate amino-transferase (A and B), phosphorus (A, B and C), total protein (B and D) and urea nitrogen (B and C).

There was a significant "treatment by sex" interaction for body weight, and significant differences between groups in the post-hoc comparisons (Table 4). Differences in change from baseline were small however: B -0.06 kg versus A in males; A -0.08 versus C in females; D -0.05 (all) and -0.08 (females) versus C.

Glomerular filtration rate (GFR)

The GFR was assessed from the CLioh. There was low variability in plasma iohexol concentrations (Fig. 1). Similar results were obtained in both studies with CLioh expressed per BWT or BSA. Final conclusions were made using BSA since *P* values for the normality of the data were higher in both studies with CLioh expressed per BSA (Tables 4 and 6).

For CLioh expressed both by BWT or BSA, there were highly significant effects of treatment, sex, "treatment by sex" and baseline in study 1 (Fig. 1, Table 4). In the post-hoc analyses, iohexol clearance was significantly greater in group D (benazepril and robenacoxib) versus the other groups (A, B and C) in all cats and in females. In addition for the BSA endpoint, the clearance was significantly higher in group B (benazepril) compared to the control (A) in females and significance was approached ($P = 0.051$) for males.

The iohexol clearance was highly significantly ($P < 0.0001$) increased compared to baseline in group D (benazepril and robenacoxib) for both BWT and BSA endpoints (all cats and females). The mean change from baseline in CLioh expressed per BSA was: -9.5 %, +12.8 %, +1.3 % and +36.1 % respectively in groups A, B, C and D.

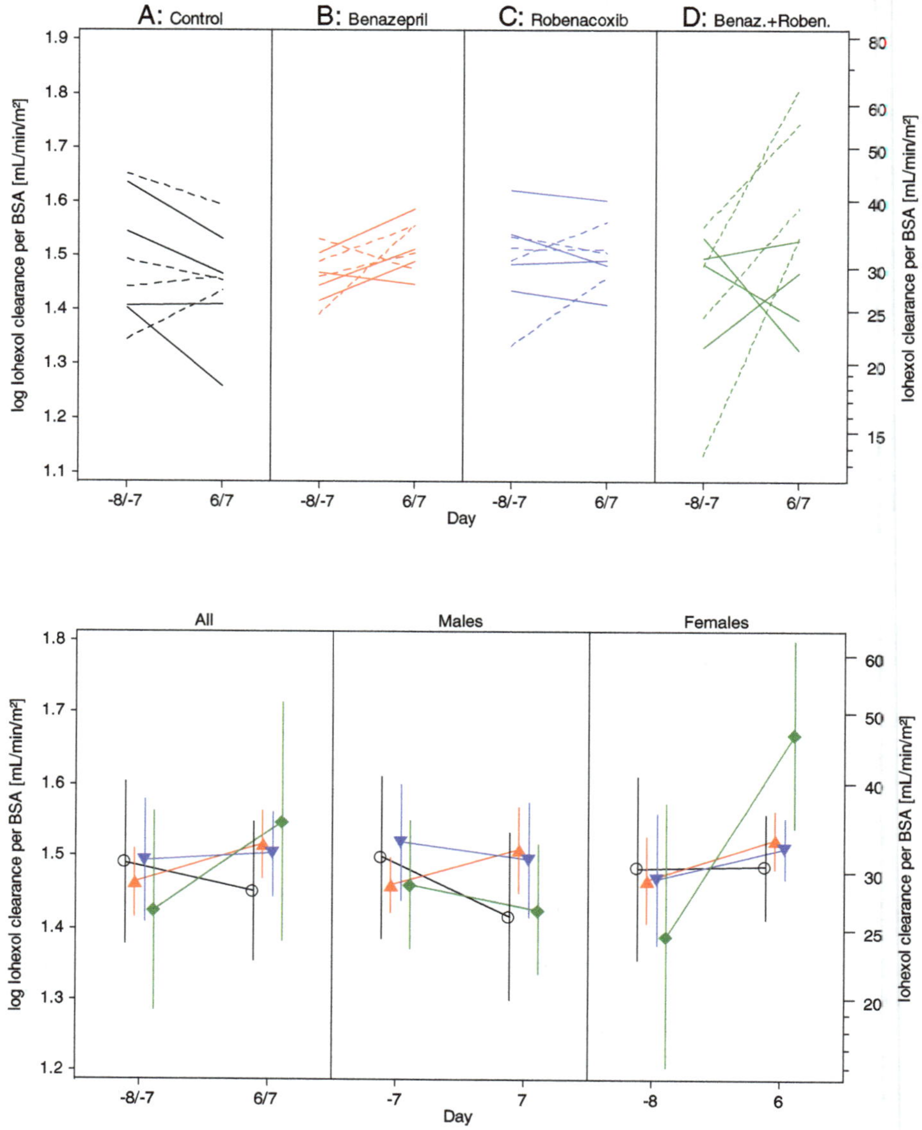

Fig. 1 Plasma clearance of iohexol, standardised to baseline body weight (BSA), as an index of glomerular filtration rate in study 1. Upper: Scatter Plots. Data are shown as solid (males) and dotted (female) lines. Lower: Mean (SD) for all cats, and separately for males and females. Control (**A**) –o–; Benazepril (**B**) –▲–; Robenacoxib (**C**) –▼–; Benazepril + Robenacoxib (**D**) –◆–

Study 2

The 32 cats were aged 1–8 years with bodyweight 2.8–7.6 kg at baseline. Groups were well matched at baseline. The mean (range) doses of the test items in mg/kg administered once orally daily alone and in combination were respectively 0.72 (0.51–0.88) and 0.79 (0.58–0.98) for benazepril hydrochloride, and 1.50 (1.02–2.14) and 1.49 (1.05–2.22) for robenacoxib. The mean (range) dose of furosemide was 0.55 (0.50–0.65) mg/kg BID by subcutaneous injection. The furosemide had the desired diuretic effect, producing a marked increase in urine volume (mean +113 %) associated with dehydration, reduced GFR and increase in plasma creatinine concentrations, and activation of the RAAS evidenced from increased PRA and aldosterone concentrations.

P values for the primary endpoint and selected (statistically significant) secondary variables are shown for change from baseline (Table 5), ANCOVA (Table 6) and RMANCOVA (Table 7) analyses.

Clinical monitoring

The test items were tolerated well. Body weight was significantly lower in the control group (A) during treatment compared to the robenacoxib group (C) (Table 6). Incidents of diarrhoea in 4 cats and vomiting in one cat were reported in the pre-test phase but not during dosing with

Table 5 *P* values for change from baseline for selected variables in study 2

Variable	Sex/time	*P* values for comparison to baseline			
		Group A: Control	Group B: Benazepril	Group C: Robenacoxib	Group D: Benazepril + Robenacoxib
Iohexol clearance per BWT	M	**0.0068 D**	**0.0003 D**	**< 0.0001 D**	**0.0002 D**
	F	**0.0033 D**	0.9475	**0.0248 D**	**0.0003 D**
	Both	**0.0001 D**	**0.0052 D**	**< 0.0001 D**	**< 0.0001 D**
Iohexol clearance per BSA	M	**0.0365 D**	**0.0006 D**	**< 0.0001 D**	**0.0002 D**
	F	**0.0005 D**	0.4843	**0.0030 D**	**< 0.0001 D**
	Both	**0.0002 D**	**0.0024 D**	**< 0.0001 D**	**< 0.0001 D**
Plasma renin activity	Day 6/13 + 2 h	**< 0.0001 I**	**< 0.0001 I**	**0.0012 D**	**< 0.0001 I**
	Day 6/13 + 6 h	**0.0002 I**	**< 0.0001 I**	**0.0166 D**	**0.0002 I**
	Day 6/13 + 12 h	0.1776	**0.0141 I**	**0.0010 D**	0.6073
	Day 6/13 + 24 h	**0.0284 I**	0.8368	**< 0.0001 D**	0.0522 (D)
Plasma aldosterone	Day 6/13 + 2 h	**0.0211 I**	**0.0012 D**	0.5563	**0.0005 D**
	Day 6/13 + 6 h	0.3873	0.0914 (D)	0.9468	**0.0022 D**
	Day 6/13 + 12 h	0.3893	0.1708	0.2046	**0.0262 D**
	Day 6/13 + 24 h	0.5757	**0.0020 D**	**0.0002 D**	**0.0054 D**
Red blood cell count		**< 0.0001 I**	**0.0093 I**	0.0816 (I)	0.0758 (I)
Haematocrit		**0.0004 I**	**0.0109 I**	0.1306	0.0771 (I)
Haemoglobin		**0.0001 I**	**0.0077 I**	0.2113	**0.0298 I**
Prothrombin time		**0.0008 D**	**0.0014 D**	**0.0238 D**	**< 0.0001 D**
Activated partial thromboplastin time		**0.0026 D**	**0.0077 D**	0.2387	0.0515 (D)
Albumin		**< 0.0001 I**	**0.0002 I**	0.1479	0.0595 (I)
Alkaline phosphatase		**0.0121 D**	**0.0001 D**	**0.0429 D**	**< 0.0001 D**
Aspartate aminotransferase		**0.0009 I**	**0.0232 I**	0.1196	**0.0276 I**
Creatinine		**< 0.0001 I**	**< 0.0001 I**	**< 0.0001 I**	**< 0.0001 I**
Total protein		**0.0004 I**	0.0510 (I)	0.9288	0.7448
Urea nitrogen		**< 0.0001 I**	**< 0.0001 I**	**< 0.0001 I**	**< 0.0001 I**
Calcium		**0.0004 I**	**0.0005 I**	**0.0045 I**	0.2532
Chloride		**< 0.0001 D**	**< 0.0001 D**	**< 0.0001 D**	**< 0.0001 D**
Magnesium		**< 0.0001 I**	**0.0003 I**	**0.0033 I**	**0.0022 I**
Potassium		**0.0010 D**	**< 0.0001 D**	**0.0081 D**	**< 0.0001 D**
Sodium		**< 0.0001 D**	**< 0.0001 D**	**0.0188 D**	**< 0.0001 D**
Water consumption		**0.0002 I**	**< 0.0001 I**	**< 0.0001 I**	**< 0.0001 I**
Urine volume		**0.0025 I**	**< 0.0001 I**	**0.0019 I**	**0.0003 I**
Urine specific gravity		**< 0.0001 D**	**< 0.0001 D**	**< 0.0001 D**	**< 0.0001 D**
Fractional excretion potassium		**0.0029 I**	**< 0.0001 I**	**0.0009 I**	**< 0.0001 I**

Only variables with at least one significant ($P < 0.05$) change from baseline are shown
BWT body weight, *BSA* body surface area, *F* female, *M* male, *h* hour
D decrease, *I* increase (in bold for $P < 0.05$). Non-bold *P* values and D or I in brackets for $P < 0.1$

the test items. Skin lesions, attributed to the repeated subcutaneous injection of furosemide or clipping of hair for blood sampling, were observed in one cat in group A and two cats in group D.

Clinical signs attributed to the furosemide included dehydration in 12 animals (4 in group A, 3 in B, 1 in C and 4 in D). Reduced appetite was observed in most cats during furosemide administration and this was reported as inappetence on one or more days for 7 cats (4 in group A, 1 in B and 2 in D). One cat (control group A) was withdrawn from the study due to decreased appetite plus dehydration and prostration.

In the control group (A) there were significant increases (% change) from baseline in: red cell count (+18.0 %),

Table 6 *P* values for selected variables in study 2 analysed by ANCOVA

Variable	Transformation	*P* values in ANCOVA				*P* value for normality	*P* < 0.05 in post-hoc tests*
		Treatment	Sex	Treatment by sex	Baseline		
Iohexol clearance per BWT	None	0.0726	0.0534*	**0.0451***	0.4365	0.2246	A < B (f), C < A (m), D < B (f & all)
Iohexol clearance per BSA	None	0.0435*	0.2698	**0.0300***	0.5357	0.6285	A < B (f), C < A (m), D < B (f & all)
Body weight	None	**0.0865***	0.2900	0.1127	< 0.0001*	0.4772	A < C
Albumin	None	**0.0066***	0.3807	0.6866	0.1354	0.3174	C & D < A
Total protein	Log	**0.0276***	0.7737	0.4227	0.0055*	0.0246*	C & D < A
Chloride	None	**0.0245***	0.9598	0.5484	0.2485	0.8120	A < C
Sodium	None	**0.0411***	0.3906	0.9749	0.8905	0.4006	A & D < C
Urine specific gravity	None	0.1205	0.4124	**0.0914***	0.0544*	0.5961	B < A (f)

Only results of variables with a significant ($P < 0.1$) treatment or "treatment by sex" effect are shown. For sex, baseline, normality and post-hoc comparisons, $P < 0.05$ was defined as significant

BWT body weight, *BSA* body surface area, *f* female, *m* male

*Results were primarily interpreted from the effect with the *P* value shown in bold

haematocrit (+19.7 %) and haemoglobin (+20.4 %); plasma concentrations of albumin (+0.88 %), creatinine (+39.1 %), total protein (+12.0 %) and urea nitrogen (+15.2 %); water consumption (+73.9 %), urine volume (+113.1 %) and FEk (+75.2 %) (Table 5). There were significant decreases in: prothrombin (-1.8 %) and activated partial thromboplastin time (-4.8 %); plasma concentrations of chloride (-14.9 %), potassium (-10.4 %) and sodium (-4.7 %); and in USG (-6.1 %).

For the variables listed above, there was a significant treatment effect for albumin, total protein, chloride and sodium (Table 6). In the post-hoc comparisons, albumin and total protein were significantly lower in groups C and D versus the control (A), while chloride and sodium were significantly higher in group C versus A.

There was a significant "treatment by sex" interaction for USG, and in the post-hoc comparisons female cats had lower USG in group B (benazepril) compared to the control (A).

Glomerular filtration rate

Similar results were obtained with CLioh expressed per BWT or BSA, with final conclusions made using BSA since the *P* value for normality was higher (Table 6). The CLioh decreased significantly from baseline in all groups (Fig. 2, Table 5), attributed to the effect of furosemide. For CLioh expressed per BSA, there were significant treatment and "treatment by sex" effects. In the post-hoc comparisons, CLioh was significantly higher in the benazepril group (B) compared to the control (A, females only) and benazepril plus robenacoxib groups (D, females and all cats). The CLioh was significantly higher in the control group (A) compared to robenacoxib (C, males only).

The mean change from baseline in CLioh expressed per BSA was: -20.4 %, -19.9 %, -31.6 % and -33.7 % respectively in groups A, B, C and D.

Plasma renin activity (PRA) and aldosterone

In the control group (A) there were significant increases from baseline in PRA (at 2, 6 and 24 h after dosing) and plasma aldosterone concentrations (at 2 h) (Figs. 3 and 4, Table 5). At peak effect (2 h), mean values were increased by +1083 % for PRA and by +519 % for aldosterone.

There were significant treatment and "treatment by time" effects for both PRA and aldosterone (Table 7). In the post-hoc analyses for PRA, values were significantly lower in group C versus groups A and D at all time points, and in group D compared to the control group A at 24 h.

In the post-hoc analyses for aldosterone, values were significantly lower at one or more time points in groups B (2 h), C (24 h) and D (2, 6 and 12 h) compared to the control group A. Values were also significantly lower in group D compared to C at 2 and 6 h. Examination of the mean values indicates, however, that all three treatment groups (B, C and D) were associated with approximately equal inhibition of the increase in plasma aldosterone induced by furosemide (Fig. 4).

Discussion

In humans concomitant administration of ACEIs and NSAIDs can potentially lead to adverse events, notably reduction in GFR and the occurrence of AKI. This risk is worsened by concomitant administration of diuretics, described as a "triple whammy" [8, 9]. In this study in healthy cats, no reduction in GFR was observed with the combination of benazepril and robenacoxib, with and without concomitant administration of the loop diuretic furosemide. Similar findings were reported recently in

Table 7 *P* values for selected variables in study 2 analysed by RMANCOVA

Variable	Transformation	*P* values in RMANCOVA				*P* value for normality	*P* < 0.05 in post-hoc tests*
		Treatment	Time	Treatment by time	Baseline		
Plasma renin activity	Log	< 0.0001*	< 0.0001*	**0.0019***	0.0048*	0.0322	C < A & D (2, 6, 12 & 24 h), D < A (24 h)
Plasma aldosterone	Log	0.0275*	0.0004 *	**0.0128***	< 0.0001*	0.1342	B < A (2 h), C < A (24 h), D < A (2, 6 & 12 h), D < C (2 & 6 h)

Only results of variables with a significant ($P < 0.1$) treatment or "treatment by time" effect are shown. For time, baseline, normality and post-hoc comparisons, $P < 0.05$ was defined as significant. There were no significant sex or "sex by treatment" interactions for these variables (data not shown)

BWT body weight, *BSA* body surface area, *h* hour

*Results were primarily interpreted from the effect with the *P* value shown in bold

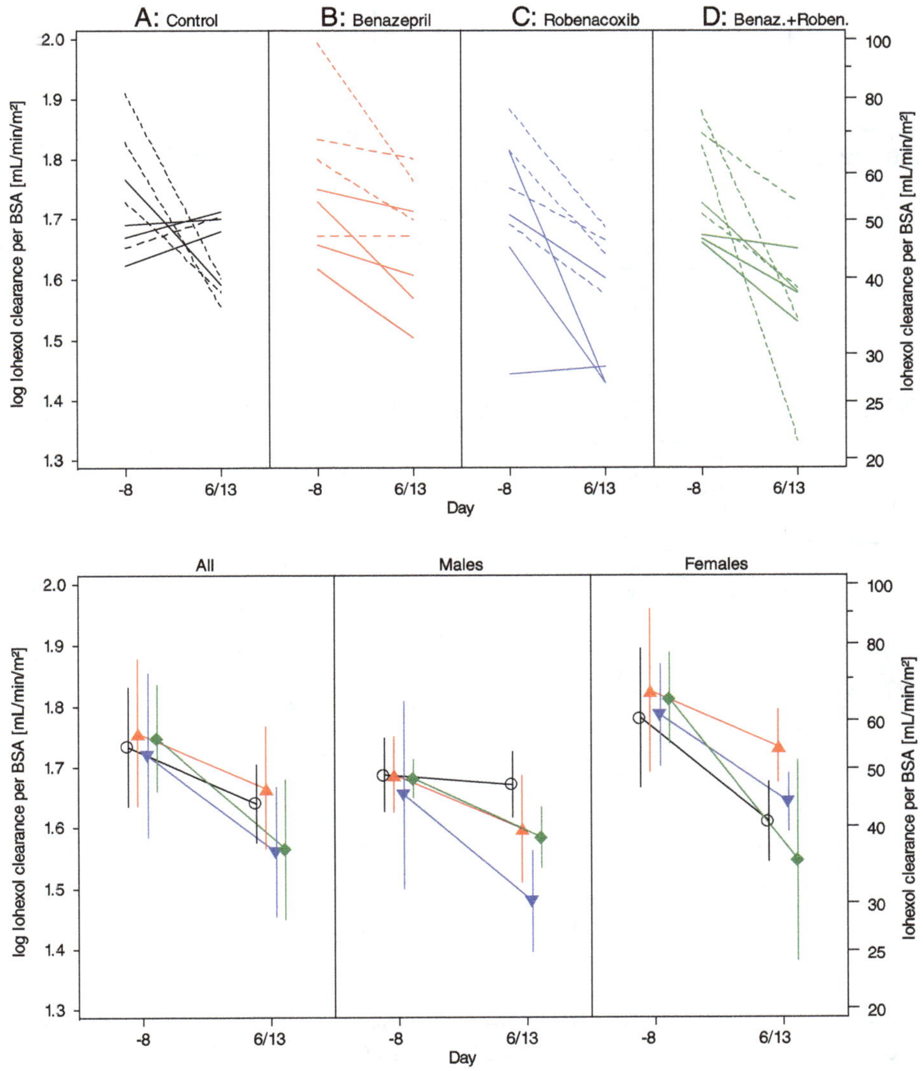

Fig. 2 Plasma clearance of iohexol, standardised to baseline body weight (BSA), as an index of glomerular filtration rate in study 2. Upper: Scatter Plots. Data are shown as solid (males) and dotted (female) lines. Lower: Mean (SD) for all cats, and separately for males and females. Control (**A**) –o–; Benazepril (**B**) –▲–; Robenacoxib (**C**) –▼–; Benazepril + Robenacoxib (**D**) –◆–

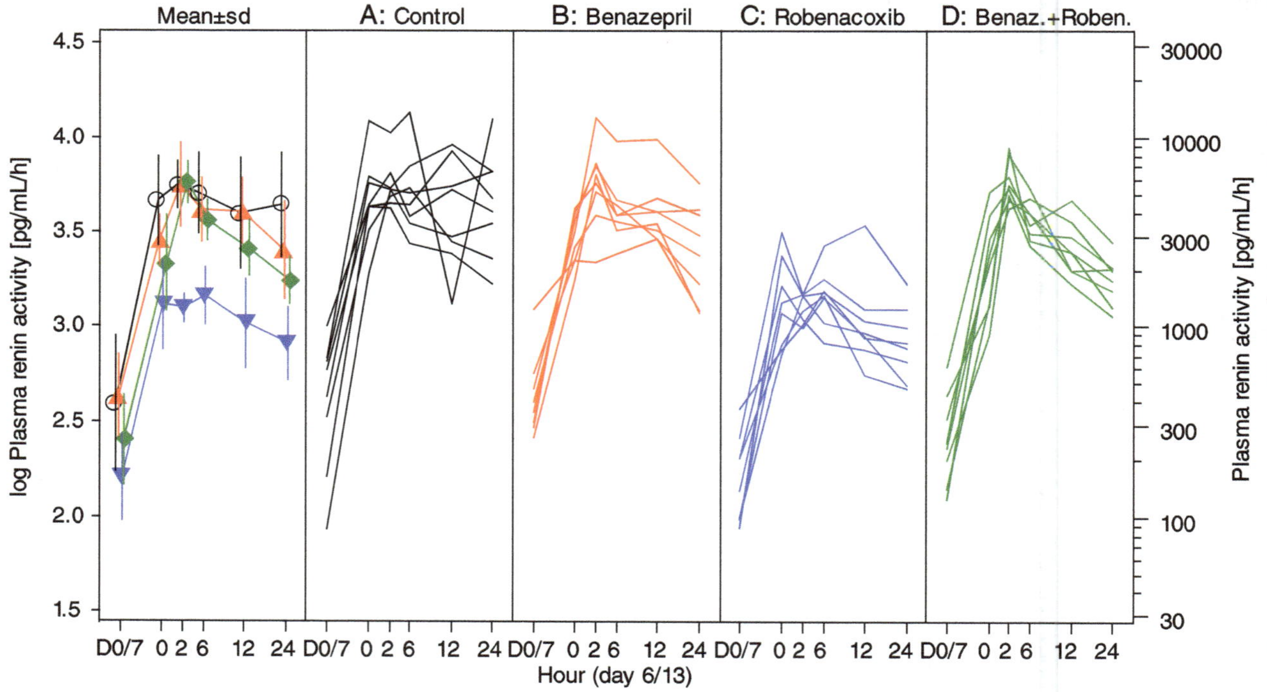

Fig. 3 Plasma renin activity (PRA) in study 2. Data are mean (SD) and scatter plots. Test items (benazepril and/or robenacoxib) plus furosemide were administered at time 0 h. D = day. Control (**A**) –o–; Benazepril (**B**) –▲–; Robenacoxib (**C**) –▼–; Benazepril + Robenacoxib (**D**) –◆–

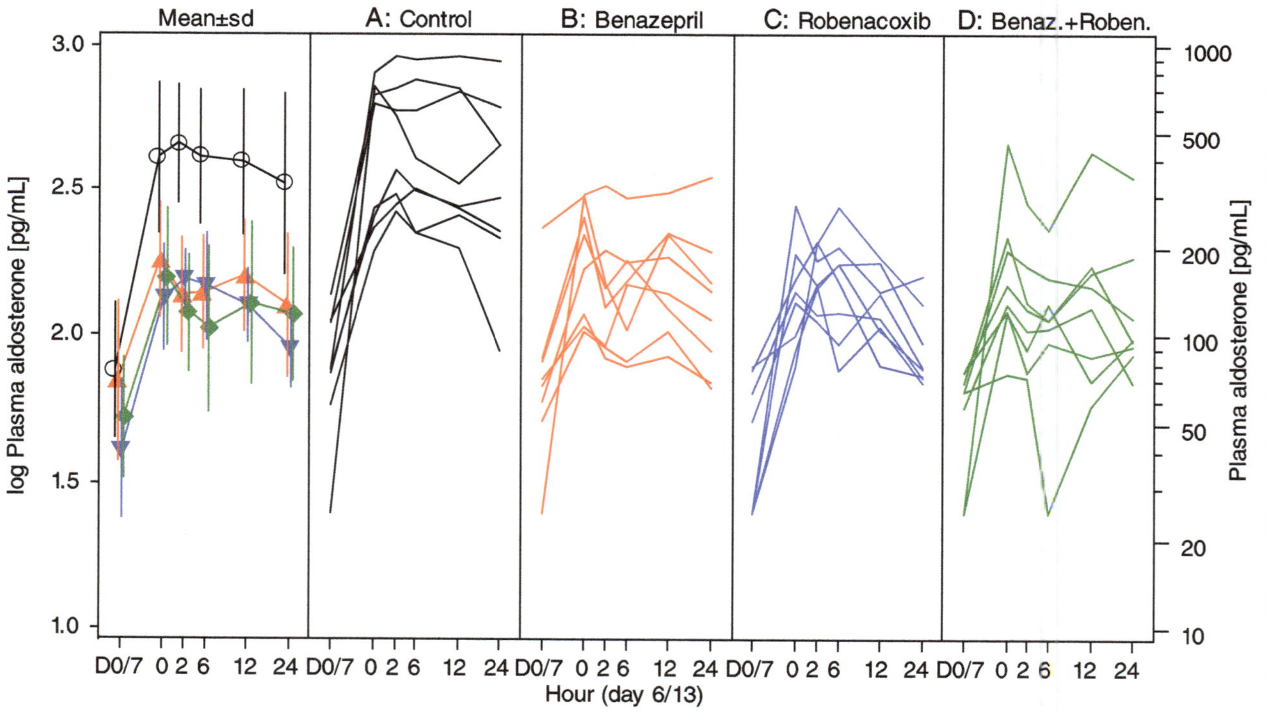

Fig. 4 Plasma aldosterone concentration in study 2. Data are mean (SD) and scatter plots. Test items (benazepril and/or robenacoxib) plus furosemide were administered at time 0 h. D = day. Control (**A**) –o–; Benazepril (**B**) –▲–; Robenacoxib (**C**) –▼–; Benazepril + Robenacoxib (**D**) –◆–

dogs [21]. The dose of furosemide administered (in study 2) was 0.5 mg/kg BID by subcutaneous injection. This is lower than the dose range of 1–5 mg/kg recommended by the manufacturer, but in pilot studies doses of 1 mg/kg BID and higher produced unacceptable loss of appetite. At the chosen dose, furosemide had the desired diuretic action in study 2, leading in the control group to a significant increase (% change from baseline) in urine volume (+113.1 %) and estimated water consumption (+73.9 %), induced dehydration (haematocrit +19.7 %, total plasma protein +12.0 %), reduced USG (-6.1 %) and renal function (plasma creatinine +39.1 %, GFR -20.4 %), and decreased prothrombin (-1.8 %) and activated partial thromboplastin (-4.8 %) times. The furosemide also led to activation of the RAAS, evidenced by significant increases in PRA and plasma aldosterone concentrations (respectively +1083 % and +519 % at peak effect). In addition, 4 of 12 cats in the control group receiving furosemide had reported inappetence and one cat had to be withdrawn from the study due to decreased appetite plus dehydration. The dose of furosemide was therefore sufficient to induce the necessary pharmacological effects needed for this study to be relevant clinically, and was the highest that could be accepted from an animal welfare perspective. Furosemide reduced GFR significantly and by a mean of 20.4 %. This is a known effect of diuretics, mediated via reduction in perfusion pressure. The diuretic action of furosemide, but with no reduction in GFR, has been demonstrated previously in cats [22].

In this investigation benazepril had no significant effect on GFR compared to the control group in all cats, although GFR was increased in female cats only in both studies 1 and 2. The PRA was increased compared to baseline by a similar extent in the control (A) and benazepril (B) groups in study 2. Increased PRA is a standard effect of ACEIs mediated by reduced synthesis of angiotensin-2 reducing the negative feedback of angiotensin-2 on renin release. The fact that benazepril did not increase PRA, an index of RAAS activation, more than that induced by furosemide alone suggests that the increase in PRA induced by the 0.5 mg/kg BID furosemide dose was already maximal. This conclusion is supported by results from the pilot study in which a dose of 1.0 mg/kg furosemide BID did not increase PRA more than 0.5 mg/kg BID. Finally, benazepril significantly inhibited the increase in plasma aldosterone induced by furosemide. Inhibition of aldosterone synthesis, secondary to reduced synthesis of angiotensin-2, is a known action of ACEIs including in cats [23].

The effects observed with benazepril, with inhibition of the RAAS and reduction of plasma aldosterone concentrations, are consistent with its demonstrated action in reducing proteinuria in cats with CKD [11]. As noted in the introduction, ACEIs as a group have the potential to reduce GFR in (human) patients with heart or kidney disease [7]. In cats with CKD however, no significant increase in plasma creatinine concentrations was observed with benazepril compared to placebo, even at the start of treatment [11], consistent with the finding in this study that benazepril did not reduce GFR. Previously Brown et al., also reported that benazepril increased GFR in cats with nephrectomy-induced chronic renal insufficiency [10].

Administration of robenacoxib without benazepril produced no consistent effects on GFR. The change from baseline in GFR in the robenacoxib versus the control group was respectively +1.3 % versus -9.5 % in study 1, and -31.6 % versus -20.4 % in study 2 (with furosemide). Differences were significantly different for males in study 2. No significant effects of robenacoxib on GFR were reported previously at a high dose (30 mg/kg) in rats [24] or at a clinically relevant dose (2 mg/kg SID or BID orally) in cats [12].

Limited studies on the effect of other NSAIDs on GFR in cats are available. Meloxicam was reported not to change GFR in healthy euvolaemic cats with reduced renal mass [25] or fed a sodium deficient diet [26]. In addition no evidence of deleterious effects on renal function, assessed from plasma creatinine and urea concentrations and lack of adverse events, was reported from field studies in cats receiving carprofen [27, 28], meloxicam [28–30] or robenacoxib [31, 32]. However, in one retrospective study, 48 cases of acute renal failure were reported in cats and 21 of these cases were attributed to the NSAIDs nimesulide (16), tolfenamic acid (3) and ketoprofen (2) [33].

Robenacoxib administered alone significantly inhibited the increase in both PRA and plasma aldosterone concentrations induced by furosemide. Similar results were reported previously with robenacoxib in dogs [21] and other NSAIDs in rats and humans [34, 35]. However no effect of robenacoxib on PRA or aldosterone compared to placebo was reported recently in healthy cats administered furosemide [12].

Many of the renal effects of furosemide are mediated by prostaglandins, and it has been shown in rats and humans that certain NSAIDs inhibit the diuretic, natriuretic and chloruretic effects of furosemide via inhibition of the reabsorption of sodium and chloride in the loop of Henle [35]. There is only weak evidence from this study that robenacoxib inhibited the diuretic action of furosemide; the significant increases from baseline in plasma albumin and total protein concentrations induced by furosemide were significantly attenuated by robenacoxib and the combination of benazepril and robenacoxib, consistent with less dehydration. In addition, robenacoxib alone inhibited the reduction in body weight (which correlated with reduced feed consumption) and plasma sodium and chloride concentrations induced by furosemide. However there were no significant or numerically visible differences between robenacoxib and placebo treated cats for other relevant variables including water consumption, urine volume and USG.

The principal objective of this study was to investigate the tolerability of the combination of benazepril and robenacoxib, notably with concomitant administration of furosemide. The triple administration of an ACEI, diuretic and an NSAID increases markedly the risk of AKI in humans [8, 9]. In this investigation, the combination of benazepril and robenacoxib was tolerated well and had no significant negative effects on GFR compared to the control group. In study 1, in fact, the combination of benazepril and robenacoxib was associated with a significant increase in GFR (+36.1 %) from baseline, compared to a 9.5 % decrease in the control. In study 2, with furosemide, the GFR was significantly lower in the benazepril and robenacoxib combination group compared to the benazepril group, but was not significantly different from the control. Therefore the results do not preclude the possibility that GFR might decline if robenacoxib was administered to a suspectible (e.g. dehydrated) cat which was previously stable with benazepril treatment.

The combination of benazepril and robenacoxib significantly inhibited plasma aldosterone concentrations compared to the control group, with mean values numerically similar to the benazepril alone group but with statistical significance at more time points (2, 6 and 12 versus 2 h). These results support the rationale for investigation of co-administration of benazepril and robenacoxib in certain diseases in cats e.g. proteinuric CKD. Aldosterone is a key mediator contributing to the progression of CHF and CKD in humans [36, 37]. Although higher aldosterone concentrations were detected in cats with hypertension [38], we are not aware of data reliably demonstrating a link between elevated aldosterone concentrations and a poor prognosis in cats. Additive effects of ACEIs and NSAIDs in reducing proteinuria have been described in humans [2, 3].

The principal limitations of the study are listed below.

First, healthy and relatively young cats were studied and the results cannot therefore be simply generalised to cats with diseases such as CKD and osteoarthritis. For example, the residence time of robenacoxib in tissues is markedly prolonged by the presence of inflammation [18] and therefore its duration of action may also be longer in the feline kidney if inflammation is present as compared to the healthy animals used in this study. In addition, the effect of the test items, including on GFR, might be different in the presence of diseases.

Second, the main endpoints in this study were orientated to safety, including GFR to assess the risk of AKI. We did not measure blood pressure, and therefore did not test for a possible interaction of robenacoxib with the anti-hypertensive efficacy of benazepril.

Third, GFR was assessed 2–4 h after dosing with the test items i.e. close to the peak concentrations of plasma benazeprilat (≤2 h) and blood robenacoxib (0.5 h) [16, 17]. The observed effects of benazepril and robenacoxib on GFR therefore presumably represent maximal or close to maximal actions, and different (probably lesser) effects might occur at other times (4–24 h) of the dosing interval.

Fourth, the cats were fed a standard diet and were dosed with the test items in the morning at approximately 8.00. Chronological differences and marked effects of feeding on the RAAS have been reported in dogs [39], and therefore different results might be obtained with other diets or different timings of feeding or dosing.

Fifth, sex and "sex by treatment" interactions were significant for several variables in both studies. The frequency of these interactions was greater in study 2, therefore the weakness in study design in study 1 (all females were included in cohort 1 and all males in cohort 2) did not appear to have a relevant impact on the results. We are not aware of previous reports of genuine gender differences in the effects of ACEIs or NSAIDs on GFR in other species. No sex differences were reported previously in the pharmacokinetics or pharmacodynamics of benazepril [16, 40, 41] or robenacoxib [17, 42] in cats. Therefore we suspect that the observed differences between genders, in addition to isolated events of statistical significance for some chemistry and haematology variables, may be type I errors associated with the multiple statistical analyses with no correction of the alpha value, rather than being genuine biological effects.

Last, the results of this study cannot be simply extrapolated to other ACEIs and NSAIDs since the pharmacology of individual agents differ. Of specific relevance to this study is fact that the active metabolite of benazepril, benazeprilat, is excreted mainly (~85 %) via the biliary rather than renal (~15 %) route in cats [41], and therefore its clearance is maintained even in the presence of moderate renal insufficiency [40]. Similar conclusions might therefore not be obtained for other ACEIs which are mainly or exclusively renally excreted. In addition robenacoxib has a short residence time in the central compartment [17, 18], and therefore is assumed to have short duration pharmacodynamic actions in the healthy kidney. Similar conclusions might therefore not be obtained with NSAIDs with longer half-lives or which are not cyclo-oxygenase (COX)-2 selective. Robenacoxib is a highly selective inhibitor of COX-2 [42], and there is some evidence in humans that the risk of AKI may be lower with selective COX-2 inhibitors compared to non-selective NSAIDs [43].

Conclusions

The combined administration of benazepril and robenacoxib was well tolerated, and either increased or had a neutral effect on GFR compared to the control group in healthy cats without or with concomitant furosemide. The combination of benazepril and robenacoxib reduced plasma aldosterone concentrations increased by furosemide and therefore might be beneficial in cats with certain diseases, notably proteinuric CKD. It is recommended to test the efficacy and clinical safety of combined administration of benazepril and robenacoxib in cats in field studies.

Abbreviations

ACE, angiotensin-converting enzyme; ACEI, angiotensin-converting enzyme inhibitor; AKI, acute kidney injury; ANCOVA, analysis of covariance; AUC: area under curve; BID, twice daily; BSA, body surface area; BWT, body weight; CKD, chronic kidney disease; CL, clearance; CLioh, plasma clearance of iohexol; CV, coefficient of variation; F, female; FE_K, fractional excretion of potassium; FE_{Na}, fractional excretion of sodium; GFR, glomerular filtration rate; IV, intravenous; LLOQ, lower limit of quantification; M, male; NSAID, nonsteroidal anti-inflammatory drug; PRA, plasma renin activity; RAAS, renin-angiotensin-aldosterone system; RMANCOVA, repeated measures analysis of covariance; USG, urine specific gravity.

Acknowledgements

We thank François Aleman for the clinical pathology, Sabine Cardinali for the plasma renin activity, Christophe Chardonnens for the aldosterone and Marlène Lacroix for the iohexol analyses. We also thank Sophie Gerber for study coordination.

Funding

The study was funded by Novartis Animal Health, now owned by Elanco Animal Health, a division of Eli-Lilly company.

Authors' contributions

The studies were designed and the results interpreted by JNK, AP, MG, GF and CD. The experimental phases were managed by AP and MG. The statistical analyses were conducted by WS. The manuscript was drafted by JNK. All authors approved the final manuscript.

Competing interests

The study was funded and all authors were employed by Novartis Animal Health, now owned by Elanco Animal Health, a division of Eli-Lilly company, which distributes and markets benazepril (Fortekor®) and robenacoxib (Onsior®).

Consent for publication

Not applicable.

Author details

[1]Companion Animal Development, Elanco Animal Health, Basel, Switzerland. [2]Preclinical, Elanco Centre de Recherche Santé Animale, St-Aubin, Switzerland. [3]Safety, Elanco Animal Health, Basel, Switzerland.

References

1. Lefebvre HP, Toutain PL. Angiotensin-converting enzyme inhibitors in the therapy of renal diseases. J Vet Pharmacol Therap. 2004;27:265–81.
2. Vogt L, Laverman GD, Navis G. Time for a comeback of NSAIDs in proteinuric chronic kidney disease? Neth J Med. 2010;68:400–7.
3. Heeg JE, de Jong PE, Vriesendorp R, de Zeeuw D. Additive antiproteinuric effect of the NSAID indomethacin and the ACE inhibitor lisinopril. Am J Nephrol. 1990;10:94–7.
4. Whelton A. Nephrotoxicity of nonsteroidal anti-inflammatory drugs: physiologic foundations and clinical implications. Am J Med. 1999;106:13S–24S.
5. Meune C, Mourad J-J, Bergmann J-F, Spaulding C. Interaction between cyclooxygenase and the renin-angiotensin-aldosterone system: rationale and clinical relevance. J Renin-Angiotensin-Aldosterone Syst. 2003;4:149–54.
6. KuKanich B, Bidgood T, Knesl O. Clinical pharmacology of nonsteroidal anti-inflammatory drugs in dogs. Vet Anaesth Analg. 2012;39:69–90.
7. Maschio G, Alberti D, Janin G, Locatelli F, Mann JFE, Motolese M, Ponticelli C, Ritz E, Zucchelli P, and the Angiotensin-Converting-Enzyme Inhibition in Progressive Renal Insufficiency Study Group. Effect of the angiotensin-converting-enzyme inhibitor benazepril on the progression of chronic renal insufficiency. N Engl J Med. 1996;334:939–45.
8. Cupp M: The "Triple Whammy". Pharmacist's Letter/Prescriber's Letter, April 2013.
9. Thomas MC. Diuretics, ACE inhibitors and NSAIDs – the triple whammy. Med J Australia. 2000;172:184–5.
10. Brown SA, Brown CA, Jacobs G, Stiles J, Hendi RS, Wilson S. Effects of the angiotensin converting enzyme inhibitor benazepril in cats with induced renal insufficiency. Am J Vet Res. 2001;62:375–83.
11. King JN, Gunn-Moore D, Tasker S, Gleadhill A, Strehlau G, BENRIC (Benazepril in Renal Insufficiency in Cats) Study Group. Tolerability and efficacy of benazepril in cats with chronic kidney disease. J Vet Intern Med. 2006;20:1054–64.
12. Pelligand L, Suemanotham N, King JN, Seewald W, Syme H, Smith K, Lees P, Elliott J: Effect of Cyclooxygenase(COX)-1 and COX-2 inhibition on furosemide-induced renal responses and isoform immunolocalization in the healthy cat kidney. BMC Vet Res 2016, accepted for publication.
13. Kilkenny C, Brown WJ, Cuthill IC, Emerson M, Altman DG. Improving bioscience research reporting: The ARRIVE Guidelines for Reporting Animal Research. PLoS Biol. 2010;8:e1000412. doi:10.1371/journal.pbio.1000412.
14. SAS 9.2.2 (SAS, 2008), SAS 9.2 Help and Documentation, Cary, NC, USA, SAS Institute Inc., Copyright 2010.
15. Giraudel JM, Gruet P, Alexander D, Seewald W, King JN. Evaluation of orally administered robenacoxib versus ketoprofen for treatment of acute pain and inflammation associated with musculoskeletal disorders in cats. Am J Vet Res. 2010;71:710–9.
16. King JN, Maurer M, Humbert-Droz E. Plasma angiotensin-converting enzyme activity and pharmacokinetics of benazepril and benazeprilat in cats after single and repeated oral administration of benazepril.HCl. J Vet Pharmacol Therap. 1999;22:360–7.
17. King JN, Jung M, Maurer MP, Schmid VB, Seewald W, Lees P. Effects of route of administration and feeding schedule on pharmacokinetics of robenacoxib in cats. Am J Vet Res. 2013;193:397–403.
18. Pelligand L, King JN, Toutain PL, Elliot J, Lees P. Pharmacokinetic/pharmacodynamics modelling of robenacoxib in a feline tissue cage model of inflammation. J Vet Pharmacol Therap. 2012;35:19–32.
19. Laroute V, Lefebvre HP, Costes G, Toutain P-L. Measurement of glomerular filtration rate and effective renal plasma flow in the conscious beagle dog by single intravenous bolus of iohexol and p-aminohippuric acid. J Pharmacol Method. 1999;41:17–25.
20. Syme HM, Fletcher MGR, Bailey SR, Elliott J. Measurement of aldosterone in feline, canine and human urine. J Small Anim Pract. 2007;48:202–8.
21. Panteri A, Kukk A, Desevaux C, Seewald W, King JN: Effect of benazepril and robenacoxib on glomerular filtration rate in dogs. J Vet Pharmacol Therap 2016, accepted for publication.
22. Friedman PA, Roch-Ramel F. Hemodynamic and natriuretic effects of bumetanide and furosemide in the cat. J Pharmacol Exp Therap. 1977;203:82–91.
23. Watanabe T, Mishina M. Effects of benazepril hydrochloride in cats with experimentally induced or spontaneously occurring chronic renal failure. J Vet Med Sci. 2007;69:1015–23.
24. King JN, Dawson J, Esser RE, Fujimoto R, Kimble EF, Maniara W, Marshall PJ, O'Byrne L, Quadros E, Toutain PL, Lees P. Preclinical pharmacology of robenacoxib: a novel selective inhibitor of cyclooxygenase-2. J Vet Pharmacol Therap. 2009;32:1–17.
25. Surdyk KK, Brown CA, Brown SA. Evaluation of glomerular filtration rate in cats with reduced renal mass and administered meloxicam and acetylsalicylic acid. Am J Vet Res. 2013;74:648–51.
26. Goodman LA, Brown SA, Torres BT, Reynolds LR, Budsberg SC. Effects of meloxicam on plasma iohexol clearance as a marker of glomerular filtration rate in conscious healthy cats. Am J Vet Res. 2009;70:826–30.
27. Lascelles BDX, Cripps P, Mirchandani S, Waterman AE. Carprofen as an analgesic for postoperative pain in cats: dose titration and assessment of efficacy in comparison to pethidine hydrochloride. J Small Anim Pract. 1995;36:535–41.
28. Slingsby LS, Waterman-Pearson AE. Comparison between meloxicam and carprofen for postoperative analgesia after feline ovariohysterectomy. J Small Anim Pract. 2002;43:286–9.

29. Carroll GL, Howe LB, Peterson KD. Analgesic efficacy of preoperative administration of meloxicam or butorphanol in onychectomized cats. J Am Vet Med Assoc. 2005;226:913–9.
30. Gunew MN, Menrath VH, Marshall RD. Long-term safety, efficacy and palatability of oral meloxicam at 0.01-0.03 mg/kg for treatment of osteoarthritic pain in cats. J Feline Med Surg. 2008;10:235–41.
31. Speranza C, Schmid V, Giraudel JM, Seewald W, King JN. Robenacoxib versus meloxicam for the control of peri-operative pain and inflammation associated with orthopaedic surgery in cats; a randomised clinical trial. BMC Vet Res. 2015;11:79.
32. King JN, King S, Budsberg SC, Lascelles BDX, Bienhoff SE, Roycroft LM, Roberts ES: Clinical safety of robenacoxib in feline osteoarthritis: results of a randomized, blinded, placebo-controlled clinical trial. J Feline Med Surg 2015, Published on line.
33. Pages JP. Nephropathies dues aux anti-inflammatoires non steroidiens (AINS) chez le Chat : 21 observations (1993-2001). Prat Med Chir Anim Comp. 2005;40:177–81.
34. Kammerl MC, Nusing RM, Schweda F, Endemann D, Stubanus M, Kees F, Lackner KJ, Fischereder M, Kramer BK. Low sodium and furosemide-induced stimulation of the renin system in man is mediated by cyclooxygenase 2. Clin Pharmacol Therap. 2001;70:468–74.
35. Besen A, Kose F, Paydas S, Gonlusen G, Inal T, Dogan A, Kibar M, Balal M. The effects of the nonsteroidal anti-inflammatory drug diclofenac sodium on the rat kidney, and alteration by furosemide. Int Urol Nephrol. 2009;41: 919–26.
36. Bianchi S, Bigazzi R, Campese VM. Long-term effects of spironolactone on proteinuria and kidney function in patients with chronic kidney disease. Kid Int. 2006;70:2116–23.
37. Pitt B, Zannad F, Remme WJ, Cody R, Castaigne A, Perez A, Palensky J, Wittes J. The effect of spironolactone on morbidity and mortality in patients with severe heart failure. Randomized Aldactone Evaluation Study Investigators. New Engl J Med. 1999;341:709–17.
38. Jensen J, Henik RA, Brownfield M, Armstrong J. Plasma renin activity and angiotensin I and aldosterone concentrations in cats with hypertension associated with chronic renal disease. Am J Vet Res. 1997;58:535–40.
39. Mochel JP, Peyrou M, Fink M, Strehlau G, Mohamed R, Giraudel JM, Ploeger B, Danhof M. Capturing the dynamics of systemic Renin-Angiotensin-Aldosterone System (RAAS) peptides heightens the understanding of the effect of benazepril in dogs. J Vet Pharmacol Therap. 2013;36:174–80.
40. King JN, Strehlau G, Wernsing J, Brown SA. Effect of renal insufficiency on the pharmacokinetics and pharmacodynamics of benazepril in cats. J Vet Pharmacol Therap. 2002;25:371–8.
41. King JN, Maurer M, Toutain PL. Pharmacokinetic/pharmacodynamic modelling of the disposition and effect of benazepril and benazeprilat in cats. J Vet Pharmacol Therap. 2003;26:213–24.
42. Schmid VB, Seewald W, Lees P, King JN. In vitro and ex vivo inhibition of COX isoforms by robenacoxib in the cat: a comparative study. J Vet Pharmacol Therap. 2010;33:444–52.
43. Lafrance J-P, Miller DR. Selective and non-selective non-steroidal anti-inflammatory drugs and the risk of acute kidney injury. Pharmacoepid DR S. 2009;18:923–31.

7

Effect of gastric acid-suppressive therapy and biological variation of serum gastrin concentrations in dogs with chronic enteropathies

Romy M. Heilmann[1,2*], Nora Berghoff[2,3], Niels Grützner[2,4], Nolie K. Parnell[1], Jan S. Suchodolski[2] and Jörg M. Steiner[2]

Abstract

Background: Serum gastrin concentration can help diagnose gastrinomas in dogs if >3–10× the upper reference limit (URL), but antisecretory therapy and other conditions can also cause hypergastrinemia. Effects of antisecretory therapy (famotidine or ranitidine, omeprazole) on serum gastrin concentration in dogs with chronic enteropathy (CE) and its biological variation (BV) are unknown. Aim of the study was to evaluate serum gastrin in acid-suppressant-treated or -naïve CE dogs; test the association between serum gastrin and histopathologic findings in acid-suppressant-naïve CE dogs; and evaluate the BV of serum gastrin in dogs not receiving any gastric acid suppressive therapy. Samples from 231 dogs were used and serum gastrin was measured by chemiluminescence assay. Gastric and duodenal histologic lesions were evaluated and graded. BV of serum gastrin was evaluated in serial samples.

Results: Serum gastrin concentrations were significantly higher in acid-suppressant-treated than acid-suppressant-naïve dogs ($P = 0.0245$), with significantly higher concentrations in proton pump inhibitor (PPI)- than H_2-antihistamine-treated patients ($P = 0.0053$). More PPI- than H_2-antihistamine-treated dogs had gastrin concentrations above URL ($P = 0.0205$), but not >3× nor >10× the URL. Serum gastrin concentrations correlated with the severity of gastric antral epithelial injury ($P = 0.0069$) but not with any other lesions or the presence/numbers of spiral bacteria in gastric biopsies. Intra- and inter-individual BV were 13.4 and 21.6%, respectively, in acid-suppressant-naïve dogs, with a reciprocal individuality index of 0. 49 and a critical difference of ≥29.5 ng/L.

Conclusions: Antisecretory (particularly PPI) treatment leads to hypergastrinemia in CE dogs, but the concentrations seen in this study are unlikely to compromise a diagnosis of gastrinoma. Use of a population-based URL for canine serum gastrin and a URL of ≤27.8 ng/L are appropriate.

Keywords: Antihistamine, Biological variation, Canine, Hypergastrinemia, Proton pump inhibitor

Background

Gastrin is a small peptide hormone that is produced by gastric and proximal duodenal G cells [1]. Gastrin acts on cells via the cholecystokinin-2 receptor stimulating gastric acid secretion and having trophic effects on the gastric mucosa [1, 2]. Measurement of serum gastrin has been suggested to be useful for the diagnosis of gastrinomas in dogs if increases in serum gastrin are in excess of three to ten times the upper limit of the reference interval (RI) [2–6].

Serum gastrin concentrations can also be affected by other conditions including hypercalcemia, chronic kidney disease, as gastrin clearance is primarily renal, administration of medications such as gastric acid-suppressants, feeding, and long distance racing[1] [1, 3, 7–12]. Serum gastrin concentrations were also approximately twice as high in a small group of dogs with moderate to severe chronic lymphocytic-plasmacytic enteritis (LPE) compared to a group of dogs without gastrointestinal disease, and were higher in dogs with severe microscopic lesions in the

* Correspondence: Romy.Heilmann@kleintierklinik.uni-leipzig.de
[1]College of Veterinary Medicine, University of Leipzig, An den Tierkliniken 23, 04103 Leipzig, DE, Germany
[2]Gastrointestinal Laboratory, Texas A&M University, TAMU 4474, College Station, TX 77843-4474, USA
Full list of author information is available at the end of the article

stomach [13]. However, the effect of antisecretory therapy on hypergastrinemia was not evaluated in this study [13].

Effects of gastric *Helicobacter* spp. on gastrin expression and release in dogs have not been definitively elucidated. While no differences in plasma gastrin concentrations were seen between dogs colonized with *Helicobacter* spp. and specific-pathogen-free, *Helicobacter* spp.-free dogs [14], an enhanced basal gastrin release from canine antral G cells was detected after incubation with *Helicobacter pylori* extracts [15], and an increase in gastrin-mRNA expression in the fundus of the stomach has been demonstrated in dogs harboring virulent strains of *Helicobacter heilmannii* [16].

Investigations in healthy dogs revealed that serum gastrin concentrations transiently increase during either histamine type-2 receptor antagonist (H2A) or proton pump inhibitor (PPI) therapy[2] [7, 10]. However, the effect of gastric acid-suppressant administration on serum gastrin concentration has not been reported in dogs with chronic enteropathies (CE).

Biological variability is an important measure in clinical pathology and consists of both intra- (within-subject) and inter-individual (between-subject) variation [17, 18]. While for most clinical chemistry analytes the components of biological variation derived from healthy subjects allows for inferences to be made in specific disease states [17, 18], for some biomarkers their interpretation can differ between health and disease [18]. To the authors' knowledge, the biological variation of serum gastrin concentrations in dogs has been reported in neither health nor disease.

The aims of the study were (i) to compare serum gastrin concentrations between dogs with CE either administered an H2A and/or PPI and dogs with CE not receiving any gastric acid-suppressive treatment, and to determine whether the serum gastrin concentrations can distinguish dogs with CE from dogs with gastrinoma; (ii) to test the possibility of an association between serum gastrin concentrations and clinical disease severity or specific microscopic lesions in the stomach and duodenum; and (iii) to evaluate the biological variability of serum gastrin concentrations in dogs with CE. We hypothesized that (i) serum gastrin concentrations are higher in acid-suppressant-treated dogs with CE compared to those dogs not receiving any antisecretory treatment, and that serum gastrin can help to separate dogs with CE from dogs with gastrinoma (historical positive controls); (ii) serum gastrin concentrations are correlated with the severity of clinical signs and with microscopic lesions in the stomach and duodenum; and (iii) use of a population-based RI for serum gastrin concentration is appropriate.

Methods

Sampling population

Dogs that presented for routine diagnostic evaluation of chronic (more than 2 weeks duration) gastrointestinal signs (i.e., vomiting, diarrhea, hypo- or anorexia, abdominal pain, weight loss), including a planned gastrointestinal endoscopy or exploratory laparotomy with collection of gastrointestinal tissue biopsies, and were diagnosed with CE [19] at the Veterinary Medical Teaching Hospitals at Texas A&M University (TAMU), Purdue University, or at one of several other referral hospitals across the United States, were prospectively enrolled between September 2009 and June 2015 (70 months) (see flow chart in Fig. 1).

The study was designed to evaluate several biomarkers, and was reviewed and approved by the Texas A&M University Institutional Animal Care and Use Committee (CRRC# 2009–06 and 2010–05, AUP# 2012-083A). The owner of each enrolled dog had to sign an informed consent form and was also asked to complete a study questionnaire, which included information about the dog's clinical signs and patient history, including any current and past medications. The attending veterinarian was asked to assess the severity of the patient's clinical signs by using a clinical disease activity scoring sheet with the nine criteria of the canine chronic enteropathy clinical activity index (CCECAI) scoring system [20].

Exclusion criteria were lack of complete patient records or clinicopathologic evidence of total hypercalcemia (>12 mg/dL) or renal azotemia (serum creatinine concentration > 2.0 mg/dL and urine specific gravity <1.030).

Follow-up data were included from patients that were clinically re-evaluated as described and complete sets of samples were collected at the time of recheck evaluation. Treatment of each individual dog, including the choice of diet, antibiotic, supplements, and/or anti-inflammatory or immunosuppressant therapy, was at the discretion of the attending clinician. Thus, gastric acid-suppressive treatment was not standardized. No interventions were performed as part of the study.

Sample collection and analyses

Whole blood, serum, and urine samples were collected from all dogs at the time of presentation for diagnostic evaluation and, if reevaluated at the same veterinary hospital, at the recheck appointment or appointments. Whole blood and serum samples were collected after withholding food for a 12-h period, and were stored refrigerated until shipped to TAMU. Within 24 h of collection, all specimens, including gastrointestinal tissue biopsies (if obtained as part of the routine diagnostic work-up), collected outside of TAMU were sent to the TAMU Gastrointestinal Laboratory overnight on ice packs. Serum samples were processed as soon as received at the TAMU Gastrointestinal Laboratory, and were kept refrigerated in between analyses.

EDTA-anticoagulated whole blood was submitted for routine hematology (either at the institution recruiting

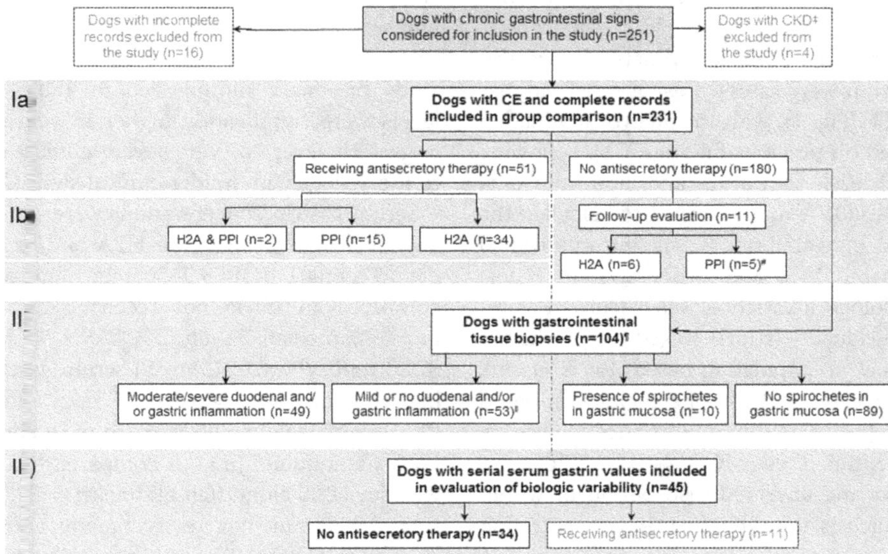

‡Crea >2.0 mg/dL and USG <1.030; #one dog receiving both H2A & PPI; ¶99 gastric and 101 duodenal biopsies; ᵗexcluded were 2 dogs with gastrointestinal neoplasia (lymphoma, mucinous adenocarcinoma)

Fig. 1 Flow chart that summarizes the subgroup allocation of all dogs (n = 231) included in the study. The three different parts of the study are indicated by the grey shaded areas: (I) evaluation of serum gastrin concentrations and antisecretory therapy in dogs with CE at the time of enrolment (Ia) and at serial evaluations (Ib); (II) evaluation of serum gastrin concentrations and histopathologic findings in dogs with CE; and (III) estimation of the biological variation of serum gastrin concentrations in dogs with CE

the dog for the study or the Texas A&M Veterinary Medical Diagnostic Laboratory). Serum was used for a chemistry profile (using an automated clinical chemistry analyzer[3]) and analysis of several biomarkers. Urine samples were submitted for routine urinalysis (either at the institution recruiting the dog for the study or the TAMU Clinical Pathology service) and, if indicated, further diagnostic testing.

Serum gastrin concentration was measured following routine laboratory procedures (i.e., within 24 h after samples were received at the laboratory) using an automated commercially available chemiluminometric assay[4,5] [21]. The lower limit of detection of the assay is 9.9 ng/L, and the intra- and inter-assay variability of the assay are <8% [21]. The upper reference limit (URL) of the assay has been previously established as ≤27.8 ng/L using serum samples from 41 healthy dogs[5].

Histopathological analysis of gastrointestinal tissue biopsies was performed by one of 7 different board-certified pathologists through the TAMU Gastrointestinal Laboratory Histopathology service (median of 10 dogs evaluated by each pathologist, range: 1–28). Tissues were evaluated according to the World Small Animal Veterinary Association Gastrointestinal Standardization scoring system [19]. The severity of inflammatory and morphologic lesions in the stomach and duodenum was recorded using a 4-point grading system (0 = normal, 1 = mild lesions, 2 = moderate lesions, and 3 = severe lesions) with individual as well as composite scores being considered for analysis.

Data analyses

All calculations and statistical analyses were performed using statistical software programs[6,7] A Shapiro-Wilk W and Brown-Forsythe test were used to assess normality and equal variances, respectively. Summary statistics are presented as medians, interquartile ranges (IQR), and ranges. A Wilcoxon rank sum test (for unrelated groups) or Wilcoxon signed-rank test (for paired data) was used for two-group comparisons. A Spearman rank sum correlation coefficient (ρ) was calculated to assess potential relationships, with a Bonferroni correction for multiple comparisons applied if indicated. A likelihood ratio test served to evaluate the association between gastric acid-suppressive therapy and serum gastrin concentrations above RI. Significance was set a $P < 0.05$. Serum gastrin concentrations below the minimum detection limit of the assay (<9.9 ng/L) were assigned a concentration of 9.9 ng/L for all statistical analyses.

Receiver operating characteristic (ROC) curves were constructed to determine the sensitivities and specificities of serum gastrin concentrations to distinguish dogs with gastrinoma (historical positive controls [4, 22–31]) from acid-suppressant-naïve and/or acid-suppressant-treated CE dogs (disease controls). The Youden index was used to establish the optimum cut-off concentrations (expressed as fold elevation of the URL established for the respective assay that was used).

Intra- and inter-individual biological variation of gastrin concentrations in serum were assessed using serial samples from 45 dogs with CE (Fig. 1), with the analytical variation (CV_A) set at 8% based on previous findings [21]. Following tests for outliers at 2 levels (i.e., intra- and inter-individual variation), a nested ANOVA model served to calculate the biologic coefficients of variation (CV): intra-individual (CV_I), inter-individual (CV_G), and total variation (CV_T) [17]. The index of biological variation was calculated as reciprocal index of individuality (rII; rII = S_G/S_{A+I}), where a rII ≤0.7 suggests that a population-based RI is useful, whereas a rII ≥1.7 indicates that use of a population-based RI is not appropriate [17]. The minimum critical difference ($MCD_{0.05}$) was determined as $MCD_{0.05} = 2.77[dk_{90}]^{1/2}$ (dk_{90} = 0.9 fractile of the observed distribution of within subject variance), which is the difference in concentration being significant at $P < 0.05$ [17].

Results

Study population

A total of 251 dogs were considered for inclusion into the study, of which 16 dogs had to be excluded due to incomplete records. An additional 4 dogs were excluded due to the presence of renal azotemia (Fig. 1), leaving a total of 231 dogs with CE (median age: 6.6 years; range: 0.3–17 years; 128 males/111 neutered and 103 females/90 spayed) included in the study. Breeds with $n \geq 5$ dogs included: mixed breed dogs (n = 36), German Shepherd dogs (n = 20), Yorkshire terriers (n = 13), Labrador retrievers (n = 12), Boxers (n = 7), and Cavalier King Charles Spaniels, Golden retrievers, Jack Russell terriers, and Pitbull terriers (each n = 5).

Clinical signs at initial presentation were diarrhea in 171/231 dogs (74%), weight loss in 139/231 dogs (60%), vomiting in 128/231 dogs (55%), and hypo- or anorexia in 100/231 dogs (43%). The CCECAI at the time of enrolment into the study ranged from 1 to 19 (median: 7). Duration of clinical signs prior to enrollment in the study was 1–90 months (median: 5 months). At least one dietary trial had been performed in 161 dogs (70%) and an antibiotic trial in 95 dogs (41%), 46 dogs (20%) were given a probiotic and 23 dogs (10%) received cobalamin supplementation. Fourteen dogs were reported to have received corticosteroids prior to enrollment.

Serum gastrin concentrations and gastric acid-suppressive therapy in dogs with CE

Serum gastrin concentrations were compared among 231 CE dogs with (H2A and/or PPI; n = 51) or without antisecretory therapy (n = 180). Serum gastrin concentrations at the time of study inclusion ranged from 9.9–571.0 ng/L (median: 10.3 ng/L, IQR: 9.9–19.6 ng/L), with an overall distribution of measurements skewed towards low serum gastrin concentrations. Information on serum gastrin concentrations and patient characteristics in this study has been summarized in Table 1. Serum gastrin levels were significantly higher in acid-suppressant-naïve dogs with severe or very severe clinical disease compared to those dogs with milder clinical signs (P = 0.0363).

Serum gastrin concentrations were significantly higher in dogs with CE receiving an H2A and/or PPI (n = 51; median: 12.4 ng/L, IQR: 9.9–36.3 ng/L, range: 9.9–490.0 ng/L) compared to those not receiving antisecretory therapy (n = 180; median: 9.9 ng/L, IQR: 9.9–17.4 ng/L, range: 9.9–571.0 ng/L; P = 0.0245), with serum gastrin concentrations being significantly higher in CE dogs administered either a PPI (omeprazole) alone (n = 15) or in combination with an H2A (famotidine) (n = 2) compared to those dogs treated with an H2A alone (famotidine: n = 32, ranitidine: n = 2; P = 0.0053) or not receiving any antisecretory therapy (P = 0.0001) (Fig. 2). Further partitioning of the group of PPI-treated dogs was not possible given the small numbers of dogs. Gastric acid-suppressive therapy was significantly associated with serum gastrin concentrations above the URL (27.8 ng/L; 16/51, 31% vs. 28/180, 16%; P = 0.0151; for acid-suppressant-treated vs untreated dogs, respectively), but not above 3 × URL (83.4 ng/L; 4/51, 8% vs. 7/180, 4%, P = 0.2689) or above 10 × URL (278 ng/L; 2/51, 4% vs. 2/180, 1%, P = 0.2165), with a larger proportion of PPI-treated CE dogs compared to those given an H2A having a serum gastrin concentration above the URL (9/17, 53% vs. 7/34, 21%; P = 0.0205) but not above 3 × URL (3/17, 18% vs. 1/34, 3%, P = 0.0748) or above 10 × URL (1/17, 6% vs. 1/34, 3%; P = 0.6200). An effect of time (i.e., the study year) on serum gastrin concentrations was not detected in canine CE patients on antisecretory treatment (P = 0.3581) nor specifically in PPI-treated dogs (P = 0.1151).

The area under the ROC curve (AUROC), optimum cut-off levels, sensitivities, and specificities for serum gastrin concentrations to diagnose a gastrinoma are summarized in Table 2.

Serum gastrin concentrations and the CCECAI scores in dogs not receiving an acid-suppressant (median: 5; IQR: 3–8, range: 1–19) were not correlated (ρ = 0.121, P = 0.1091). Also, no association was identified between serum gastrin concentrations and the presence of vomiting (P = 0.0675), diarrhea (P = 0.3646), weight loss (P = 0.1510), or hypo- or anorexia (P = 0.9416) in acid-suppressant-naïve dogs. Furthermore, serum gastrin concentration was not correlated with serum creatinine (median: 0.8 mg/dL; IQR: 0.6–1.0 mg/dL, range: 0.3–1.8 mg/dL; ρ = 0.0180, P = 0.8263) or serum total calcium concentrations (median: 9.6 mg/dL; IQR: 8.6–10.3 mg/dL, range: 3.4–13.0 mg/dL; ρ = −0.0437, P = 0.5928).

Paired serum gastrin concentrations were evaluated in 11 initially acid-suppressant-naïve CE dogs that had received

Table 1 Summary of the serum gastrin concentrations and characteristics of the study population

Patient characteristics	Serum gastrin (in ng/L) in acid-suppressant-naïve dogs	*P*	Serum gastrin (in ng/L) in acid-suppressant-treated dogs	*P*
Age				
< 6 years	9.9 [9.9–14.9]	0.0770	10.6 [9.9–43.9]	0.5496
> 6 years	10.8 [9.9–22.8]		18.0 [9.9–34.4]	
Sex				
Female	9.9 [9.9–15.3]	0.5102	11.2 [9.9–31.8]	0.4276
Male	10.0 [9.9–19.4]		13.5 [9.9–44.6]	
Breed				
Purebred	10.1 [9.9–19.4]	0.1744	11.4 [9.9–35.0]	0.7206
Mixed breed	9.9 [9.9–14.4]		15.8 [9.9–46.9]	
German Shepherd (GSD)	12.1 [9.9–15.1]	0.8011	N/A	N/A
Non-GSD	9.9 [9.9–20.0]		11.4 [9.9–35.0]	
Yorkshire Terrier (YT)	11.3 [9.9–14.8]	0.6147	9.9 [9.9–9.9]	0.1202
Non-YT	10.1 [9.9–19.5]		13.5 [9.9–36.3]	
Clinical disease severity (CCECAI score)				
Mild to moderate	9.9 [9.9–14.8]	***0.0363***	11.2 [9.9–39.8]	0.9911
Severe to very severe	12.8 [9.9–25.0]		17.6 [9.9–31.2]	
Clinical signs				
Vomiting	9.9 [9.9–18.0]	0.6869	10.8 [9.9–33.1]	0.1354
No vomiting	9.9 [9.9–17.3]		22.8 [10.3–48.2]	
Diarrhea	10.0 [9.9–17.5]	0.5810	24.5 [9.9–12.4]	***0.0090***
No diarrhea	9.9 [9.9–16.3]		24.5 [9.9–50.0]	
Weight loss	9.9 [9.9–19.3]	0.6704	19.2 [9.9–44.7]	0.2113
No weight loss	10.3 [9.9–15.1]		10.7 [9.9–27.1]	
Hypo–/anorexia	10.4 [9.9–23.0]	0.5200	15.2 [9.9–31.8]	0.4983
No hypo–/anorexia	9.9 [9.9–16.1]		11.4 [9.9–47.5]	

P values in boldface and italicized indicate significance at $P < 0.05$

an H2A or a PPI alone or in combination with an H2A when rechecked 2–35 weeks (median: 13 weeks) after initiation of treatment. Dogs that were resampled had a median change (decrease) in CCECAI score of 83% (70% in H2A-treated dogs and 88% in dogs receiving a PPI with or without H2A). Serum gastrin concentrations did numerically increase in those dogs receiving a PPI alone or in combination with an H2A, but the difference did not reach significance ($P = 0.1563$) (Fig. 3); and no differences were seen in dogs given an H2A ($P = 0.5938$). There was no correlation between the change in CCECAI scores and the change in serum gastrin concentrations ($\rho = -0.073$, $P = 0.8302$), neither was an improvement in the CCECAI score associated with a normalization of serum gastrin concentration ($P = 0.3852$).

Serum gastrin concentrations and histopathologic results in acid-suppressant-naïve dogs with CE

Gastrointestinal tissues were available for 104 dogs: endoscopic biopsies from 88 dogs (median number of gastric biopsies: 12, range: 2–34; median number of duodenal biopsies: 12, range: 2–29) and surgical biopsies from 16 dogs (median number of gastric biopsies: 2, range: 1–4; median number of duodenal biopsies: 1, range: 1–3). Two dogs were excluded from this part of the study due to the diagnosis of gastrointestinal lymphoma or a gastric mucinous adenocarcinoma.

No difference in serum gastrin concentrations were detected between acid-suppressant-naïve CE dogs with moderate or severe histologic lesions in the stomach ($n = 22$; median: 9.9 ng/L, IQR: 9.9–25.7 ng/L, range: 9.9–571.0 ng/L) and those dogs with none or mild gastric lesions ($n = 75$; median: 10.2 ng/L, IQR: 9.9–14.9 ng/L, range: 9.9–104.0 ng/L; $P = 0.9815$). Serum gastrin concentrations were slightly higher in dogs with moderate or severe microscopic lesions in the duodenum ($n = 38$; median: 12.1 ng/L, IQR: 9.9–32.7 ng/L, range: 9.9–111.0 ng/L) or stomach/duodenum combined ($n = 49$; median: 11.4 ng/L, IQR: 9.9–30.5 ng/L, range: 9.9–571.0 ng/L) compared to dogs with only mild or no such lesions

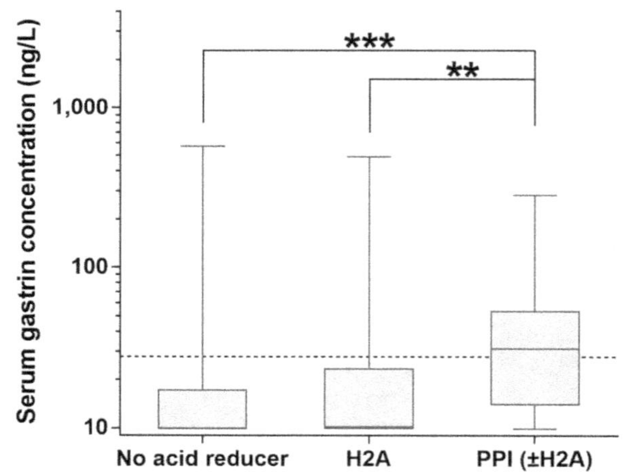

Fig. 2 Serum gastrin concentrations and gastric acid-suppressive (PPI and/or H2A)-treatment in dogs with CE. Serum gastrin concentrations were significantly higher in dogs with CE administered either a PPI alone (n = 15) or in combination (n = 2) with an H2A (group PPI (±H2A); median: 31.2 ng/L, IQR: 14.0–54.1 ng/L, range: 9.9–282.0 ng/L) compared to CE dogs treated with an H2A alone (group H2A; n = 34; median: 10.2 ng/L, IQR: 9.9–23.7 ng/L, range: 9.9–490.0 ng/L; P = 0.0053) and those not receiving any gastric acid-suppressive treatment (group No acid reducer; n = 180; median: 9.9 ng/L, IQR: 9.9–17.4 ng/L, range: 9.9–571.0 ng/L; P = 0.0001). No significant difference was seen between H2A-treated CE dogs and dogs receiving no antisecretory treatment (P = 0.7312). Boxes: interquartile range (IQR), vertical lines within boxes: medians, whiskers: minimum to maximum data points; dashed line: upper limit of the RI (≤27.8 ng/L)

(duodenum: n = 61, median = 9.9 ng/L, IQR = 9.9–14.3 ng/L, range = 9.9–571.0 ng/L; stomach/duodenum: n = 53; median = 9.9 ng/L, IQR = 9.9–13.5 ng/L, range = 9.9–72.3 ng/L) but neither difference reached statistical significance (P = 0.0543 and 0.0726, respectively). Serum gastrin concentration demonstrated a moderate positive correlation with the severity of surface epithelial injury in the gastric antrum (ρ = 0.324; unadjusted P = 0.0023, adjusted P = 0.0069), but was not correlated with any other morphologic or inflammatory microscopic findings (Table 3). Histopathologic evidence of atrophic gastritis was not reported in any of the dogs included in this study. A weak positive correlation with the composite duodenal lesion score did not reach statistical significance (ρ = 0.211; unadjusted P = 0.0362, adjusted P = 0.0724).

Also, no significant difference in serum gastrin concentrations was seen between acid-suppressant-naïve CE dogs with spiral bacteria present in gastric biopsies (n = 10; median: 11.3 ng/L, IQR: 9.9–16.1 ng/L, range: 9.9–28.5 ng/L) and those dogs without (n = 89; median: 9.9 ng/L, IQR: 9.9–17.1 ng/L, range: 9.9–571.0 ng/L; P = 0.9154); nor was there a difference between dogs with large numbers of spiral bacteria (n = 5; median: 13.4 ng/L, IQR: 11.3–21.7 ng/L, range: 9.9–28.5 ng/L) and those with small numbers of spiral bacteria in gastric biopsies (n = 5; median: 9.9 ng/L, IQR: 9.9–14.8 ng/L, range: 9.9–19.6 ng/L; P = 0.1812). Presence and numbers of spiral bacteria in gastric biopsies were also not associated with the severity of microscopic lesions in the stomach (P = 0.5708 and 0.4870, respectively) nor in the duodenum (P = 0.6944 and 0.3406, respectively).

Biological variation of serum gastrin concentrations in dogs with CE

Biologic variability of serum gastrin concentrations was evaluated on an average of 2.3 serial specimens from 34 CE dogs (46 rechecks within 2–72 weeks, median: 7 weeks) not receiving any gastric acid-suppressive therapy (median age: 6.0 years; range: 0.3–12 years; 23 males/21 neutered and 11 females/9 spayed): 4 samples from 2 dogs, 3 samples from 8 dogs, and 2 samples each from 24 dogs. One within-subject outlier and two between-subject outliers were excluded from the dataset, resulting in a total of 73 mildly skewed data points and a

Table 2 Sensitivities and specificities at the optimal cut-off concentrations (expressed as the fold elevation above the respective URL for the assay) and area under the ROC curve (AUROC) for serum gastrin concentrations to distinguish acid-suppressant (H2A and/or PPI)-treated or acid-suppressant-naïve dogs with CE from dogs diagnosed with gastrinoma (n = 14 historical positive controls)

Group comparison	AUROC	Cut-off	Sensitivity	Specificity
all CE dogs vs. gastrinoma[a]	97%	>1.8 × URL	100%	90%
		>3.2 × URL	93%	95%
acid-suppressant-naïve CE dogs vs. gastrinoma[a]	98%	>1.8 × URL	100%	92%
		>3.2 × URL	93%	97%
acid-suppressant-treated CE dogs vs. gastrinoma[a]	95%	>1.8 × URL	100%	82%
		>10.3 × URL	57%	95%
H2A-treated CE dogs vs. gastrinoma[a]	97%	>1.8 × URL	100%	90%
		>3.2 × URL	93%	95%
PPI-treated CE dogs vs. gastrinoma[a]	91%	>3.2 × URL	93%	77%
		>10.3 × URL	57%	95%

AUROC area under the ROC curve, *CE* chronic enteropathy, *H2A* histamine type-2 receptor antagonist, *PPI* proton pump inhibitor, *URL* upper reference limit
[a]historical positive controls [4, 21–30]

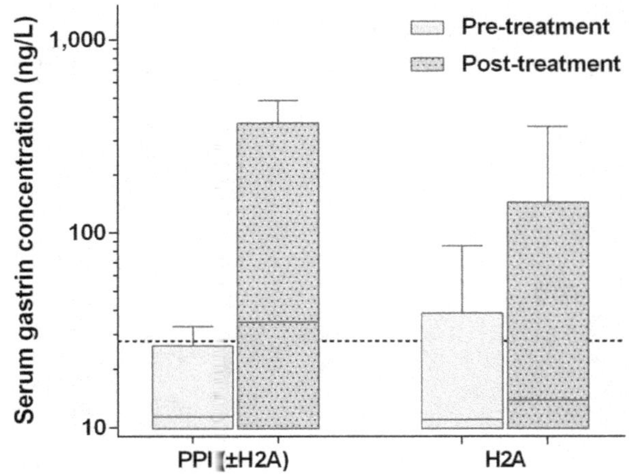

Fig. 3 Paired serum gastrin concentrations were evaluated in initially acid-suppressant-naïve CE dogs that received either an H2A (n = 6) or a PPI alone or in combination with an H2A (n = 5) at their next recheck. Serum gastrin concentrations did numerically increase in those dogs receiving a PPI alone or in combination with an H2A (prior to antisecretory therapy: median = 11.4 ng/L, IQR = 9.9–19.6 ng/L, range = 9.9–33.1 ng/L; receiving gastric acid-suppressive therapy: median = 34.8 ng/L, IQR = 9.9–254.0 ng/L, range = 9.9–485.0 ng/L), but the difference did not reach significance (P = 0.1563). No difference in serum gastrin concentrations was seen in dogs given an H2A alone (prior to antisecretory therapy: median = 11.0 ng/L, IQR = 9.9–20.2 ng/L, range = 9.9–85.5 ng/L; receiving acid-suppressant therapy: median = 13.9 ng/L, IQR = 9.9–59.6 ng/L, range: 9.9–355.0 ng/L; P = 0.5938). Boxes: interquartile range (IQR), vertical lines within boxes: medians, whiskers: minimum to maximum data points; dashed line: upper limit of the RI (≤27.8 ng/L)

narrow range of serum gastrin concentrations in individual dogs (Fig. 4a). CV_I was calculated as 43.4% and CV_G as 21.6%, resulting in an estimated CV_T of 73.0% and a rII of 0.49. Relevant serum gastrin concentration changes (as assessed by the $MCD_{0.05}$) were calculated as ≥29.5 ng/L. The desirable analytical goal of estimated $CV_A \leq ½ \times CV_I$ was achieved (maximum allowable imprecision $½ \times CV_I$ = 21.7%).

Biologic variability could not be assessed in acid-suppressant-treated dogs (median age: 6.1 years; range: 2–12 years; 7 males/6 neutered and 4 females/4 spayed) due to the small number of data points (4 samples from 3 dogs, 3 samples from 2 dogs, and 2 samples each from 6 dogs) remaining for analysis after 2 between-subject outliers were excluded from the dataset.

Discussion

This study evaluated serum gastrin concentrations in acid-suppressant-naïve CE dogs and CE dogs receiving gastric acid-suppressive therapy, and it is reasonable to assume that the findings of this study are likely to also translate to other species.

Antisecretory treatment with a PPI was associated with an approximately 3-fold increase (though not statistically significant) in serum gastrin concentrations (in contrast to an increase of only 1.3-fold in dogs receiving an H2A) in this population of dogs. This finding is consistent with the 3- to 5-fold increase seen in people taking a PPI [32]. The hypergastrinemia seen with H2A/PPI treatment can be explained by the reduction in gastric acidity, which inhibits the negative feedback on gastrin secretion [1].

Compared to Parente et al. [10], serum gastrin concentrations more than three-fold above the URL were rare in acid-suppressant-naïve (7/180, 4%) and H2A-treated CE dogs (1/34, 3%), but were seen in almost every fifth PPI-treated dog (3/17, 18%). This is consistent with PPIs being more potent at reducing gastric acid production by inhibiting all stimulatory effects through binding to the luminal α-subunit of the proton pump compared to H2A that block only the effect of histamine (but not gastrin and acetylcholine) as stimulators [1, 33]. Whether the length of PPI treatment or PPI dosing could also have an effect on serum gastrin concentration is unknown and cannot be clarified by the results of this study.

Serum gastrin concentrations in our study were comparable to those obtained in a small study in dogs with CE [13] but were slightly lower compared to serum gastrin concentrations measured in an experimental study in healthy dogs [10]. A possible explanation for the difference in measured concentrations is the use of different assays (a radioimmunoassay was used in the study by Parente et al. [10] whereas a chemiluminometric assay was used in the present study) as immunoassays depend on antigen-antibody binding and thus are not truly quantitative. An alternative explanation could be a difference in the length of antisecretory therapy as H2A administration has been shown to cause a transient hypergastrinemia in healthy dogs [10]. Our findings also agree with the hypergastrinemia seen in people with Crohn's disease [34] whereas they are in contrast with another study that found systemic gastrin concentrations to be normal in Crohn's disease patients [35]. The increase in serum gastrin concentrations in dogs with CE has been speculated to be due to either the gastric lesions per se or the stimulation of gastric G cells resulting from a decreased acidity in the gastric antrum [13]. However, the hypergastrinemia seen in CE dogs may also be associated with the inflammation as tumor-necrosis factor-α has been shown to affect gastrin concentrations [36, 37]. Whether decreased gastrin-releasing peptide receptor expression as seen in patients with Crohn's disease [38] also affects the extent of the hypergastrinemia seen in dogs with CE has not been determined. While atrophic gastritis as a cause of hypergastrinemia [26] can be ruled out by histopathology (none of the dogs included in this study had histopathologic evidence of atrophic gastritis), the possibility of antral G-cell hyperplasia [33] (a condition that has not been reported in

Table 3 Correlation of serum gastrin with variables of the histologic score for canine CE

Histologic findings correlated with		serum gastrin concentration (ng/L)		
	N	Spearman ρ	unadjusted $P^{\dagger}$	adjusted $P^{\#}$
Stomach (composite score)	97	−0.1291	0.2075	0.4150
Fundus: Morphologic criteria (sum)	92	0.0885	0.4014	ns
- Surface epithelial injury	92	0.0517	0.6248	ns
- Gastric pit epithelial injury	92	0.0151	0.8866	ns
- Mucosal fibrosis	92	0.0167	0.8741	ns
Fundus: Inflammatory criteria (sum)	92	−0.0902	0.3923	ns
- Intraepithelial lymphocytes	92	−0.0434	0.6815	ns
- Lamina propria LPC	92	−0.1358	0.1966	ns
- Lamina propria eosinophils	92	0.0408	0.6993	ns
- Lamina propria neutrophils	92	−0.0938	0.3740	ns
- Lamina propria macrophages	92	−0.0938	0.3740	ns
- Lymphoid follicular hyperplasia	92	0.0079	0.9401	ns
Antrum: Morphologic criteria (sum)	86	0.0299	0.7844	ns
- Surface epithelial injury	86	0.3241	***0.0023***	***0.0069***
- Gastric pit epithelial injury	86	−0.1258	0.2483	ns
- Mucosal fibrosis	86	−0.0968	0.3754	ns
Antrum: Inflammatory criteria (sum)	86	−0.1489	0.1737	0.6948
- Intraepithelial lymphocytes	86	−0.0474	0.6650	ns
- Lamina propria LPC	86	−0.1969	0.0691	0.4146
- Lamina propria eosinophils	86	0.0140	0.8990	ns
- Lamina propria neutrophils	86	−0.1933	0.0745	0.4470
- Lamina propria macrophages	86	−0.0651	0.5512	ns
- Lymphoid follicular hyperplasia	86	−0.0815	0.4557	ns
Duodenum (composite score)	100	0.2108	***0.0362***	0.0724
Morphologic criteria (sum)	100	0.1178	0.2432	0.4864
- Villus stunting	100	0.1130	0.2629	ns
- Epithelial injury	100	0.0452	0.6554	ns
- Crypt distension	100	0.0966	0.3391	ns
- Lacteal dilation	100	0.1320	0.1906	0.9530
- Mucosal fibrosis	100	−0.0467	0.6444	ns
Inflammatory criteria (sum)	100	0.1239	0.2218	0.4436
- Intraepithelial lymphocytes	100	−0.0877	0.3855	ns
- Lamina propria LPC	100	0.0680	0.5013	ns
- Lamina propria eosinophils	100	0.1927	0.0560	0.2800
- Lamina propria neutrophils	100	0.1096	0.2779	ns
- Lamina propria macrophages	100	0.0663	0.5121	ns

Relationship between serum gastrin concentrations and the severity of morphologic and inflammatory histologic lesions of the stomach and duodenum in dogs with CE (n = 102)

CE chronic enteropathy, *LPC* lymphocytes/plasma cells, *N* sample size, *ns* non-significant with P = 1.0000; †without correction ($P < 0.05$); #after Holm-Bonferroni correction (n = 2, 4, or 5)

P values in boldface and italicized indicate significance at $P < 0.05$

dogs to date) or an effect of antral distention associated with delayed gastric emptying or even gastric outlet obstruction on serum gastrin concentrations in individual dogs cannot be excluded in our study.

Clinical signs of dogs with gastrinoma can include vomiting, weight loss, abdominal pain, hypo- or anorexia, diarrhea, melena and/or hematochezia [3, 4, 22, 24, 26–31, 39, 40] and thus can mimic the clinical presentation of dogs

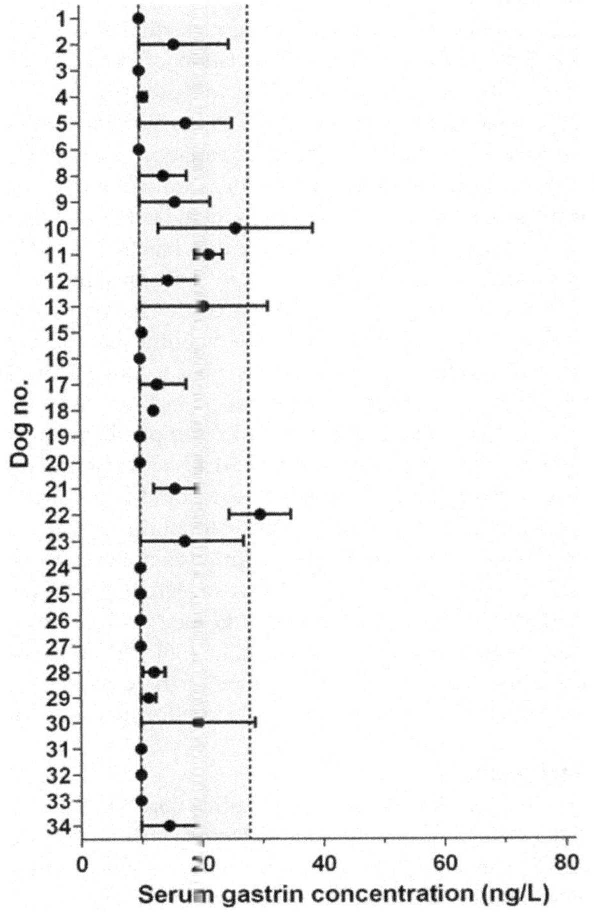

Fig. 4 Biological variability of serum gastrin concentrations in dogs with CE that did not receive gastric acid-suppressive therapy. Serum gastrin concentrations ranged from 9.9–38.5 ng/L (mean: 13.5 ng/L) in 32 dogs with CE not receiving an acid-suppressant. A total of 44 measurements (60%) were at or below the detection limit of the gastrin assay and 4 (6%) were above URL. Closed circles: mean serum gastrin concentrations, horizontal bars: range of serum gastrin concentrations in individual dogs; gray shaded area (delineated by dashed vertical lines): RI (left dashed vertical line: lower reference limit coinciding with the lower detection limit of the assay

with CE [13, 19, 20, 26]. Serum gastrin concentrations >3× or >10× above the URL (the currently used criteria for the diagnosis of gastrinoma) were rare in all dogs with CE (acid-suppressant-treated: 8% and 4%, respectively; untreated: 4% and 1%, respectively) in this study. Thus, the hypergastrinemia associated with CE and antisecretory therapy appears unlikely to compromise a diagnosis of gastrinoma in dogs, which differs from studies in people where a substantial overlap among those patient groups has been seen [41] and treatment with a PPI or H2A was associated with plasma gastrin concentrations being more than 20-fold higher than in acid-suppressant-naïve patients. Nonetheless, it is reasonable to assume that false positive results can also occur in dogs. Our findings also contrast an experimental study in dogs where supratherapeutic PPI doses caused up to 20-fold elevations of serum gastrin concentrations[2].

Although the use of historical controls is controversial, with canine gastrinoma it was deemed necessary in order to determine the sensitivity and specificity of the gastrin assay due to the very low prevalence of this neoplastic condition [2–4, 29]. In the 14 canine gastrinoma cases reported in the literature to date where serum gastrin was measured [4, 22–31], the respective concentrations ranged from 72 to 2780 ng/L (median: 519 ng/L, IQR: 370–1020 ng/L; central 95th percentile: 90–2705 ng/L). Because the radioimmunoassays used in these 14 cases do not yield comparable results that could be used interchangeably with the chemiluminometric (Immulite®) method used in our study, the fold elevation of serum gastrin concentrations above the respective URL of the assay used in that study was evaluated and distinguished canine gastrinoma patients from both acid-suppressant-naïve and acid-suppressant-treated CE dogs with a high sensitivity and specificity. The best sensitivity was seen with cut-off serum gastrin elevations of 2- to 3-fold the URL, whereas a cut-off of 3- to 10-fold above the URL yielded the best specificity. However, the diagnostic performance of the serum gastrin assay in dogs with gastrinoma cannot be determined as the overall prevalence of the condition in dogs is unknown. Also, the impact of the use of PPIs on potentially delaying a diagnosis of gastrinoma or resulting in a false diagnosis of gastrinoma [42] in our canine population cannot be determined based on the results of this investigation. The optimal diagnostic algorithm to arrive at a diagnosis of gastrinoma [32, 43] in dogs will also require further study.

Consistent with our findings is the lack of a correlation between serum gastrin concentration and clinical disease activity seen in people with Crohn's disease [34]. In contrast to a previous study in dogs that revealed significantly higher serum gastrin concentrations in dogs with severe gastric lesions compared to those dogs with no lesions in the stomach [13], serum gastrin concentrations correlated significantly only with the severity of surface epithelial injury in the gastric antrum but not with any other lesions in our study. A possible explanation for this discrepancy could be the different histologic lesion scores used or the selection of the patient population as only patients with moderate or severe gastric lesions were included in the study by García-Sancho et al. [13]. However, the possibility of an effect of the patient population, differences in assay methodology (e.g., radioimmunoassays are often more sensitive than chemiluminometric assays), or an effect of antisecretory drugs that was not considered in the study by García-Sancho et al. [13] cannot be excluded. Also, consistent with our results is the lack of a significant difference in serum gastrin concentrations between dogs with gastric carcinoma and healthy control dogs [44].

Only one dog with a large number of spiral bacteria had a serum gastrin concentration slightly above the URL (28.5 ng/L) but none of the dogs with spiral bacteria present had a serum gastrin concentration > 10× above URL in this study. Lack of an effect of spiral bacteria on serum gastrin concentrations and the presence of gastric or duodenal lesions is consistent with previous studies in dogs [14, 45] and also in cats [46]. This finding suggests that *Helicobacter*-like organisms in dogs may not inhibit the gastric proton pump (H^+/K^+-ATPase) as does *Helicobacter pylori* in people [1]. An interesting finding of our study is the normogastrinemia in one dog with gastric lymphoma (14.5 ng/L) and a dog with gastric mucinous adenocarcinoma (9.9 ng/L), which is in contrast to a previous case report [47]. Further, the prevalence of gastric spiral bacteria was lower in this study when compared to previous investigations [48, 49], but the prevalence of such organisms has been shown to vary with the patient population and method of detection [48]. An effect of prior antibiotic (given in 95 dogs included in this study) or probiotic administration (given to 46 of the dogs) on the prevalence of *Helicobacter*-like organisms [50–52] could also be possible.

Being a small peptide hormone, the serum half-life of gastrin is short (10–20 min) [1, 53] and the biological variation is important for the interpretation of serum gastrin concentrations. With the narrow range of serum gastrin concentrations in individual dogs with CE not receiving antisecretory therapy and the low rII, use of a population-based RI for serum gastrin concentrations appears justified. A relevant change in serum gastrin concentration of ≥29.5 ng/L indicates that the currently used URL in dogs (≤27.8 ng/L) is also appropriate.

This study had some limitations. First, while ultrasound evaluation (if performed as part of the diagnostic work-up) did not reveal any pancreatic masses (85% of dogs with a diagnosis of gastrinoma have pancreatic masses [3, 4, 25, 27, 30, 31] or evidence of metastatic disease [3, 29, 40]), a diagnosis of gastrinoma could not be definitively ruled out in all CE dogs. Also, gastric acid output was not determined as part of this study rendering the possibility of hypergastrinemia to exist in the face of either hypochlorhydria (appropriate hypergastrinemia) or hyperchlorhydria (gastric acid hypersecretion) unclear. Second, gastric acid-suppressive treatment was not standardized in dogs with CE enrolled in this study and the potency of gastric acid reducers (especially PPIs) has been shown to vary with the temporal relation to food intake [54] as well as the dose and dosing interval [1]. Thus, it is possible that most dogs were sampled at through. Furthermore, no constraints were placed on additional treatments in this study and a potential effect of supplements with reducing capacity (e.g., glutathione) on the potency of PPI [55] cannot be excluded. Third, involvement of different pathologists in the histopathological evaluation of tissue biopsies and of different attending veterinarians assessing the severity of the patients' clinical signs in this study may potentially introduce an additional degree of variation. Not blinding the pathologist for the patient history, clinical, and/or clinicopathological findings is also a limitation. Fourth, serum samples could not be analyzed in one batch due to concerns about the stability of gastrin in these specimens over the 70-months study period. This practice has the potential to inflate the overall variation in the quantification of serum gastrin. Further, clear instructions on specimen handling procedures were given to participating institutions, but an effect of even slight differences in sample handling on serum gastrin concentrations cannot be entirely excluded. Lastly, a possible effect of undiagnosed mild hypercalcemia on serum gastrin concentrations cannot be entirely excluded as blood free (ionized) calcium was not measured in the dogs in this study. However, correcting the calcium concentration for serum albumin and total protein concentration, although of questionable value [56], did not change the results (data not shown) as none of the dogs were hypercalcemic after applying the correction formula.

Conclusions

We conclude that, as seen in healthy dogs, antisecretory (particularly PPI) therapy leads to hypergastrinemia in dogs with CE, especially dogs with more severe duodenal and/or gastric lesions. However, the hypergastrinemia associated with gastric acid-suppressive therapy in CE dogs is unlikely to compromise a diagnosis of gastrinoma in dogs. Use of a population-based URL for serum gastrin and the currently used URL in dogs (≤27.8 ng/L) are appropriate.

Endnotes

[1]Bregazzi VS, Fettman MJ, Twedt DC. Hypergastrinemia associated with hypercalcemia in the dog. J Vet Intern Med 2000; 14(3): 389 (abstract).

[2]Dossin O, Jones K, Ridgway M, et al. Effect of omeprazole on serum gastrin concentrations and calcium metabolism in healthy dogs. J Vet Intern Med 2011; 25(3): 688 (abstract).

[3]LiquiColor, Sirrus, Stanbio Laboratory, Boerne, TX, USA.

[4]Immulite® 2000 Gastrin immunoassay, Siemens Healthcare Diagnostics Ltd., Deerfield, IL, USA.

[5]Steiner JM, Findlay KM, Suchodolski JS. Analytical validation of a commercial immunoassay for the measurement of serum gastrin concentrations in dogs. J Vet Intern Med 2007; 21(6): 1438 (abstract).

[6]JMP® v13.0, SAS Institute, Cary, NC, USA.

[7]GraphPad Prism® v6.0, GraphPad Software, San Diego, CA, USA.

Abbreviations

AUROC: Area under the ROC curve; CCECAI: Canine chronic enteropathy clinical activity index; CE: Chronic enteropathy; CI: Confidence interval; CV: Coefficient of variation; CV_A: Analytical variation; CV_G: Inter-individual variation; CV_I: Intra-individual variation; CV_T: Total variation; H2A: Histamine type-2 receptor antagonist; IQR: Interquartile range; $MCD_{0.05}$: Minimum critical difference; PPI: Proton pump inhibitor; RI: Reference interval; rII: Reciprocal index of individuality; ROC: Receiver operating characteristic; TAMU: Texas A&M University; URL: Upper reference limit

Acknowledgements

The authors acknowledge the help of Dr. Tomomi Minamoto and Dr. Panpicha Sattasathuchana with the collection and processing of samples. Part of the data were presented at the 26th Annual Congress of the European College of Veterinary Internal Medicine (ECVIM), Gothenburg, Sweden (8–10 September, 2016).

Funding

This study was not supported by a grant or otherwise.

Authors' contributions

RMH, NB, NG, NKP, and JMS designed the study and enrolled patients into the study. RMH, NB, and NG analyzed the specimens from dogs enrolled in the study. RMH, NG, NKP, JSS, and JMS analyzed and interpreted the patient and biomarker data. All authors read and approved the final manuscript.

Consent for publication

Not applicable.

Competing interests

JSS and JMS are employed at the Gastrointestinal Laboratory at Texas A&M University where measurement of serum gastrin concentrations is performed on a fee-for-service basis. No other conflicts of interest have been declared.

Author details

[1]College of Veterinary Medicine, University of Leipzig, An den Tierkliniken 23, 04103 Leipzig, DE, Germany. [2]Gastrointestinal Laboratory, Texas A&M University, TAMU 4474, College Station, TX 77843-4474, USA. [3]Department of Pathobiology & Diagnostic Investigation, College of Veterinary Medicine, Michigan State University, 784 Wilson Rd, East Lansing, MI 48824, USA. [4]Farm Animal Clinic, Vetsuisse Faculty, University of Bern, Bremgartenstrasse 109a, CH, 3012 Bern, BE, Switzerland.

References

1. Schubert ML, Kaunitz JD. Gastric secretion. In: Feldman M, Friedman LS, Brandt LJ, editors. Sleisenger and Fordtran's gastrointestinal and liver disease – pathophysiology, diagnosis, management. Philadelphia: Saunders; 2010. p. 818–32.
2. Steiner JM. Neuroendocrine tumors of the gastrointestinal tract. In: Steiner JM, editor. Small animal gastroenterology. Hannover: Schattauer; 2008. p. 337–51.
3. Shaw DH. Gastrinoma (Zollinger-Ellison syndrome) in the dog and cat. Can Vet J. 1988;29(5):448–52.
4. Hughes SM. Canine gastrinoma: a case study and literature review of therapeutic options. N Z Vet J. 2006;54(5):242–7.
5. Kim S, Hosoya K, Takagi S, Okumura M. Treatment of gastrin-secreting tumor with sustained-release octreotide acetate in a dog. J Am Anim Hosp Assoc. 2015;51(6):407–12.
6. Ward CR. Gastrointestinal endocrine disease. In: Ettinger SJ, Feldman EC, editors. Textbook of veterinary internal medicine. Philadelphia: Saunders; 2010. p. 1857–65.
7. Mordecai A, Sellon RK, Mealey KL. Normal dogs treated with famotidine for 14 days have only transient increases in serum gastrin concentrations. J Vet Intern Med. 2011;25(6):1248–52.
8. Schenck PA, Chew DJ, Nagode LA, Rosol TJ. Disorders of calcium: Hypercalcemia and hypocalcemia. In: DiBartola SP, editor. Fluid, electrolyte, and acid-base disorders in small animal practice. Philadelphia: Saunders; 2012. p. 120–94.
9. McLeland SM, Lunn KF, Duncan CG, et al. Relationship among serum creatinine, serum gastrin, calcium-phosphorus product, and uremic gastropathy in cats with chronic kidney disease. J Vet Intern Med. 2014;28(3):827–37.
10. Parente NL, Bari Oliver N, Refsal KR, Johnson CA. Serum concentrations of gastrin after famotidine and omeprazole administration to dogs. J Vet Intern Med. 2014;28(5):1465–70.
11. James FE, Mansfield CS, Steiner JM, Williams DA, Robertson ID. Pancreatic response in healthy dogs fed diets of various fat compositions. Am J Vet Res. 2009;70(5):614–8.
12. Fergestad ME, Jahr TH, Krontveit RI, Skancke E. Serum concentration of gastrin, cortisol and C-reactive protein in a group of Norwegian sled dogs during training and after endurance racing: a retrospective cohort study. Acta Vet Scand. 2016;58:24.
13. García-Sancho M, Rodríguez-Franco F, Sainz A, et al. Serum gastrin in canine chronic lymphocytic-plasmacytic enteritis. Can Vet J. 2005;46(7):630–4.
14. Simpson KW, Strauss-Ayali D, McDonough PL, et al. Gastric function in dogs with naturally acquired gastric *Helicobacter* spp. infection. J Vet Intern Med. 1999;13(6):507–15.
15. Beales IL, Calam J. *Helicobacter pylori* increases gastrin release from cultured canine antral G-cells. Eur J Gastroenterol Hepatol. 2000;12(6):641–4.
16. Joosten M, Blaecher C, Flahou B, et al. Diversity in bacterium-host interaction within the species *Helicobacter heilmannii* sensu stricto. Vet Res. 2013;44:65.
17. Fraser CG, Harris EK. Generation and application of data on biological variation in clinical chemistry. Crit Rev Clin Lab Sci. 1989;27(5):409–37.
18. Ricós C, Iglesias N, García-Lario JV, et al. Within-subject biological variation in disease: collated data and clinical consequences. Ann Clin Biochem. 2007; 44(Pt 4):343–52.
19. Washabau RJ, Day MJ, Willard MD, et al. WSAVA international gastrointestinal standardization group. Endoscopic, biopsy, and histopathologic guidelines for the evaluation of gastrointestinal inflammation in companion animals. J Vet Intern Med. 2010;24(1):10–26.
20. Allenspach K, Wieland B, Gröne A, Gaschen F. Chronic enteropathies in dogs: evaluation of risk factors for negative outcome. J Vet Intern Med. 2007;21(4):700–8.
21. Eastvold ML, Wallinder HW, Preissner CM, et al. A two-center international evaluation of the Immulite 2000 automated serum gastrin assay. Clin Biochem. 2006;39(4):387–90.
22. Jones BR, Nicholls MR, Badman R. Peptic ulceration in a dog associated with an islet cell carcinoma of the pancreas and an elevated plasma gastrin level. J Small Anim Pract. 1976;17(9):593–8.
23. Straus E, Johnson GF, Yalow RS. Canine Zollinger-Ellison syndrome. Gastroenterology. 1877;72(2):380–1.
24. Happé RP, van der Gaag I, Lamers CB, et al. Zollinger-Ellison syndrome in three dogs. Vet Pathol. 1980;17(2):177–86.
25. Drazner FH. Canine gastrinoma: a condition analogous to Zollinger-Ellison syndrome in man. Calif Vet. 1981;35:6–11.
26. Breitschwerdt EB, Turk JR, Turnwald GH. Hypergastrinemia in canine gastrointestinal disease. J Am Vet Med Assoc. 1986;22(5):585–92.
27. Altschul M, Simpson KW, Dykes NL, et al. Evaluation of somatostatin analogues for the detection and treatment of gastrinoma in a dog. J Small Anim Pract. 1997;38(7):286–1.
28. Brooks D, Watson GL. Omeprazole in a dog with gastrinoma. J Vet Intern Med. 1997;11(6):379–81.
29. Green RA, Gartrell CL. Gastrinoma: a retrospective study of four cases (1985–1995). J Am Vet Med Assoc. 1997;33(6):524–7.
30. Fukushima R, Ichikawa K, Hirabayashi M, et al. A case of canine gastrinoma. J Vet Med Sci. 2004;66(8):993–5.
31. Fukushima U, Sato M, Okano S, et al. A case of gastrinoma in a Shih-Tzu dog. J Vet Med Sci. 2004;66(3):311–3.
32. Jensen RT, Norton JA. Endocrine tumors of the pancreas and gastrointestinal tract. In: Feldman M, Friedman LS, Brandt LJ, editors. Sleisenger and Fordtran's gastrointestinal and liver disease – pathophysiology, diagnosis, management. Philadelphia: Saunders; 2010. p. 491–523.
33. Dacha S, Razvi M, Massaad J, et al. Hypergastrinemia. Gastroenterology Report. 2015;3(3):201–8.
34. Triantafillidis JK, Tzourmakliotis D, Peros G, et al. Serum gastrin levels in

patients with inflammatory bowel disease. Hepatogastroenterology. 2003;50(Suppl2):cccxv–cccxvii.
35. Besterman HS, Mallinson CN, Modigliani R, et al. Gut hormones in inflammatory bowel disease. Scand J Gastroenterol. 1983;18(7):845–52.
36. Suzuki T, Grand E, Bowman C, et al. TNF-alpha and interleukin 1 activate gastrin expression via MAPK- and PKC-dependent mechanism. Am J Physiol Gastrointest Liver Physiol. 2001;281(6):G145–1412.
37. Hopman WP, de Jong DJ, Naber AH, Jansen JB. Tumor necrosis factor alpha antibody affects gastrin release in Crohn disease. Scand J Gastroenterol. 2003;38(5):522–5.
38. ter Beek WP, Muller ESM, van Hogezand RA, et al. Gastrin releasing peptide receptor expression is decreased in patients with Crohn's disease but not in ulcerative colitis. J Clin Pathol. 2004;57(10):1047–51.
39. Vergine M, Pozzo S, Pogliani E, et al. Common bile duct obstruction due to a duodenal gastrinoma in a dog. Vet J. 2005;170(1):141–3.
40. Lunn KF, Page RL. Tumors of the endocrine system. In: Withrow SJ, Vail DM, Page RL, editors. Withrow and MacEwen's small animal clinical oncology. St. Louis: Elsevier; 2012. p. 504–31.
41. Dhillo WS, Jayasena CN, Lewis CJ, et al. Plasma gastrin measurement cannot be used to diagnose a gastrinoma in patients on either proton pump inhibitors or histamine type-2 receptor antagonists. Ann Clin Biochem. 2006;43(Pt 2):153–5.
42. Corleto VD, Annibale B, Gibril F, et al. Does the widespread use of proton pump inhibitors mask, complicate and/or delay the diagnosis of Zollinger-Ellison syndrome? Aliment Pharmacol Ther. 2001;15(10):1555–61.
43. Jensen RT, Niederle B, Mitry E, et al. Frascati consensus conference; European neuroendocrine tumor society. Gastrinoma (duodenal and pancreatic). Neuroendocrinology. 2006;84(3):173–82.
44. Seim-Wikse T, Kolbjørnson Ø, Jörundsson E, et al. Tumour gastrin expression and serum gastrin concentrations in dogs with gastric carcinoma are poor diagnostic indicators. J Comp Pathol. 2014;151(2–3):207–11.
45. Simpson KW, McDonough PL, Strauss-Ayali D, et al. *Helicobacter felis* infection in dogs: effect on gastric structure and functions. Vet Pathol. 1999;36(3):237–48.
46. Simpson KW, Strauss-Ayali D, Scanziani E, et al. *Helicobacter felis* infection is associated with lymphoid follicular hyperplasia and mild gastritis but normal gastric secretory function in cats. Infect Immun. 2000;68(2):779–90.
47. De Brito Galvao JF, Pressler BM, Freeman LJ, et al. Mucinous gastric carcinoma with abdominal carcinomatosis and hypergastrinemia in a dog. J Am Anim Hosp Assoc. 2009;45(4):197–202.
48. Neiger R, Simpson KW. Helicobacter infection in dogs and cats: facts and fiction. J Vet Intern Med. 2000;14(2):125–33.
49. Yamasaki K, Suematsu H, Takahashi T. Comparison of gastric lesions in dogs and cats with and without gastric spiral organisms. J Am Vet Med Assoc. 1998;212(4):529–33.
50. Gatta L, Di Mario F, Vaira D, et al. Quantification of serum levels of pepsinogens and gastrin to assess eradication of helicobacter pylori. Clin Gastroenterol Hepatol. 2011;9(5):440–2.
51. Francavilla R, Polimeno L, Demichina A, et al. Lactobacillus reuteri strain combination in helicobacter pylori infection: a randomized, double-blind, placebo-controlled study. J Clin Gastroenterol. 2014;48(5):407–13.
52. Myllyluoma E, Kajander K, Mikkola H, et al. Probiotic intervention decreases serum gastrin-17 in helicobacter pylori infection. Dig Liver Dis. 2007;39(6):516–23.
53. Gabbert NH, Nachreiner RF, Holmes-Wood P, Kivela JH. Serum immunoreactive gastrin concentrations in the dog: basal and postprandial values measured by radioimmunoassay. Am J Vet Res. 1984;45(11):2351–3.
54. Hatlebakk JG, Katz PO, Camacho-Lobato L, Castell DO. Protein pump inhibitors: better acid suppression when taken before a meal than without a meal. Aliment Pharmacol Therapeut. 2000;14(10):1267–72.
55. Shin JM, Sachs G. Restoration of acid secretion following treatment with proton pump inhibitors. Gastroenterology. 2002;123(5):281–90.
56. Sharp CR, Kerl ME, Mann FA. A comparison of total calcium, corrected calcium, and ionized calcium concentrations as indicators of calcium homeostasis among hypoalbuminemic dogs requiring intensive care. J Vet Emerg Crit Care. 2009;19(6):571–8.

Antimicrobial drug use in food-producing animals and associated human health risks: what, and how strong, is the evidence?

Karin Hoelzer*, Nora Wong, Joe Thomas, Kathy Talkington, Elizabeth Jungman and Allan Coukell

Abstract

Background: Antimicrobial resistance is a public health threat. Because antimicrobial consumption in food-producing animals contributes to the problem, policies restricting the inappropriate or unnecessary agricultural use of antimicrobial drugs are important. However, this link between agricultural antibiotic use and antibiotic resistance has remained contested by some, with potentially disruptive effects on efforts to move towards the judicious or prudent use of these drugs.

Main text: The goal of this review is to systematically evaluate the types of evidence available for each step in the causal pathway from antimicrobial use on farms to human public health risk, and to evaluate the strength of evidence within a 'Grades of Recommendations Assessment, Development and Evaluation'(GRADE) framework. The review clearly demonstrates that there is compelling scientific evidence available to support each step in the causal pathway, from antimicrobial use on farms to a public health burden caused by infections with resistant pathogens. Importantly, the pathogen, antimicrobial drug and treatment regimen, and general setting (e.g., feed type) can have significant impacts on how quickly resistance emerges or spreads, for how long resistance may persist after antimicrobial exposures cease, and what public health impacts may be associated with antimicrobial use on farms. Therefore an exact quantification of the public health burden attributable to antimicrobial drug use in animal agriculture compared to other sources remains challenging.

Conclusions: Even though more research is needed to close existing data gaps, obtain a better understanding of how antimicrobial drugs are actually used on farms or feedlots, and quantify the risk associated with antimicrobial use in animal agriculture, these findings reinforce the need to act now and restrict antibiotic use in animal agriculture to those instances necessary to ensure the health and well-being of the animals.

Keywords: Antimicrobial drug use, Farm animals, Antimicrobial resistance, Public health risk

Background

Antimicrobial use and resistance in animal agriculture

Antimicrobial resistance is a global public health threat, reflected in at least 2 million resistant infections and at least 23,000 deaths in the United States each year [1]. Antimicrobial drug use is considered to be the single most important factor leading to resistance [1]. However, effective policy interventions are hindered by the fact that the emergence and spread of antimicrobial resistance is complex and the underlying dynamics incompletely understood [2, 3]. Antimicrobial drugs are used in a variety of settings including hospitals, outpatient clinics, and long-term care facilities as well as animal-associated settings such as veterinary clinics, farms, and feedlots. There is general scientific consensus that antimicrobial drug use in a variety of settings contributes to the burden of antimicrobial resistance [2, 3]. However, the relative contribution of different antimicrobial uses to the overall burden has so far remained unclear. Moreover, despite decades of research and a considerable body of scientific evidence, the link between antimicrobial drug use on farms and antimicrobial resistant infections in humans remains contested by critics, primarily in the U.S. [3]. This dispute is

* Correspondence: khoelzer@pewtrusts.org
The Pew Charitable Trusts, 901 E Street NW, Washington, DC 20004, USA

disruptive to the debate around judicious use of antimicrobial drugs in animal agriculture, and has the potential to slow the implementation of policies aimed at assuring the responsible and prudent use of antibiotics in animal agriculture. Notably, various organizations including the World Health Organization for Animals (OIE), U.S. Food and Drug Administration, and the British and American Veterinary Medical Associations, have defined the concept of responsible, prudent or judicious antimicrobial use in animal agriculture. Optimizing therapeutic efficacy and minimizing antimicrobial resistance are key objectives underpinning all of these definitions, despite some definitional differences. For the purposes of this study, judicious antimicrobial use shall be equivalent to OIE's 'responsible and prudent use' definition of 'improv[ing]animal health and animal welfare while preventing or reducing the selection, emergence and spread of antimicrobial-resistant bacteria in animals and humans.'

Policy solutions to ensure judicious antimicrobial use in animal agriculture

Around the world, policy efforts to ensure judicious antimicrobial use in animal agriculture have generally, as a first step, focused on restricting the use of those antimicrobial drugs important for human medicine for 'growth promotion' purposes. For the purposes of this article, the Codex Alimentarius definition of growth promotion shall be used, where 'growth promotion refers to the use of antimicrobial substances to increase the rate of weight gain and/or the efficiency of feed utilization in animals by other than purely nutritional means' and antimicrobials are thus administered to healthy animals with the primary goal of increasing growth rates and enhancing feed conversion efficiency [4].

As early as 1969, a report by the U.K. Joint Committee on the Use of Antibiotics in Animal Husbandry, known as the 'Swann Report', motivated by concerns about the emergence of antimicrobial resistance, called for the ban of medically important (i.e., shared between humans and animals) antimicrobials for growth promotion purposes [3]. However, it took nearly another two decades before governments took concrete action and individual countries differ drastically in their responsiveness on the issue [3]. Sweden outlawed the use of all antimicrobial drugs for growth promotion in 1986 and Denmark banned the use of the two medically important antimicrobials, avoparcin and virginiamycin, as growth promoters in 1995 [5]. Avoparcin was banned for growth promoting purposes across the European Union in 1997 and growth promotion uses of the remaining four medically important antibiotics (as defined by the World Health Organization [6]) bacitracin, spiramycin, tylosin and virginiamycin were banned in 1999 [5]. Following the precautionary principle, the use of any antimicrobial drug for growth promotion, including antimicrobial drug classes not used in human medicine, has been banned in Europe since 2006 [7]. In the U.S., the use of medically important antimicrobial drugs (as defined by the U.S. Food and Drug Administration [8]) for growth promotion was phased out on January 1, 2017. In fact, according to data collected by the OIE for 2015, more than 70% of member countries that responded to the survey did not authorize antimicrobial drugs for growth promotion purposes [9]. However, outlawing the use of medically important antimicrobial drugs for growth promotion is only the first step towards assuring their judicious use in animal agriculture. Several European countries have taken concrete next steps towards curtailing the emergence and spread of antimicrobial resistance by assuring antimicrobial drugs are used judiciously and only when necessary to ensure the health and well-being of the animal, and the U.S. Food and Drug Administration has recently announced plans to examine potential actions to that effect [10].

The dynamics of antimicrobial resistance and their relevance for this study

For the purpose of this study, antimicrobial resistance is defined as 'microbiological resistance' and refers to the increased resistance of a bacterium in vitro compared to a population of wild-type bacteria which can be expressed, for instance, as an increase in minimal inhibitory concentration (MIC). Infections with bacteria that meet this definition of resistance may in fact on occasion still respond to treatments with the antimicrobial drug. In this respect, microbiological resistance is different from the concept of 'clinical resistance', which is focused on treatment failures and considers clinical factors such as the therapeutic concentration that can be reached at the site of infection. To evaluate clinical resistance, MIC values can be compared to clinical breakpoints, which should be specific to the animal species and site of infection [11]. However, for many situations encountered in veterinary medicine specific breakpoints have not been established and extrapolations from existing breakpoints can be challenging.

This study focuses on the emergence and spread of acquired antimicrobial resistance. This resistance can emerge through point mutations, usually associated with a progression from low-level to high-level resistance as sequential mutations occur [12], or through horizontal gene transfer (HGT), which usually shows immediate high-level resistance as resistance genes are shared among bacteria [12]. HGT can occur through several mechanisms [12]; for instance, plasmids that carry resistance genes can be shared among bacterial strains, bacteriophages can transfer resistance genes from one bacterium to another, and bacteria can take up naked DNA (e.g., genes originating from dead bacteria). Notably, the relative importance of each resistance pathway appears to at least partially depend on the bacterial species [12]. Acquired resistance has to be distinguished from inherent resistance. Some bacteria are inherently resistant to a drug because the bacterium is outside of the drug's spectrum of action, for example because the bacterium lacks the drug target. In addition, some bacteria can be transiently resistant to a drug without a corresponding genetic change, probably because of a transient dormant state in which the bacterium's metabolism is lowered to a point where it virtually ceases to function. These resistance types are generally believed not to be affected by antimicrobial use and will not be considered here.

The analysis of the link between antibiotic use on farms and human health risk is complicated by the fact that the evolutionary dynamics of antimicrobial resistance do not followed a simple 'necessary and sufficient' [13] model of epidemiological causation, where the presence of antimicrobial drug use would be both necessary and sufficient for the emergence of resistance. In many cases, the same acquired antimicrobial resistance type or trait can be encoded by more than one genetic mechanism. Resistance traits often, although not always, carry a fitness cost, at least in in vitro experimental systems, and fitness costs may differ for the same resistance trait based on the determining genetic changes [12]. If there is a fitness cost associated with a resistance trait, resistant strains are selected *against* in antimicrobial-free environments and selected *for* in the presence of antimicrobials. The fitness cost may be higher for chromosomally-mediated than plasmid-mediated mutations, may differ by resistance mechanism (e.g., whether resistance is conferred by modification of a metabolic pathway, alteration of a target site, or upregulation of membrane channels), and may increase with the number of point mutations required to express the trait [12]. In some cases, however, the fitness cost is very low. Moreover, compensatory mutations that correct the fitness loss brought about by the resistance-conferring mutations are possible. It is unknown how closely fitness costs under in vitro conditions track those experienced in vivo – for instance, multi-drug resistance may be associated with a lower fitness cost in vivo than predicted based on in vitro data [14].

Antimicrobial resistance is not a new phenomenon. There is strong scientific evidence for the pre-existence of some antimicrobial resistance genes (e.g., beta-lactamase genes) in the absence of any antimicrobial use [14]. In fact, many antimicrobial drugs are naturally produced by fungi or bacteria to stave off competition from other bacteria; some resistance genes are necessary to allow these antimicrobial-producing microbes to survive, and others have emerged as an adaptation to the natural presence of these antimicrobial compounds in the environment, primarily in soil [15]. The term 'resistome' has been proposed to describe the ecology of resistance genes, broadly encompassing all resistance genes circulating in pathogenic and non-pathogenic bacteria, be they from soil, animals, humans, or other sources [15]. A comprehensive knowledge of the resistome and adequate phylogenetic analysis is necessary to determine whether a newly-detected resistance gene truly emerged recently, has been present for a while but recently became more prevalent, or simply has not been detected previously.

The evolutionary dynamics of antimicrobial resistance are further complicated by the potential for cross-resistance (the simultaneous resistance to multiple related drugs that share a drug target) and co-resistance (where several genes are transferred together, for instance on one plasmid, and selection for one of the genes indirectly selects for the others as well). Moreover, antimicrobial resistance to a given drug can be mediated by multiple genetic changes, with potentially different evolutionary dynamics, and bacterial mutation rates vary, potentially pre-disposing some bacteria (i.e., 'hypermutators') to the more rapid emergence of resistance-conferring mutations than others.

For all of these reasons, the exact dynamics between antimicrobial use and resistance development may differ by bacterial species, drug or drug target, and resistance-conferring mutation, and may be influenced by external factors such as the selection pressures exerted by the use of related drugs. Even if antimicrobial use decreases or ceases, this may not necessarily translate into a direct, measurable drop in antimicrobial resistance, and the impact of introducing, restraining or eliminating antimicrobial use may vary by bacterial strain, bacterial target and environment (e.g., as a result of different resistance mechanisms with different evolutionary and ecological properties). Perhaps most importantly, resistance may not in all cases be reversible by discontinuing antimicrobial use alone. As is also clear from this discussion, there are many aspects about the emergence, ecology and evolution of antimicrobial resistance genes that are not yet fully understood. For these reasons it is difficult to extrapolate from individual research studies to other settings, and to adequately evaluate all direct and indirect impacts of antimicrobial use on the emergence of resistance.

Because antimicrobial drug use and the emergence of resistance may not follow a direct cause and effect relationship, it can be very difficult to establish causality outside of tightly controlled experimental settings. However, many chronic diseases also do not follow a direct cause and effect relationship and research methods developed to address these challenges may be applicable to antimicrobial resistance. One widely used epidemiological model of causation that fits these chronic diseases and antimicrobial resistance is that of 'sufficient-component causes,' first articulated by Rothman [16]. According to this model, a sufficient cause can be made up of multiple components, each of which needs to occur in order for the sufficient condition to occur. For example, in order for a certain bacterium in a certain environment and with a given genetic make-up to acquire antimicrobial resistance both exposure to an antimicrobial drug and external factors such as contact with bacteria carrying a plasmid with resistance against the antimicrobial drug have to occur. In addition, there can be more than one sufficient condition for a cause. For example, another bacterium with a different genetic predisposition or exposed to other environmental conditions may not require exposure to the antimicrobial drug to develop resistance, for instance because of co-selection for heavy-metal resistance. While antimicrobial exposure may be a necessary condition for resistance in one situation, it may not be necessary in all situations, depending on the genetic predisposition and external factors. This model of causation, which is widely accepted by epidemiologists, will be used here. It provides a useful framework for the assessment of causality, including in instances with seemingly contradictory study findings. Moreover, it demonstrates the challenge associated with quantifying the proportion of antimicrobial resistant bacteria associated with different causes: if each cause in fact consists of multiple component causes each occurrence of antimicrobial resistant bacteria could be attributed to each of the component causes.

Study aims and objectives

The goal of this review is to provide an objective methodical summary of the available scientific evidence for or against a relationship between antimicrobial drug use on farms and antimicrobial resistant human infections. Because this nexus remains contested by some groups, particularly in the U.S., relevant antibiotic use policies and restrictions in the U.S. are highlighted where relevant. To achieve this, we review the scientific evidence supporting or refuting each step in the causal pathways from on-farm antimicrobial use to human public health risk, placing particular emphasis on the strengths and limitations of the available scientific evidence. Breaking down the exceedingly complex pathway from farm to public health risk into discrete intermediary steps considerably reduces complexity and allows for a hypothesis-driven approach. The goal of this study is to characterize the link between antimicrobial use on farms and human infections with resistant bacteria, rather than quantifying the relative importance of this link compared to antimicrobial drug use in other settings even though that quantification will ultimately be important to guide public health policy and data gaps that complicate or prevent quantification are highlighted. Similarly, quantifying the relative importance of different transmission routes from farm to humans is important but beyond the scope of this study.

Pathways from antimicrobial drug use on farms to resistant infections in humans

There are different pathways that can lead from antimicrobial use on farms to a public health risk, including foodborne and non-foodborne routes. (Drug residues are a separate public health concern not considered in this study.) Regardless of pathway, four distinct factors have to be understood to characterize the public health risk associated with antimicrobial drug use in animal agriculture.

Antimicrobial drug use on farms and feedlots

How antimicrobial drugs are used on farms and feedlots is central to understanding the emergence of antimicrobial resistance. Unfortunately, the amount of information available on actual antimicrobial drug use on farms and feedlots differs considerably across countries and is in many cases insufficient for understanding antimicrobial exposures.

Risk of resistance emergence as a result of antimicrobial exposure on farms and feedlots

This question concerns foodborne and zoonotic pathogens as well animal pathogens and commensal bacteria (i.e., the very large number of naturally occurring microorganisms that usually inhabit the body surfaces of humans and animals [17]). Resistance in commensal or animal pathogens poses a human health risk only if the resistance genes can be transferred to human pathogens; this is regardless of whether the transfer occurs in the gut of farm animals, in the environment – be that on farms or off - or within the human gut. Horizontal gene transfer between human commensals and human pathogens has been widely demonstrated [18]. Therefore, evidence of resistance gene transfer from animal-associated bacteria to human commensals can be regarded as indirect evidence for a potential transmission to human pathogens and therefore a public health risk.

Risk of infection due to resistant bacteria that emerged on the farm

Bacteria, including foodborne or zoonotic pathogens, can be transferred from food producing animals to humans through direct contact, or indirectly through food or the environment. In addition to contact with the environment in which the animals are raised, indirect transmission may also include exposure to agricultural operations through manure run-offs, airborne particles, or other environmental exposures, even though these transmission routes are considerably less well understood and documented than the other possible transmission routes [19–21]. Some evidence further suggests that humans can transmit bacteria that originated on farms to other humans through direct contact, food contamination during processing, or contamination of shared environments, but, again, the evidence is limited and often circumstantial, the underlying dynamics are not well understood, and at least some animal-associated bacteria may be poorly equipped to be transmitted from human to human [22–24].

In some cases (e.g., foodborne outbreaks) the directionality of infection is quite obvious, but this is not always true. The question of directionality has to be considered in evaluations of the available scientific evidence. However, even if directionality may not always be clear, such studies imply a shared host range, which makes cross-species transmissions likely.

Excess morbidity and mortality caused by antimicrobial resistance traits that emerged on farms

Several specific mechanisms by which antimicrobial resistance can have adverse human health impacts have been identified in the literature, of which at least three are directly relevant to resistance that emerged in animal agriculture [25]:

1. Linkage of virulence and resistance traits, leading to drug-resistant strains with increased virulence
2. Treatment delay because initial treatments are ineffective
3. Necessity to choose less desirable treatment options because of resistance to more desirable antimicrobial drugs

Observational studies on the topic can be complicated by the presence of potential confounders such as differences in age or underlying disease among patient groups [26, 27]; the choice of reference group can also have significant impacts on study findings [28]; in addition, bacterial strains can differ in the severity of associated health outcomes independent of antimicrobial resistance [29], thus potentially introducing another source of confounding.

Given the vast amount of literature published on the subject, this review does not strive to be comprehensive in reviewing the available literature associated with the topic. Rather, for each step in the pathway a selected number of studies that exemplify each relevant study type are discussed together with a general discussion of the strength and limitations of the available evidence. Unanswered questions and areas requiring further study are clearly highlighted. Therefore, this study documents the current scientific understanding about the link between antimicrobial drug use on farms and human health risks associated with antimicrobial resistant infections, highlighting what is known and what remains to be determined.

Main text

A modified GRADE approach for evaluating the strength of scientific evidence

The approach for evaluating the scientific evidence for a link between antimicrobial use in food producing animals, antimicrobial resistance, and a resulting human health risk is based on the principles guiding the GRADE (Grades of Recommendation, Assessment, Development and Evaluation) approach to systematic reviews. The fundamental notion underpinning this approach is that scientific studies vary in the strength of evidence they provide, or, as stated by the Cochrane Collaboration, the 'extent to which one can be confident that an estimate of effect or association is close to the quantity of specific interest'. The GRADE approach considers the study type as well as factors relevant to study quality that are specific to an individual study (e.g., width of confidence intervals, inconsistency of results) to arrive at a quality rating for each study. The grade approach considers three basic types of evidence [30]:

1. **Controlled trials** are intervention studies where subjects are allocated by the investigators into treatment and control groups, ideally randomly but occasionally based on another allocation scheme. The GRADE approach classifies randomized controlled trials (RCTs) as 'high quality of evidence' because further research is unlikely to change the confidence in the effect estimate. However, as detailed below, the presence of specific study limitations can cause the quality of evidence to be downgraded.
2. **Observational studies** include epidemiological study designs such as cohort, case-control and cross-sectional studies; contrary to RCTs the investigators do not allocate subjects to specific exposures, but compare outcomes among exposed and comparable unexposed population subgroups. The GRADE approach classifies observational studies as 'low quality of evidence'. Because allocation of individuals to different exposures cannot be controlled, biases are more difficult to control than in RCTs and therefore further research is likely to have an important impact on the confidence in the effect estimate and is likely to change the estimate. The presence of

specific study characteristics can cause the quality of evidence to be up- or downgraded.

3. **Any other evidence** is classified in the GRADE approach as 'very low quality of evidence' because any effect estimate is uncertain; however, specific study characteristics can cause the quality of evidence to be upgraded, and a variety of study types in this category can provide useful information, including for example molecular subtyping studies, phylogenetic analyses, and case studies or outbreak investigations that lack a proper control group.

In the GRADE approach, the evidence ratings can be up- or downgraded based on a variety of study characteristics that impact study quality, including [31]:

1. **Study limitations** and risk of **bias**
2. **Directness of evidence** (i.e., the extent to which the subjects, interventions and outcome measures are similar to those of interest)
3. **Consistency of results** (i.e., similarity of effect estimates across studies)
4. **Precision of estimates** (e.g., width of confidence intervals around effect estimates)
5. Risk of **residual confounding** and **publication bias**

Finally, the strength of recommendations based on this evidence is affected by [31]:

1. **Quality of evidence**
2. Uncertainty about the **balance between desirable and undesirable effects**
3. Uncertainty or variability in **values and preferences**
4. Uncertainty about whether the intervention represents a **wise use of resources**

Importantly, practical as well as ethical considerations can restrict the type of evidence that can be collected to address a specific research question in a meaningful way [32]. For instance, a randomized controlled trial to evaluate human health outcomes associated with exposure to drug resistant foodborne pathogens would in most cases be unethical.

In the following sections, each step in the causal pathway from antimicrobial use in food producing animals to public health risks caused by infections with antimicrobial drug resistant pathogens is described and the strength of the available evidence is evaluated. A similar approach has been used by the Australian government to review the scientific literature on antimicrobial resistance in animal bacteria and human disease in a study completed in 1999 [33].

Notably, because a number of somewhat different definitions have been used in different scientific disciplines it is important to clearly define the terms 'antimicrobial drug' and 'antibiotic'. For the purpose of his study, and following similar definitions in other authoritative publications [34], we use the term 'antimicrobial drug' to refer to 'antibacterial agents classically used for therapy, prophylaxis, or growth promotion' as adapted from EFSA [34]. The effects of disinfectants, biocides, antiviral, antifungal or antiparasitic drugs will not be considered while synthetic antibacterial agents will be considered. For the purposes of this study and following the definitions herein, the terms 'antimicrobial drug' and 'antibiotic' will be used synonymously.

Evaluating the link between antimicrobial use on farms to the emergence of antimicrobial resistant human infections

Antimicrobial drugs use on farms and feedlots

Intervention studies are not applicable for measuring antimicrobial use but a number of observational studies have been conducted. Many follow a cross-sectional design where antibiotic consumption is recorded at one point in time, even though longitudinal designs have also been used and may be preferable to address certain research questions (see for instance [35]). As the examples in Table 1 demonstrate, a number of different data sources are available that contain information regarding on-farm antimicrobial drug use. Data should ideally be based directly on a review of treatment and/or prescription records (e.g., [35–39]). However, this data source may not be readily available or the data collection may be cost-prohibitive. In these cases, more indirect sources may be used, for instance questionnaires administered to veterinarians [40], producers [41–43] or both [44]. In addition, other data sources such as antimicrobial sales data reported by drug manufacturers (e.g., data reported in the U.S. under section 105 of the Animal Drug User Fee Act) may be used albeit the information collected in these cases is less direct and detailed, and consequently less informative. In some cases, it may be possible to collect data from each relevant operation – for instance every producer in the target area (see for instance [36]). Often, however, this is impossible and a subset of operations must be sampled. Ideally, the sampling design should lead to nationally representative estimates (for example [35, 40]). Realistically, it may be possible only to collect data that is representative of a subset of operations, for instance operations representing a segment of the animal agriculture industry such as dairy herds [41] or broiler chicken and turkey flocks [35]. Similarly, studies may focus on operations located in a specific geographic region such as the densest pig production area in Belgium [37], Vietnam's Tien Giang province [42] or Germany's state of Northrhine-Westfalia [39]. Regardless of study scope, a robust sampling frame and an

Table 1 Examples of select studies available for evaluating antimicrobial consumption in animal agriculture

Reference	Study			Data source	Population; no. of farms or producers or veterinarians	Nationally representative	Directness of evidence	Information regarding			Study timing / period
	Country	Setting	Goals or focus					dosage	duration	reason for use	
				GRADE level: observational study							
[35]	France	government	antibiotic consumption metrics	treatment records (reviewed medication purchases, daily records, forms submitted at slaughter; conducted farmer interviews)	Turkey and chicken broiler flocks ($n = 106$; 57 turkey & 49 chicken flocks)	Restricted to western France	actual treatment records	yes	yes	limited	one time
[36]	Denmark	government	antibiotic consumption	treatment records (data collected from pharmacies, veterinarians and feed mills)	all farm animal operations (all prescriptions)	Yes	actual treatment records	yes	yes	yes	annual
[37]	Belgium	academic	antibiotic consumption	treatment records	Pig herds in Belgium's densest pig production area	Restricted to key pig production area	actual treatment records	yes	yes	limited	one time
[38]	Canada	academic	antibiotic use practices	treatment records & producer questionnaires	Beef herds in western Canada ($n = 203$)	Restricted to western Canada	actual treatment records	yes	yes	yes	one time
[39]	Germany	academic	antibiotic use practices	treatment & prescription records	Cattle farms in Northrhine-Westfalia ($n = 47$)	Restricted to one geographic area	actual treatment records	yes	yes	yes	one time
[40]	Finland	academic	antibiotic use practices	veterinarian questionnaires	Veterinarians in Finland	Yes	response to survey	yes	yes	yes	one time
[41]	U.S.	academic	antibiotic use and farm management practices on conventional & organic operations	producer questionnaire	Dairy farms in 4 U.S. states ($n = 99$ conventional and $n = 32$ organic)	No	response to survey	no	no	yes	one time
[44]	Vietnam	academic	antibiotic use practices and farm management	producer, veterinarian or technical staff questionnaires	Pig and poultry operations in 3 locations in Vietnam ($n = 270$)	Restricted to red river delta	response to survey	no	no	limited	one time
[42]	Vietnam	academic	quantify antibiotic use; identify risk factors for use	producer questionnaire	Chicken farms in Vietnam's Tien Giang province ($n = 208$)	Restricted to one province	response to survey	yes	yes	limited	one time
[43]	U.S.	government	farm management	producer questionnaire	U.S. operations[a]	Yes	responses to survey; trained interviewer	no	limited	limited	periodic *every 5–7 years*
[45]	U.S.	government	farm financials	producer questionnaire	U.S. operations	Yes	responses to survey; trained interviewer	no	no	no	annual
				GRADE level: other							
[129]	U.S.	government	antibiotic sales & distribution	annual reporting of antibiotic sales by drug sponsors	All U.S. drug sponsors	Yes	Sales data	no	no	limited	annual

[a]Survey specific to species and production class (e.g., cow-calf, feedlot); conducted on rotational basis; approximately every 5–7 years

appropriate sample size are needed to ensure the study will be representative of the target population, and extrapolations beyond that population may be challenging.

Studies of antimicrobial consumption can be conducted for surveillance or research purposes. Surveillance studies are typically conducted by governmental organizations (e.g., [36, 43]) and research studies more commonly done by academic investigators (e.g., [37–42, 44]). In some cases, a study goal may for instance be to evaluate different antibiotic use metrics (e.g., [35]), but more common research questions involve evaluating antibiotic use practices ([38, 39]) or comparing antibiotic use and farm management practices across different types of operations, such as conventional and organic operations [41]. The study goals have important implications for which study aspects to prioritize if resource limitations force trade-offs among them. For instance, for surveillance purposes it may be more important to collect nationally representative data and to repeat the data collection periodically to evaluate temporal trends ([36, 43, 45]) than to collect highly granular and detailed data on related issues such as correlation of antibiotic use with farm management practices. In contrast, some research questions may require the collection of comprehensive and highly detailed data on study operations but funding may not be available to repeat the study periodically (e.g., [38, 40, 41]). Regardless of purpose, though, information on antimicrobial dosage, duration and reason for use are key determinants of antimicrobial use patterns and necessary to evalaute antibiotic exposures. This information should be collected in surveillance as well as research studies where possible. Unfortunately, this information is not consistently collected in all studies (see Table 1) and for instance in the U.S. this data is currently very scarce.

Antimicrobial sales data are the only nationally representative, annually available data source in the U.S. However, these data do not directly capture antimicrobial use on farms, and are currently not specific to individual species, even though drug companies are required to estimate sales for the major food-producing species (i.e., cattle, swine, chicken and turkey) separately starting with the reporting of the 2016 data. Other nationally representative data sources in the U.S. are surveys conducted as part of the National Animal Health Monitoring System, which are focused on farm management practices, not quantitative with respect to dosage and duration, and currently only conducted every 5 to 7 years; and surveys conducted as part of the Agricultural Resource Management Survey, which are focused on farm finances. Despite these data limitations it is clear that antimicrobial drugs are used on U.S. farms and feedlots. According to the most recent available sales data, almost 10 million kilograms of medically important antibiotics approved for food-producing species were sold in the U.S. in 2015, including 6.9 million kilograms of tetracyclines, 900 thousand kilograms of penicillin and 600 thousand kilograms of macrolides. Also sold were drugs in a number of other classes including aminoglycosides, amphenicoles, cephalosporins, fluoroquinolones, lincosamides, and sulfonamides. While it is thus not currently possible to sufficiently characterize antibiotic exposures on U.S. farms and feedlots they undoubtedly occur.

Risk of resistance emergence as a result of antimicrobial exposure on farms and feedlots

Data based on studies in foodborne and zoonotic pathogens

Data on the emergence of resistance in foodborne or zoonotic pathogens is directly relevant for human health but studies have more commonly focused on commensal bacteria or animal pathogens. Yet, as shown in Table 2, a variety of study types are available that evaluate the link between antimicrobial use on farms and the emergence of resistance in foodborne or zoonotic pathogens. These include controlled trials, various observational study types, and other studies such as microbiological studies comparing resistance levels across production types.

Among the controlled trials allocation to treatment or control groups should ideally be random and often is ([46–48]), but this is unfortunately not in all studies sufficiently described [49, 50]. Treatment and control animals are often experimentally challenged with foodborne pathogens such as *Campylobacter* [46, 49] or *Salmonella* [47, 48, 51]. In these cases bacterial strains used for the inoculum are well-characterized and the emergence of resistance can easily be detected. However experimental challenges may differ from naturally occuring infections in important ways including for instance the types and diversity of bacterial strains used for infection, the metabolic profiles of the bacteria at the time of infection, and the bacterial quantities used for challenge. Naturally occuring bacterial populations of *Campylobacter* have also been investigated [50], and in some cases naturally occuring populations of *E. coli* have been analyzed together with experimentally inoculated human pathogens [48, 51]. In most cases, the outcome of interest is phenotypic resistance measured by dilution or, more rarely, disc diffusion test but phenotypic methods have also been combined with genotyping, which provides more detailed information about the emerging resistance traits [51].

A number of controlled studies have demonstrated the emergence of resistance in *Campylobacter* isolates after exposure to antimicrobial drugs . For instance, one study experimentally infected groups of 15 broiler chicken each on day 19 of life with a quinolone-sensitive *Campylobacter* strain, and exposed the birds to enrofloxacin flumequine at low (15 ppm) or high (50 ppm) dosages in

Table 2 Examples of studies evaluating the emergence of resistance in foodborne pathogens after food producing animals were exposed to antimicrobial drugs

Reference	Study									Key findings
	Type[a]	species	bacterial target	antimicrobial drug	administration route	study outcomes related to antimicrobial resistance	study design	susceptibility testing	controls	
					Grade level: Controlled trial					
[46]	RCT	broiler chicken	*Campylobacter* experimental infection with 5 susceptible strains on day 16 or 24 of life	fluoroquinolones enrofloxacin, sarafloxacin, ciprofloxacin; treated for 5 days, starting on day 30 of life	drinking water	emergence of resistance	2 groups; 25 or 50 chicks per group (half treated)	Phenotypic *agar dilution*	negative controls	resistance emerged rapidly in isolates from treated birds and, for birds treated with enrofloxacin, resistance was retained throughout the sampling period; resistance remained low in untreated controls throughout the study
[47]	RCT	pigs	*Salmonella* Typhimurium DT104; native *E. coli* population monitored; experimental infection with 5 strains isolated from apparently healthy pigs (pentaresistant phenotype)	aureomycin, standard or subtherapeutic dose, treated for 7 days starting 48 h after inoculation	feed	emergence of resistance	3 groups; 6 pigs per group	Phenotypic *agar dilution*	negative controls	resistance emerged in native *E. coli* populations from treated animals and increased resistance persisted for 2 weeks after treatment; treated pigs shed higher numbers of *Salmonella* Typhimurium DT104 than untreated pigs.
[48]	RCT	pigs	*Salmonella* Typhimurium; native *E. coli* population; experimental challenge of piglets 2 days after weaning	aparamycin in different dosing schemes, in some cases followed by sulfamethazine and carbadox or gentamicin and neomycin; treatment initiated 7 days after infection, for 14 days	feed or drinking water	emergence of resistance	2 trials; 6 groups of 8 pigs each	Phenotypic *dilution test*	negative controls	resistance of *Salmonella* isolates was not impacted by treatment regimen; resistance emerged in native *E. coli* populations and was effected by treatment regimen; use of similar antibiotics in rotation resulted in greater resistance than if dissimilar antibiotics were used
[49]	CT	broiler chicken	*Campylobacter;* experimental infection with susceptible strain on day 19 of life	fluoroquinolones: enrofloxacin or flumequine in different concentrations; treated for 4 days, beginning 7 days after infection (or on day 1 of the experiment for one group)	drinking water	emergence of resistance	8 groups; 15 chicks per group	Phenotypic *disc diffusion*	negative controls	resistance emerged in *Campylobacter* isolates from enrofloxacin treated birds (isolates from all other groups remained susceptible)
[50]	CT	beef cattle	*Campylobacter;* naturally occurring bacterial populations	chlortetracycline with or without sulfamethazine; virginiamycin; monensin; or tylosin; treated for 56 days, starting 18 days after arrival at feedlot; antimicrobials removed for 91 days, reintroduced for 42 days	feed	emergence of resistance	30 groups; 10 steers per group	Phenotypic *agar dilution*	negative controls	administration of antimicrobial drugs increased the carriage rate for resistant isolates, but results differed by antimicrobial drug and *Campylobacter* species

Table 2 Examples of studies evaluating the emergence of resistance in foodborne pathogens after food producing animals were exposed to antimicrobial drugs *(Continued)*

[51]	RCT	pigs	*Salmonella* Typhimurium with nalidixic acid resistance; native *E. coli* population; experimental challenge of piglets (from treated or untreated sows)	oxytetracycline, aparamycin; sows treated prior to farrowing	feed	emergence of resistance (in piglets after treatment of sows)	3 groups of pigs	Phenotypic *dilution test* Genotypic *PCR-based*	negative controls	Exposure of sows to oxytetracycline associated with increased resistance in bacterial isolates from pigs
[52]	RCT	Pigs	*Campylobacter;* naturally occurring populations	enrofloxacin; treated with standard therapeutic dose for 5 days	per os	emergence of resistance	2 groups of pigs; 6 pigs per group	Phenotypic *agar dilution*	negative controls	exposure to enrofloxacin resulted in *Campylobacter* isolates resistant to nalidixic acid and ciprofloxacin (no quinolone resistance detected prior to antibiotic exposure); resistant isolates detected for up to 35 days
[53]	RCT	Pigs	*Salmonella* Typhimurium; experimental challenge with marked strain containing nalidixic acid resistance marker	ceftiofur, aparamycin, or carbadox, followed by oxytetracycline; Treated starting 2 days post inoculation	feed (i.m. for ceftiofur)	emergence of resistance	4 groups of pigs; 12 pigs per group	Phenotypic *Disc diffusion*	negative controls	frequency of antimicrobial resistance varied over time – resistance was lowest on day 4 post inoculation but increased steadily afterwards and was highest on the last day of sampling; continued increase of select antimicrobial resistance after exposure was discontinued
					Grade level: observational study					
[54]	Cohort period: 2000–2001	dairy cattle	*Salmonella*	various used on conventional farms	n/a	antimicrobial resistance levels	95 farms: 26 organic and 69 conventional	Phenotypic *broth dilution*	organic vs. conventional	results differed by antibiotic; for most antimicrobial drugs, resistance levels were not significantly different; resistance to streptomycin and sulfamethoxazole was greater on conventional farms.
[55]	CS	dairy cattle	*Campylobacter*	various used on conventional farms	n/a	antimicrobial resistance levels	60 farms: 30 organic and 30 neighboring conventional	Phenotypic *disk diffusion*	organic vs. conventional	no statistically significant difference in resistance rates for organic vs. neighboring conventional dairy herds
[56]	CS	broiler chicken and turkey	*Campylobacter*	various used on conventional farms (gentamicin, lincomycin, bacitracin, virginiamycin, etc.)	feed and water	antimicrobial resistance levels	30 farms: 10 organic, 20 conventional	Phenotypic *agar dilution*	organic vs. conventional	antimicrobial resistance rates were significantly higher in isolates from conventional than organic farms, and conventional isolates were significantly more likely to be multi-drug resistant; resistance levels varied across antimicrobial drugs
					Grade level: other					
[57]	Longitudinal study	broiler chicken	*Campylobacter*	fluoroquinolones; difloxacin or enroflaxcin; treatment for 5 days to treat clinically relevant infection; bacterial samples taken before, during and after treatment of flocks	drinking water	prevalence of antimicrobial resistance	5 commercial flocks	Phenotypic *agar dilution* Genotypic *PCR-based*	resistance before, during and after treatment	prevalence of resistant strains increased during treatment and remained elevated after treatment

Table 2 Examples of studies evaluating the emergence of resistance in foodborne pathogens after food producing animals were exposed to antimicrobial drugs *(Continued)*

[58]	bacterial samples at slaughter	broiler chicken	*Campylobacter*	various used on conventional farms	various	prevalence of antimicrobial resistance at slaughter	$n = 600$ ceacal samples from chicken	Phenotypic *dilution method*	resistance levels at slaughter as a function of production type and antimicrobial use history	antimicrobial resistance levels differed significantly by production type and antimicrobial administration history
[59]	bacterial samples of retail meats	Chicken meat	*Campylobacter*	fluoroquinolone	presumably water	Prevalence of resistance	5 producers, meats sampled at retail for 20 consecutive weeks in 2004 and 15 consecutive weeks in 2006	Phenotypic	NAE vs. conventional	No statistically significant difference in fluoroquinolone resistance levels after use was reportedly discontinued (no sample collection or validation at the farm or producer level)
[60]	bacterial samples	chicken and turkey meat; healthy human volunteers	*Enterococci;* VanA-type vancomycin resistant (VRE)	avoparcin use for growth promotion phased out during study period	various	levels of VRE prevalence	convenience samples	N/A	VRE carrier rates before and after the ban	VRE detection in poultry meat and intestinal bacteria of healthy volunteers decreased after the ban
[61]	bacterial samples	humans and poultry products	*Campylobacter*	fluroquinolones	n/a	prevalence of resistance	convenience sample, collected from 1982 to 1989	Phenotypic *disk diffusion*	prevalence of resistance over time	prevalence of quinolone resistance increased from 0 to 14% in poultry products and from 0 to 11% in human samples
[62]	bacterial samples at slaughter	broiler chicken	*Campylobacter*	various used on conventional farms; 1992–1996 time period falls before ban for antibiotic growth promoters, 2001–2002 period does not	various	prevalence of antimicrobial resistance at slaughter	22 flocks; 10 chickens per flock	Phenotypic *agar dilution*	resistance levels at slaughter as a function of production type (free-range or standard) and study period	antimicrobial resistance was more likely in isolates from standard than free-range chicken, differed by *Campylobacter* strain, and for many antimicrobial drugs and strains resistance increased over time
[63]	correlation study	isolates from chicken meat and humans	*Salmonella* Heidelberg, ceftiofur resistant commensal *E. coli*	2003–2008	n/a	prevalence of ceftiofur-resistance in bacterial isolates from chicken meat and human cases	Correlation across provinces and time periods	Phenotypic *broth dilution*	Resistance levels before, during, and after a voluntary discontinuation of ceftiofur use in hatcheries in Quebec	Statistically significant correlation between prevalence of ceftiofur-resistant *Salmonella* Heidelberg on retail chicken and human infections; in Quebec, levels of ceftiofur use in hatcheries during study period seemed correlated with ceftiofur resistance in chicken *Salmonella* and *E. coli* isolates.
[64]	Longitudinal study	pigs	*Enterococcus faecium*	tylosin; resistance to erythromycin, spiramycin, clindamycin, penicillin, tetracycline, chloramphenicol, streptomycin, gentamycin	feed	prevalence of antimicrobial resistance	16 farms; 13 farms were examined again 183 to 287 days later	Phenotypic *disk diffusion*	resistance before and after the ban of tylosin as a growth promoter	Resistance to macrolides, lincosamides and tetracyclines decreased after the use of tylosin for growth promotion was banned.

[a]*CT* controlled trial (allocation scheme not clearly described), *RCT* randomized controlled trial, *CS* cross-sectional study

drinking water for 4 days, beginning on day 26 of life, 7 days after infection [49]. On days 29, 33 and at slaughter on day 43, *Campylobacter* isolates from both exposed groups harbored resistance to enrofloxacin as well as nalidixic acid and flumequine, while those from unexposed control groups remained sensitive to these drugs and non-infected control groups did not yield *Campylobacter* isolates, making introduction of other *Campylobacter* strains from outside sources unlikely. In another trial, broiler chicken were experimentally infected with susceptible *Campylobacter* strains on days 16 or 24 of life and exposed to enrofloxacin or sarafloxacin in drinking water for 5 days, starting on day 30 of life [46]. Flurquinolone resistance emerged rapidly in *Campylobacter* isolates from exposed birds, and, for birds treated with enrofloxacin, resistance was retained throughout the sampling period. Another controlled trial evaluated the impact of a single enrofloxacin exposure on naturally occuring *Campylobacter* populations isolated from pigs. Before exposure, all 867 collected isolates were susceptible to nalidixic acid and ciprofloxacin. After treatment, isolates with high resistance to nalidixic acid and ciprofloxacin were detected in the exposed groups, up to 35 days after treatment [52]. Similar observations have also been made for naturally occuring *Campylobacter* populations in beef cattle. In this study, steers were exposed to a variety of antimicrobial treatments (i.e., chlortetracycline with or without sulfamethazione, virginiamycin, monensin and tylosin) in feed for 56 days, and then again for 42 days after 91 days without any antimicrobial exposures [50]. Exposure to antimicrobials resulted in an increased carriage rate for resistant *Campylobacter* isolates but the authors noted marked differences among antimicrobial drugs and *Campylobacter species*. For *Campylobacter jejuni*, administration of antimicrobials significiantly increased resistance rates to ampicillin and tetracycline but not erythromycin. In contrast, for *Campylobacter hyointestinalis*, results were not statistically signficiant for ampicillin and erythromycin resistance was statistically signficiant only in cattle fed tetracycline, highlighting the potentially important differences among antimicrobial drugs and bacterial species.

In fact, studies for *Salmonella* have yielded somewhat different results. A randomized controlled trial investigating the impact of different treatment regimen administered to pigs through feed or drinking water failed to find a statistically significant impact of antimicrobial exposure on resistance in the *Salmonella* Typhimurium isolates used in the experimental challenge, but did find an impact on resistance in the native *E. coli* population which was effected by treatment regimen [48]. In that study, piglets were experimentally challenged with *Salmonella* two days after weaning and treatement through feed or drinking water was initiated 7 days after infection, for 14 days. Notably, data for *Salmonella* Typhimurium were not actually presented in the study and isolation rates were not reported. Still, the reasons for this apparent difference in results for *Salmonella* compared to native *E. coli* are not clear. In another controlled trial, sows were treated with oxytetracycline prior to farrowing (or not), their piglets challenged with *Salmonella* Typhimurium, and then piglets were treated with oxytetracycline or apramycin (or not at all) [51]. Resistance levels in the *Salmonella* isolates were not significantly effected by the treatment regimen, but resistance to both aparamycin and oxytetracycline was reportedly highest in *E. coli* isolates from pigs that nursed sows treated with oxytetracycline prior to farrowing. In yet another randomized controlled trial, piglets were experimentally infected with *Salmonella* Typhimurium and exposed to aureomycin fourty-eight hours after challenge. Exposed pigs consistently shed statistically significantly higher numbers of *Salmonella* than unexposed controls but resistance was not reported for *Salmonella* isolates. On the contrary, in another randomized controlled trial pigs were experimentally challenged with a *Salmonella* Typhimurium strain carrying a nalidixic acid resistance marker and then exposed to ceftiofur and oxytetracycline, aparamycin and oxytetracycline, or carbadox and oxytetracycline [53]. Resistance levels varied over the study period and differed by antibiotic treatment but for all treatments were highest on the last day of the study. Notably, for aparamycin, carbadox and ceftiofur, resistance continued to increase after the antimicrobial exposure was discontinued.

Evidence from observational studies supports a risk of resistance emergence in foodborne pathogens exposed to antimicrobial drugs on farms but also reinforces the complexity of the issue. For instance, one cohort study during the years 2000 and 2001 compared phenotypic resistance to various antimicrobial drugs in *Salmonella* isolates from 69 conventional and 26 organic daries. Results differed by antibiotic. Resistance to streptomycin and sulfamethoxazole was greater on conventional farms while for most antimicrobial drugs, resistance levels were not significantly different [54]. In contrast, a cross-sectional study of *Campylobacter* resistance in insolates from 30 organic dairies and 30 neighboring conventional operations failed to find a statistically significant difference in resistance rates [55]. Yet another cross-sectional study of *Campylobacter* resistance in conventional and organic broiler chicken and turkey flocks found signficiantly higher antimicrobial resistance rates in isolates from conventional compared to organic farms [56]. In addition, isolates from conventional farms were significantly more likely to be multi-drug resistance, and resistance levels varied across drugs.

A variety of other study designs have also been used to investigate the issue and generally support a risk of resistance emergence after exposure, even though the strength of evidence is significantly lower compared to that from controlled trials or observational studies. For instance, one study investigated the prevalence of antimicrobial resistance in *Campylobacter* isolates from 5 commercial broiler flocks before, during and after they were exposed to difloxacin or enrofloxacin in the drinking water [57]. Even though this study lacks proper control groups it was conducted in commercial flocks and therefore provides a valuable complement to the controlled trials discussed above. The prevalence of resistant strains increased significantly during treatment and remained elevated after treatment. Other studies have compared rates of resistance across production systems [58, 59], over time periods that coincided with the introduction or ban of certain antimicrobials [60, 61], or both [62]. These studies generally support a risk of antimicrobial resistance emergence after on-farm exposure. A drop in *vanA* –type vancomycin resistance in *Enterococci* from poultry meat and health volunteers, for instance, coincided with a ban of avoparcin as growth promoter [62], ceftiofur resistance levels in *Salmonella* Heidelberg from retail chicken and human cases decreased while ceftiofur use in hatcheries was temporarily discontinued and increased when it was reinstated [63], and a rise in fluoroquinolone resistant *Campylobacter* coincided with the introductin of enrofloxacin [61]. Notably, another study failed to find a statistically significant drop in fluoroquinolone resistance among *Campylobacter* isolates after their use was supposedly discontinued [59].

Taken together, these studies provide evidence that antimicrobial use on farms can and does lead to an increase in resistance among foodborne pathogens isolated from the exposed animals. How quickly resistance emerges seems to depend on many factors, including the pathogen species, strain and drug treatment of interest. In some instances, discontinuation of use may lead to a rapid decrease in resistance; for example, a decrease in vancomycin-resistant *Enterococci* (VRE) coincided with a ban of avoparcin as growth promoter [60], and a decrease in vancomycin resistance was demonstrated on individual farms after the ban of antimicrobial growth promoters [64]. In other cases, however, resistance levels have remained increased for extended periods of time after antibiotic uses were discontinued. For example, in a longitudinal study of farms that discontinued fluoroquinolone use as well as control farms, resistance rates in *Campylobacter* isolates remained high for years after use was discontinued [59]. Similarly, vancomycin resistance in *Enterococci* isolates from pigs did not decrease in response to a discontinuation of use until the use of tylosin, a macrolide, was also discontinued, because both resistance traits were genetically linked [2]. Also notably, antimicrobial exposure does not always lead to a statistically significant increase in resistance rates during the studied time periods [54]. Similarly, resistance levels in bacteria associated with operations that do not use antimicrobial drugs are not in all cases significantly lower than those associated with operations that do [55]. Therefore, while exposure of foodborne pathogens to antimicrobial drugs on farms or feedlots clearly poses a risk of resistance emergence that risk is currently difficult to quantify.

Data based on studies in animal pathogens or commensal bacteria

Bacteria can readily share their genetic material. The emergence of antimicrobial resistance in commensal bacteria or animal pathogens contributes to the abundance of resistance genes that may subsequently be transferred to human pathogens. Because commensal bacteria are ubiquitous in the environment and their study tends to be easier than that of foodborne or zoonotic pathogens, considerably more studies have focused on the impact of antimicrobial exposure on commensal bacteria than foodborne or zoonotic pathogens. Only a few representative studies are highlighted in Table 3, as illustrative examples. Additional examples are provided in other reviews, including that performed by the Joint Expert Technical Advisory Committee on Antibiotic Resistance (JETACAR) [32].

As shown in Table 3, a variety of study types are available that investigate the emergence of resistance in commensal bacteria in response to antimicrobial exposure. These include controlled trials, observational studies, and correlation studies that compare bacterial populations across settings. Similar to the situation described in the preceding section, most studies rely on phenotypic methods to evaluate resistance levels, and studies vary vastly in the amount of control they exert on treatment allocation and antimicrobial exposures. Because the primary focus is on commensal bacteria, studies typically follow naturally-occurring bacterial populations, even though, as described in the preceding section, in some cases animals are experimentally challenged with pathogens and both pathogens and commensals are followed over time.

A number of randomized controlled trials have demonstrated an increase in the prevalence of antimicrobial resistant bacteria following antimicrobial exposure. For instance, in one study feedlot steers were fed chlortetracycline with or without sulfamethazine, monensin, tylosin or virginiamycin for 61 days in a silage-based diet, followed by 86 days without antimicrobials, and then another 42 days of exposure while being on a grain-based

Table 3 Examples of study types evaluating the emergence of antimicrobial resistance in natural bacterial background populations after food producing animals were exposed to antimicrobial drugs

Reference	Study Type[a]	species	bacterial target	antimicrobial drug	administration route	study outcomes related to antimicrobial resistance	study design	susceptibility testing	controls	Key findings
						Grade level: Controlled trial				
[65]	RCT	cattle	*E. coli*	chlortetracycline (with or without sulfamethazine), monensin, tylosin, virginiamycin; all as growth promoters	feed	emergence of antimicrobial resistance	6 treatments, 5 pens per treatment, 10 steer per pen	Phenotypic agar dilution	negative control	exposure to chlortetracycline and sulfamethazine increased the prevalence of resistance; diet had an important impact on shedding of resistant strains
[66]	RCT	cattle	*E. coli*	florfenicol	s.c. injection	emergence of antimicrobial resistance	42 pens (8–10 cows per pen), 2 cows per pen enrolled in study	Phenotypic *disk diffusion*	negative control	after antimicrobial treatment, increased antimicrobial resistance; prior treatment predictive of resistance; animal source and previous management impact results
[67]	RCT	Cattle	fecal bacteria	ceftiofur, tetracycline	s.c. injection	antimicrobial resistance	176 steers; 2 replicates of 88 steers each, 8 pens of 11 steers per replicate; total of 4 treatment groups	Genotypic *PCR based*	positive and negative controls	Initial and subsequent antimicrobial treatments led to increased frequency of resistance genes
[68]	RCT	pigs	*Enterococci Staphylococcus hyicus*	tylosin (as growth promoter)	feed	erythromycin resistance levels	2 trials a 10 pigs, $n = 5$ per group	Phenotypic	negative control	Prevalence of resistance in enterococci immediately increased 2.4× in response to tylosin exposure; resistance in *Staphylococcus hyicus* occurred more gradually, at a rate of 8% per day and 5× over 20 days
[130]	RCT	pigs	*aerobic gram negative bacteria; Salmonella*	chlortetracycline	feed	antimicrobial resistance	3 farms (convenience sample); 12, 2 and 8 barns per farm	Phenotypic *broth dilution*	negative control	antimicrobial exposure was associated with increased prevalence of resistance in aerobic gram-negative bacteria
						GRADE level: observational study				
[69]	cohort	pigs	coliform bacteria	olaquindox	feed	emergence of resistance	12 farms	Phenotypic	neighboring farms that do not use olaquindox	prevalence and level of resistance increased on farms that used it, and to lesser extent on adjacent farms
[70]	CS	pigs	*E. coli*	various	feed	emergence of antimicrobial resistance	34 farms	Phenotypic	negative control	antimicrobial use increases the emergence of resistance

Table 3 Examples of study types evaluating the emergence of antimicrobial resistance in natural bacterial background populations after food producing animals were exposed to antimicrobial drugs *(Continued)*

[71]	CS	pigs	*E. coli*	various	various	antimicrobial resistance	47 farms	Phenotypic	negative control	antimicrobial use (in weaner rather than finisher pigs) was associated with resistance; some evidence for cross-resistance and co-selection
						GRADE level: other				
[72]	correlation study	pigs, cattle, poultry	*E. coli*	various	various	correlation between antimicrobial use and resistance	7 countries	phenotypic	comparison across countries	use of antimicrobial drugs is strongly correlated with resistance in *E. coli*
[73]	correlation study	Poultry	*Enterococci, Vancomycin-resistant*	avoparcin	various	Comparison of resistance prevalence before and after avoparcin ban	Italy	phenotypic	comparison over time	prevalence of vancomycin-resistant *Enterococci* decreased in poultry meat samples after the avoparcin ban

[a] *CT* controlled trial (allocation scheme not clearly described), *RCT* randomized controlled trial, *CS* cross-sectional study

diet [65]. Expsoure to antimicrobial drugs significantly incrased the prevalence of steers shedding resistant baceria and the data suggested a potential genetic link between tetracycline and ampicillin resistance. Notably, the type of feed significantly impacted shedding rates with higher rates associated with the grain-based diet, emphasizing the importance of external factors. In another randomized controlled trial, feedlot steers were exposed to a single dose of florfenicol by subcutaneous injection and resistance in fecal *E. coli* populations were measured before and immediately after exposure, and up to a month later [66]. Notably, treated and control animals were housed in the same pen together with other steers. Immediately after treatment, all isolates from treated animals were resistant to multiple antimicrobial drugs including chloramphenicol, and resistance persisted in later samplings. The source of the animals and their previous management were found to have a statistically significant impact on the resistance dynamics. Yet another study used a metagenomic approach [67]. Feedlot steers were exposed to chlortetracycline – administering the drug either to one or all steers in the pen – followed by administration of chlortetracycline (or no antimicrobial drugs). Fecal bacterial communities were analyzed for common resistance genes (*i.e.*, bla_{CMY-2}, bla_{CTX-M}, tet(A) and tet(B)) by real-time PCR. A determination of the bacterial species carrying the resistance genes was not performed but 16S rRNA gene quantity was determined to standardize the number of resistance gene copies. The frequency of ceftiofur resistance genes increased significantly when all steers received ceftiofur while tetracycline resistance decreased at the same time, likely indicating a shift in the composition of the microbial community. In response to subsequent chlortetracycline exposure both ceftiofur and tetracycline resistance genes increased.

Similar results have also been observed in pigs. In one trial, for instance, pigs on 3 farms were exposed to chlortetracycline in the feed and resistance was evaluated in their aerobic gram negative bacteria as well as *Salmonella*. Antimicrobial exposure was associated with increased prevalence of resistance in aerobic gram-negative bacteria. In another study, pigs were fed tylosin and weekly samples were taken to evaluate macrolide resistance in fecal enterococci and skin staphylococci [68]. The prevalence of resistance in enterococci immediately increased 2.4 times in response to tylosin exposure. By comparison, resistance in *Staphylococcus hyicus* occurred more gradually, at a rate of 8% per day and 5 times over 20 days.

As shown in Table 3, there is also strong evidence from observational studies as well as the analysis of convenience samples that antimicrobial use on farms leads to an increase in resistance among commensals and animal pathogens isolated from the exposed animals. In one cohort study, for instance, the impact of olaquindox exposure on coliform bacteria from pigs was analyzed and compared to resistance in coliform bacteria from pigs on neighboring farms not exposed to olaquindox [69]. Both the prevalence and level of resistance increased on farms that used olaquindox, and to lesser extent on adjacent farms. Two cross-sectional studies of 34 and 47 pig farms provide further evidence for a risk of resistance in response to antimicrobial exposure [70, 71]. Notably, one of the studies provided some evidence for co-resistance and cross-selection, and noted that antimicrobial use in weaners was associated with incrased resistance [71]. In addition, a study of *E. coli* convenience samples across 7 countries revealed a correlation between antimicrobial use and resistance [72] and an analysis of *Enterococci* from poultry samples collected before and after the avoparcin ban found the prevalence of vancomycin-resistant *Enterococci* decreased in poultry meat samples after the avoparcin ban [73].

Taken together there is ample evidence supporting a risk of resistance emergence in commensal bacteria after exposure to antimicrobial drugs. How quickly resistance emerges is affected by a variety of factors, including the bacterial species and the antimicrobial treatment choice as well as potential preceding antimicrobial exposures [66, 68]. A variety of external factors, such as the type of feed chosen, can also influence the emergence of resistance [65]. Resistance may be reversible [73], but can remain at elevated levels after use is discontinued [47], and a single exposure can lead to increased resistance in the commensal bacterial population [66]. Therefore, while exposure to antimicrobial drugs on farms or feedlots clearly poses a risk of resistance emergence in commensal bacteria that risk is currently difficult to quantify.

Data based on studies in humans, laboratory animal models or in vitro systems

Data on the correlation between antimicrobial use and the emergence of antimicrobial resistance have also been collected in human healthcare, laboratory animal models and in vitro systems. Results collected in these settings are generally consistent with the observations made in agricultural settings. As shown in Table 4, a variety of study types are available, including RCTs, observational studies, and other types of evidence. Many of the scientific studies have analyzed the emergence of resistance in humans during treatment, monitoring the resistance of bacteria isolated from the patients over time. In some cases, patients were randomly allocated to treatment arms, whereas other studies compared isolates from patients that received treatments with different antimicrobial drugs or treatment regimen. Yet other studies

Table 4 Examples of studies evaluating the emergence of antimicrobial resistance in response to antimicrobial exposure

Reference	Study: Type[a]	study population	drug of concern	bacterial target	endpoint or outcome relevant to antimicrobial resistance	controls	period of concern[b]	Key findings
				Grade level: Controlled trial				
[74]	SR of RCTs; $n = 46$ studies	pneumonia patients	imipenem	*Pseudomonas aeruginosa*	initial resistance; resistance emergence on treatment	other antimicrobials: beta-lactams, aminoglycosides, vancomycin, fluoroquinolone	1993–2008	resistance emerged: imipenem: 38.7% (range: 5.6–77.8%) of isolates comparator groups: 21.9% (range: 4.8–56.5%)
[75]	MA of RCTs; $n = 8$ studies	patients with various infections	beta-lactam	various	emergence of antimicrobial resistance	other antimicrobials: beta-lactam and aminoglycoside combination	1980–2004	resistance emerged in various bacterial species (up to 20% of isolates); no significant difference between the two treatment arms in resistance emergence
[85]	RCT; $n = 313$ patients	patients with nosocomial pneumonia, sepsis, or severe diffuse peritonitis	imipenem	*Pseudomonas aeruginosa*	emergence of antimicrobial resistance	imipenem plus netilmicin	1988–1992	resistance to imipenem occurred in monotherapy ($n = 8$) and combination therapy ($n = 13$) patients
				Grade level: Observational study				
[76]	SR & MA of RCTs and OS; $n = 24$ studies	patients with various infections and healthy volunteers	various	various	resistance emergence under treatment	other antimicrobials	1955–2009	prescription of antibiotics in primary care is associated with resistance in bacteria
[77]	cohort study; $n = 271$ patients	hospitalized patients with lab-confirmed *Pseudomonas* infection where initial isolate was susceptible	ceftazidime ciprofloxacin imipenem piperacillin	*Pseudomonas aeruginosa*	emergence of resistance during treatment	compare patients with resistance emergence to those without	1994–1996	resistance emerged in 10% of patients ($n = 28$); risk differed by antimicrobial drug
[78]	cohort study; $n = 2641$ patients	coronary artery bypass graft surgery patients	Various; short vs. prolonged antibiotic prophylaxis	*Enterobacteriaceae* (cephalosporin resistant); *Enterococci* (vancomycin resistant)	emergence of resistance during prophylaxis	compare patients with acquired antibiotic resistance to those without	1993–1997	Prolonged antibiotic prophylaxis was associated with an increased risk of acquired antibiotic resistance
[79]	CC study	patients with lab-confirmed bacteremia, resistant *Pseudomonas*	Piperacillin, ceftazidime, imipenem, ciprofloxacin, gentamicin, amikacin	*Pseudomonas aeruginosa*	odds of previous antibiotic treatment	patients with lab-confirmed bacteremia caused by susceptible *Pseudomonas* strains	1989–1998	previous exposure to antimicrobial monotherapy is associated with increased risk of subsequent resistance to that antimicrobial
				Grade level: Other				
[80]	in vivo trial	mice experimentally challenged with bacteria	amikacin, ceftriaxone, perfloxacin or their combination	*Pseudomonas aeruginosa, Klebsiella pneumoniae,*	resistance emergence after treatment	other antimicrobials (single vs. combination therapy)	1986	resistance emerged in response to treatment; the frequency of resistance emergence varied by pathogen and antibiotic / combination

Table 4 Examples of studies evaluating the emergence of antimicrobial resistance in response to antimicrobial exposure *(Continued)*

				Enterobacter cloacae, Serratia marcescens				
[81]	in vitro trial (lab evolution system)	bacteria experimentally exposed to antimicrobial	colistin (different treatment regimen)	*Acinetobacter baumannii*	resistance emergence after exposure	negative control	2007	extensive resistance emerged during re-growth (as early as 6 h after treatment)
[82]	Cross-national database study (26 countries in Europe)	antibiotic use in outpatient settings (calculated as defined daily dose per 1000 inhabitants) and antibiotic resistance rates	various	various	correlation between antibiotic use and resistance across countries	n/a	1997–2002	rates of antibiotic resistance are higher in high consuming countries

[a] *SR* systematic review, *MA* meta-analysis, *RCT* randomized controlled trial, *OS* observational study, *CC* case-control study
[b] For experimental laboratory studies that do not specify the date of the experiments the publication date is substituted

followed bacterial populations in laboratory animals or in vitro systems, or evaluated correlations between antibiotic use practices and the prevalence of resistance.

A systematic review of randomized controlled trials in pneumonia patients with initially sensitive *Pseudomonas aeruginosa* infection, for instance, found that resistance emerged readily *de novo* in response to imipenem exposure, with an average of 38.7% of isolates (range: 5.6–77.8%) acquiring resistance [74]. Notably, *de novo* resistance emergence was less likely in the comparator group treated with other antimicrobials (i.e., beta-lactams, aminoglycosides, vancomycin, or fluoroquinolone), where resistance emerged in an average of 21.9% of isolates (range 6.8–56.5%). Another meta-analysis of human patients with various types of infections treated with beta-lactam antibiotics or a combination of beta-lactams and aminoglycosides found that resistance rapidly emerged *de novo*, with up to 20% of isolates becoming resistant, and there was no statistically significant difference between the two treatments [75]. Results from a variety of observational studies as well as meta-analyses of individual observational studies also support a risk of resistance emergence in response to antimicrobial exposure [76–79]. Studies in laboratory animals and in vitro models have also demonstrated for a number of different bacteria and drugs that antimicrobial resistance readily emerges in response to exposure, sometimes very quickly, even though the dynamics of that resistance depend on the specific bacterium and drug [80, 81]. Similar to the situation in animal agriculture [72], a cross-national study has demonstrated a correlation between antibiotic use patterns and resistance levels, showing that rates of antimicrobial resistance are higher in high-consuming countries [82].

Together, these data further support that antimicrobial drug use can and does lead to the emergence of resistance in exposed bacteria. The data also suggest that in general, longer exposure periods and preceding antimicrobial exposure tend to be associated with an increased risk of resistance compared to short exposure times [78, 79, 83]. However, how quickly resistance emerges depends on the pathogen, drug, and resistance mechanism, among other factors [80, 83]; exposure to a drug can also select for resistance to a related drug due to cross-selection, and some resistance may be maintained in the absence of antimicrobial selection, for instance due to co-selection [84]. The data further suggest that certain treatment regimens may be associated with an increased risk of resistance compared to others (see for instance [77, 78, 85]), but more data are needed to allow the optimization of treatment regimen to minimize the risk [83, 86] and data specific to animal agriculture are needed to determine how to translate the information to optimize treatments in this regard in veterinary settings.

Risk of infection due to resistant bacteria that emerged on the farm

Transmission of foodborne or zoonotic pathogens to humans

Because of ethical considerations, RCTs that evaluate the risk of pathogen transmission from animals to humans are generally not feasible. However, there is considerable evidence from observational studies, as well as other study types, such as outbreak investigations, case reports, and bacterial studies of correlation among bacteria from different sources that foodborne or zoonotic pathogens carrying antimicrobial resistance genes are shared between animals and humans (Table 5). Many of the studies have focused on *Salmonella* or methicillin-resistant *Staphylococcus aureus* (MRSA), and many are based on case-control studies that compare risk factors for infections with resistant or susceptible isolates retrospectively. In at least some studies, the directionality of transfer remains unknown; and for at least some pathogens and settings, cross-species transfers may be relatively infrequent. Moreover, in some instance the study analyzed colonization with a potential human pathogen such as MRSA, rather than actual infection that led to clinical disease. While colonization with these potential pathogens clearly demonstrates transmission, the associated public health risk is less clear.

A number of observational studies have evaluated the human health risk posed by infections with antimicrobial resistant foodborne or zoonotic pathogens. A retrospective case-control study in New England (U.S.), for instance, evaluated risk factors for infections with a multidrug-resistant *Salmonella* Newport strain (MDR AmpC), comparing 34 case patients to 37 controls infected with susceptible *Salmonella* Newport strains and 94 healthy community controls [87]. Infections with the multidrug-resistant *Salmonella* Newport strain were significantly associated with dairy farm exposure.

(Adjusted odd ratio 12.2; 95% Confidence Interval: 1.2–640). Investigation of two regional dairy farms where the *Salmonella* Newport strain had recently been identified detected the strain in animals and ill farm workers. In fact, bacterial isolates from humans and cattle were indistinguishable or closely related based on antibiotic resistance profiles and PFGE patterns. Another case-control study, also focusing on *Salmonella* Newport MDR AmpC in the U.S. but national in scope and comparing 54 case patients to 146 controls infected with pan-susceptible *Salmonella* Newport strains and 1154 healthy community controls, identified consumption of uncooked ground beef or home prepared runny scrambled eggs or omelets during the 5 days prior to illness onset as a significant risk factor [88]. A third case-control study of *Salmonella* Newport MDR AmpC, comparing 268 cases from Wisconsin to 402 controls from

Table 5 Examples of study types evaluating the human health risk posed by infections with antimicrobial resistant foodborne or zoonotic pathogens

Reference	Study Type[a]	subjects	country	time period	bacterial target	relevant study outcomes	sample size	controls	comments	Key findings relevant to antimicrobial resistance
GRADE level: Controlled trial										
Not applicable because of ethical concerns										
GRADE level: observational study										
[87]	CC	human patients	U.S.	1999–2001	*Salmonella* Newport; MDRAmpC resistant	risk factors for infection	34 cases; 37 infected controls and 94 community controls	*Salmonella* patients with susceptible Newport infection; healthy community controls	followed up by investigation of cattle isolates and risk factors for shedding on dairy farms; regional in scope (New England)	Association of infection with *Salmonella* Newport MDRAmpC with dairy farm exposure; bacterial isolates from humans and cattle were indistinguishable or closely related (based on antibiotic resistance profile and PFGE pattern)
[88]	CC	human patients	U.S.	2002–2003	*Salmonella* Newport; MDRAmpC resistant	risk factors for infection	215 case patients; 54 with MDRAmpC resistant strain and 146 pansusceptible; 1154 community controls	healthy community controls; volunteers without diarrhea in the previous 28 days	FoodNet study; national in scope (8 of 9 FoodNet sites)	Association of infection with *Salmonella* Newport MDRAmpC with consumption of uncooked ground beef or home prepared runny scrambled eggs or omelets during the 5 days before onset of illness
[89]	CC	human patients in Wisconsin	U.S.	2003–2005	*Salmonella* Newport MDR AmpC	associations between antimicrobial resistance and reported exposures	268 isolates from Wisconsin and 402 from the remaining U.S.	Cases in Wisconsin vs. rest of the U.S.	Controls were collected 2003–2004	Infections with multidrug-resistant *Salmonella* Newport strains were associated with exposures to cattle, farms and unpasteurized milk
[90]	CC	human patients in California	U.S.	1985	*Salmonella* Newport (chloramphenicol resistant)	risk factors for infection	45 patients and 89 matched controls	healthy volunteers	Epidemic *Salmonella* strain was isolated from hamburger products eaten by cases, as well as the abattoirs where the animals were slaughtered, dairies that sent the animals to slaughter, and ill dairy cows.	Association of infection with resistant *Salmonella* Newport isolates with eating ground beef during the week before onset and penicillin and tetracycline use during the month before onset of symptoms; chloramphenicol resistant *Salmonella* from dairy farms were associated with chloramphenicol use on those dairies

Table 5 Examples of study types evaluating the human health risk posed by infections with antimicrobial resistant foodborne or zoonotic pathogens *(Continued)*

[91]	CC	human patients from national database	Netherlands	2003–2005	MRSA (non-typable)	risk factors for infection	35 cases, 76 controls	MRSA infections with other strains	Analysis aimed to exclude secondary cases	Living in rural areas and contact with pigs and cattle were associated with case patients
[92]	CS	veal calf farmers	Netherlands	2007–2008	MRSA ST 398	risk factors for carriage	102 farms, 390 questionnaires, 2151 nasal swabs from calves	farmers negative for MRSA ST 398	nasal swabs taken from farmers and farm calves; farms randomly selected	Human MRSA ST 398 carriage was associated with intensity of animal contact and number of positive animals on farm; calves were more likely to be carriers when treated with antibiotics, and good farm hygiene had a protective effect.
[93]	CS	swine farmers	Belgium	2007	MRSA ST 398	risk factors for carriage	49 swine farms, 127 persons on the farms participated and 1500 pigs were sampled	farmers negative for MRSA ST 398	nasal swabs and wound samples; farms randomly collected	MRSA ST 398 carriage by farmers was associated with prevalence among pigs on the farm, having regular contact with pigs, dogs, and horses, and use of protective equipment.
						GRADE level: other				
[22]	phylogenetic study	bacterial isolates	various	1997–2011	MRSA CC398	evolution and transmission dynamics including transmission between species	n/a	none	Phylogenetic and population genetic analysis	human and animal populations of CC398 are separate, but with multiple transfers back and forth; same data suggesting onward transmission of animal-associated strains in community settings (e.g., hospitals); different tetracycline resistance genes showed different evolutionary patterns
[94]	outbreak	human patients with rare strain	Denmark	1998	*Salmonella* Typhimurium DT104	source of multidrug resistant infection outbreak	27 cases	none	rare strain isolated from patients and pork samples; pork samples were traced back to herd; resistant infections in humans were more difficult to treat	A swine herd was the likely source of a human outbreak with MDR *Salmonella* Typhimurium DT104
[95]	outbreak	human patients infected with rare strains	U.S.	1983	*Salmonella* Newport	source of multidrug resistant infection outbreak	18 cases	none	rare isolate strain found in human patients and cattle	hamburger from beef cattle fed sub therapeutic chlortetracycline for growth promotion likely outbreak source

Table 5 Examples of study types evaluating the human health risk posed by infections with antimicrobial resistant foodborne or zoonotic pathogens *(Continued)*

[96]	human case report	human patient infected with rare strain	U.S.	1998	*Salmonella* Typhimurium	source of multidrug resistant infection	1 case	none	Infection traced back to farm;	The farm was identified as the source of a multidrug resistant *Salmonella* isolate from a human case patient
[97]	human case report	MRSA cluster around pig farmer	Netherlands	2004	MRSA	source of multidrug resistant infection	pig farmer, family and co-workers, pigs	none	animals on farm sampled	Infection with MRSA traced back to farm, onward transmission in farm family
[98]	correlation study	Isolates from swine and swine workers	U.S.	Unspecified	MRSA	risk factors for MRSA colonization	20 workers and 299 swine	none	animals and humans sampled	Colonization with MRSA ST 398 was very common in swine herds, similar isolates in humans and animals
[99]	correlation study	isolates from farm personnel and milk samples	Hungary	2002–2004	MRSA	risk factors for MRSA colonization	1 farm, 12 workers sampled, 595 milk samples	none	MRSA strains were subtyped	MRSA isolates from workers in close contact with cows were indistinguishable from cow isolates

[a]*CC* case-control study (or case-case study where controls are cases of infection with other strains), *CS* cross-sectional study

the remaining U.S. found infections with *Salmonella* Newport MDR AmpC significantly associated with exposure to cattle, farms and unpasteurized milk [89]. Yet another case-control study of 45 case patients infected with *Salmonella* Newport strains carrying chloramphenicol resistance and 89 matched healthy controls identified eating ground beef during the week before illness onset and penicillin and tetracycline use during the month before onset of symptoms as significant risk factors [90]. Notably, the same *Salmonella* strain was isolated from hamburger products eaten by case patients, as well as the abattoirs where the animals were slaughtered, dairies that sent the animals to slaughter, and ill dairy cows. Chloramphenicol resistant *Salmonella* from dairy farms were associated with chloramphenicol use on those dairies. In addition, case-control [91] and cross-sectional [92, 93] studies in the Netherlands and Belgium have identified animal contacts as risk factors for carriage or infections with MRSA. In one study of veal calf farmers in the Netherlands, human MRSA ST 398 carriage was associated with intensity of animal contact and number of positive animals on farm; calves were more likely to be carriers when treated with antibiotics, and good farm hygiene had a protective effect [92]. In another study of swine farmers in Belgium, MRSA ST 398 carriage by farmers was associated with prevalence among pigs on the farm, having regular contact with pigs, dogs, and horses, and use of protective equipment [93]. A case-control study of human infections with non-typable MRSA in the Netherlands, comparing 35 cases to 76 controls based on a national database of human patients, identified living in rural areas and contact with pigs and cattle as significantly associated with case patients [91].

In addition, *Salmonella* outbreaks have been traced back to farm animals. For instance, an outbreak of multidrug-resistant *Salmonella* Typhimurium DT104 that occurred in Denmark in 1998 was traced back to a swine herd [94]. The outbreak strain was a rare strain, simplifying the trace-back. In fact, the same rare strain was isolated from patients and pork samples and pork samples were traced back to the swine herd of origin. Notable, the resistant infections in humans were more difficult to treat due to the resistance profile. In another outbreak involving a rare strain of *Salmonella* Newport that occurred in the U.S., hamburgers from beef cattle fed chlortetracycline were identified as the likely outbreak source [95]. Trace-back investigations revealed the same rare *Salmonella* strain found in human patients was shed by cattle. Human case reports have identified farm exposures as the likely source of infections with multidrug resistant *Salmonella* Typhimurium in the U.S. [96] and MRSA in the Netherlands [97]. In fact, in the latter case infection with MRSA was traced back a pig farm, where it was isolated from the pigs and coworkers, and onward transmission to the farm family was documented [97]. Correlation studies and phylogenetic analyses also provide evidence supporting a transmisison of MRSA between animals and human contacts [22, 98, 99]. In Canada, the rate of ceftiofur-resistant *Salmonella* Heidelberg infections was statistically significantly associated with contamination rates on retail chicken [63].

Taken together, the evidence for a link between foodborne or zoonotic bacteria with antimicrobial resistance genes on farms or feedlots and human health risks is undisputable. Exposure to farms, consumption of raw or undercooked foods of animal origin, and living in rural areas have been identified as risk factors for infections with those foodborne pathogens that carry antimicrobial resistance genes [87, 88, 90, 91]. Outbreaks of foodborne illness associated with resistant bacteria have been traced back to the farm of origin [94–96]; identical bacterial strains have been identified in animals and humans in contact with them or the food they produce [97–99]. And in at least some cases, increased intensity of animal contact led to a measurably increased risk of human infection with resistant strains [92, 93]. While the magnitude of the risk may vary across pathogens and circumstance, it is clear that foodborne or zoonotic bacteria on farms or feedlots that carry resistance genes pose a human health risk.

Transmission of commensal bacteria from food-producing animals to humans

Most of the research on the emergence of resistance as a result of on-farm use of antimicrobial drugs has been conducted on commensal bacteria, and observations from studies which simultaneously analyzed resistance emergence in foodborne as well as commensal bacteria suggest that resistance may emerge more quickly in the latter. The question of whether the emergence of resistance among commensal or animal pathogens on farms poses a human public health risk is therefore an important one.

As shown in Table 6, a variety of studies have evaluated the link between antimicrobial resistance in animal commensals and human health risks. The available evidence types include observational studies and other study designs such as correspondence of bacterial strains from different sources. Notably, because of the complexity of the events evaluated, study designs are often intricate and may include, for instance, a randomized controlled trial of chicken exposed to antimicrobials, paired with an observational study evaluating the colonization of their human caretakers [100]. While some studies choose prevalence of resistance as study outcome, others also include degree of resistance, expressed for instance as MIC. Farm workers as well as

Table 6 Examples of study types evaluating the human health risk posed by antimicrobial resistance genes that emerged in animal pathogens or commensal bacteria

Reference	Study Type[a]	subjects	country	time period	bacterial target	relevant study outcomes	sample size	controls	comments	Key findings relevant to antimicrobial resistance
GRADE level: Controlled trial										
Not available										
GRADE level: observational study										
[100]	CC	poultry workers	Nigeria	published in 1989	*E. coli*, nalidixic acid resistant	colonization of poultry workers with challenge *E. coli* strain	Complex study design: - Birds were experimentally inoculated with challenge strain of *E. coli* (*n* = 36 birds on university farm, and *n* = 16 on commercial farm) - Poultry works in direct contact with challenged birds were sampled for colonization with challenge strain - This was compared to control workers with or without direct contact to control birds, and to samples collected from the exposed workers prior to exposure - birds were sampled for colonization			after birds were challenged, the poultry workers in direct contact with challenged birds were colonized; results were similar on the university and commercial farm
[101]	CC	poultry farmers	U.S.	published in 1978	aerobic bacterial cultures, tetracycline resistance	resistance in bacterial microflora of chicken and contact farmers	Complex study design: - RCT of chicken, *n* = 50 chicken per group, test chicken were exposed to tetracycline in feed, controls were not; emergence of resistance was tested in commensal bacteria - farm family in contact with chicken was tested for emergence of resistance in background microflora - farm family was compared to other farm families in proximity, and to medical students			antimicrobial resistance emerged in exposed chicken and farm contacts
[102]	cohort	poultry farmers	U.S.	published in 1976	intestinal bacterial flora, tetracycline resistance	resistance in bacterial microflora of chicken and contact farmers	*n* = 11 farm members, 24 neighbors	neighbors	birds were exposed to tetracycline in feed, emergence of resistance was traced in birds and contact humans, and compared to neighbors	antimicrobial resistance emerged under exposure on the farm; the prevalence of antimicrobial resistance was higher in bacteria from exposed farm families than in neighbors;
[103]	CS	pig farmers and abattoir workers	Netherlands	published in 1994	*E. coli*	Prevalence of resistance	*n* = 290 pig farmers; *n* = 316 abattoir workers; *n* = 160 urban/suburban residents	urban/suburban residents	fecal *E. coli* from the three human groups were tested for resistance to multiple antimicrobial drugs	Pig farmers had the highest percentage of resistant *E. coli*, and urban/suburban residents had the lowest
[104]	CC	turkey, broiler and layer farmers and slaughterers	Netherlands	published in 2001	*E. coli*	Prevalence and degree of resistance	*n* = 47 turkey farmers and their flocks; *n* = 51 broiler farmers and *n* = 50 broiler flocks; 25 layer farmers and	comparison across human (and corresponding animal) populations; ciprofloxacin-resistant isolates were further subtyped; meat	humans and birds sampled; antibiotic use on farms recorded	Prevalence of resistance significantly higher in turkey and broiler samples than laying hens (which correlated with antibiotic use);

Table 6 Examples of study types evaluating the human health risk posed by antimicrobial resistance genes that emerged in animal pathogens or commensal bacteria *(Continued)*

							their flocks; $n = 46$ poultry slaughterers	samples were collected immediately after slaughter		prevalence of resistance was higher in turkey and broiler farmers and slaughterers than in laying hen farmers; isolates from farmers/ slaughterers and birds / meat seemed to match, despite variability across farms
						GRADE level: other				
[63]	correlation study	isolates from chicken meat and humans	Canada	2003–2008	*Salmonella* Heidelberg, *E. coli*	Prevalence of ceftiofur-resistance in chicken samples and human cases	Correlation across provinces and time periods	n/a	n/a	Statistically significant correlation between ceftiofur-resistant *Salmonella* Heidelberg on retail chicken and human infections; in Quebec, changing levels of ceftiofur use in hatcheries during study period seemed to impact dynamics from before voluntary withdrawal to reintroduction.
[105]	uncontrolled transmission study	farmers, livestock and environment	U.S.	published in 1990	*E. coli*	Spread of resistant bacteria on farm; emergence of resistance	2 trials with $n = 2$ cattle each; $n = 4$ pigs, $n = 5$ mice per cage; bovine experiments repeated in indoor / outdoor settings one challenged pig exchanged with one unchallenged pig from unchallenged pen	N/A; study monitored contact animals, mice in pens of challenged and non-challenged pig or cow, environment including flies, and human caretakers study also evaluated impact of chlortetracycline use on emergence of resistance	one pig and one cow were inoculated with marked strains of *E. coli* with resistance; contact animals (pigs or cows and mice) were sampled for the *E. coli* strain, as were human caretakers and the environment	Contact animals, mice, flies and caretakers excreted challenge strain of *E. coli*; length of colonization varied, but in several cases exceeded 4 weeks; *E. coli* strain was found in environment and housing system impacted spread; chlortetracycline use led to increased resistance; transfer of resistance plasmid to other bacteria not detected
[106]			US		*E. coli*		1 trial	N/A		

Table 6 Examples of study types evaluating the human health risk posed by antimicrobial resistance genes that emerged in animal pathogens or commensal bacteria *(Continued)*

	uncontrolled transmission study	Consumer handling chicken carcasses		published in 1977		spread of resistant bacteria from contaminated carcass to volunteer handling it				Bacterial strain with antibiotic resistance transferred from chicken carcass to human volunteer handling it
[107]	Conjugation study	Transfer of resistance genes among bacteria of different origin	Norway	Published in 1994	*E. coli* as well as *Vibrio, Aeromonas*	Conjugation frequencies across bacteria and environmental settings	Conjugation was studied in multiple environments (e.g., seawater, hand towel, meat)	N/A		Plasmids were readily transferred from one bacterium to another, across bacterial species and in a number of different environments
[108]	Conjugation study	Transfer of resistance genes between *Enterobacteriaceae*	UK	Published in 2003	*Commensal E. coli, E. coil O157, Salmonella*	Conjugation across bacterial species	Conjugation across a number of bacterial pairs was evaluated under conditions in the gut (i.e., ileum)	N/A		Antibiotic resistance genes were readily transferred from one bacterial strain to another
[109]	Conjugation study	Transfer of resistance genes among *Enterococci* in the mouse gut	France	Published in 2003	*Enterococcus faecium isolates from humans and pigs*	Conjugation across *Enterococci* of different origin	In the gut of mice	N/A	mice were gnotobiotic (i.e. reared under conditions so that colonization with bacteria is fully known)	Vancomycin resistance was readily transferred from porcine to human isolates in the gut of mice; tylosin exposure (through drinking water) favored colonization due to conjugation.
[110]	Conjugation study	Transfer of resistance genes between *Enterococci* strains	Sweden	Published in 2006	*Enterococci faecium of human and animal origin*	Conjugation across *Enterococci* of different origin	In vitro and in the gut of mice	N/A	Mice were germ-free	Vancomycin resistance was readily transferred among *Enterococci* of different origin; conjugation frequency was higher in the mouse gut than in the environment; in most cases resistance disappeared within 3 days but one of the bacterial strains persisted for more than 20 days without antibiotic selection

Table 6 Examples of study types evaluating the human health risk posed by antimicrobial resistance genes that emerged in animal pathogens or commensal bacteria *(Continued)*

[111]	Conjugation study	Transfer of resistance genes in the gut of human volunteer	Denmark	Published in 2006	*Enterococcus faecium*	Conjugation between *Enterococcus faecium* of chicken and human origin	n = 6 volunteers	n/a	In the gut of human volunteers	Resistance genes were readily transferred from chicken to human isolates in the gut of human volunteers; in one volunteer, additional resistance genes were transferred
[112]	Conjugation study	Transfer of resistance from *Klebsiella* to *E. coli* in the mouse intestine	Denmark	Published in 2008	*Klebsiella* and *E. coli*	Conjugation between *Klebsiella* and *E. coli*	In vitro and in the gut of mice	n/a	Some mice were exposed to antimicrobial treatment	Resistance genes were readily transferred in vitro and in vivo. Antimicrobial treatment selected for resistant strains, which rapidly disappeared in the guts of mice not exposed to antibiotics.
[113]	uncontrolled transmission study	Calves and humans in contact with them	US	published in 1978	*E. coli*	Spread of resistant bacteria from calves to human contacts, and impact of tetracycline exposure on risk	1 trial repeated 3 times	N/A	calves were inoculated with rare *E. coli* strain carrying resistance genes	Bacteria were transferred from calves to human contacts; no statistically significant impact of tetracycline exposure on transmission risk; exposure of calves to tetracycline did not result in statistically significant differences in resistance levels of bacteria in human volunteers
[114]	correlation study	Cattle and human contacts	Norway	1996	*E. coli*	Presence of drug-resistant *E. coli* in animals and human contacts	n = 13 cattle; n = 3 family members; n = 1 veterinarian (sampling of humans repeated after 1 year, and samples from 4 other veterinarians added)	N/A	study of concurrence of *E. coli* strains	Multi-drug resistant *E. coli* were found in the animals and human contacts.

Table 6 Examples of study types evaluating the human health risk posed by antimicrobial resistance genes that emerged in animal pathogens or commensal bacteria *(Continued)*

[115]	correlation study	Poultry farmers and their birds	Norway	1998	*Enterococcus faecium (VRE)*	Genetic relatedness of human and animal isolates	*n* = 5 farmers and *n* = 7 broiler chicken	N/A	study of concurrence of *E. coli* strains	On one of the farms, human and animal bacteria were genetically closely related; genetically unrelated strains shared related vancomycin resistance genes, suggesting HGT
[116]	correlation study	farm families and their animals (i.e., cattle or swine)	US	Published in 1975	*E. coli*	Genetic relatedness of human and animal isolates	*n* = 14 farm families	N/A	Farm families in Missouri; impact of factors such as animal contact	Frequency of animal contact was not significantly correlated with genetic relatedness of human and animal isolates; consumption of home-raised beef appears to be associated with concordance between human and animal isolates
[118]	Conjugation study	Transfer of resistance genes from *E.coli* from pig to those from human gut	Denmark	2007–2008	*E. coli*	Conjugation between resistance genes among *E.coli* of pig and human origin	*n* = 9 human volunteers;	n/a	donor strain of *E.coli* from Danish pig; recipient strain *E.coli* of human origin	Transfer of resistance genes between *E.coli* bacteria in human intestine
[119]	Conjugation study	Transfer of mobile genetic elements associated with MRSA	UK	Published in 2014	*Staphylococcus aureus* bacterial populations	Frequency of horizontal gene transfer of pig and human origins	Gnotobiotic piglets	n/a	Co-colonization with human and pig associated variants of MRSA	High frequency of horizontal gene transfer; transfer of mobile genetic elements from pig to human within 4 h of co-colonization
[120]	Phylogenetic study	Presence of tetQ resistance gene in different bacteria	US	Published in 1994	*Bacteroides*	Sequence comparison for tetQ resistance gene	n/a	n/a	Presence of identical or closely related resistance genes across distantly related bacteria	Virtually identical resistance genes found in different bacterial species and isolates of different geographic origin

[a]*CC* case-control study (or case-case study where controls are cases of infection with other strains), *CS* cross-sectional study, *ET* experimental trial (i.e., no randomization and no controls)

workers in slaughterhouses tend to be the primary population subgroups of concern in these studies, even though consumers handling potentially contaminated carcasses, as well as animals in contact with infected animals have also been considered in some studies [100–106]. Studies also vary in the bacterial population of concern and range from narrowly defined, for instance *E. coli* carrying nalidixic acid resistance [100] to broad, for example anaerobic bacterial populations in general [107]. Conjugation studies are a special study type relevant in this context, which evaluates the transfer rates of bacterial resistance genes between bacterial populations in vivo, in the gut of animals or human volunteers [108–112], or in vitro [107].

A number of observational studies have investigated the effect of antimicrobial exposures on farms on resistance in commensal bacteria isolated from farm animals and human contacts. In one cohort study in the U.S., for instance, when broiler chicken were exposed to tetracycline in the feed, the emergence of tetracycline resistance was traced in the intestinal bacteria isolated from the birds, and in commensal bacteria isolated from 11 members of the farms where the exposed birds were housed [102]. Resistance to tetracycline in the intestinal bacteria from farm members in contact with the exposed birds was compared to that of 24 neighbors. Antimicrobial resistance emerged under exposure on the farm and the prevalence of antimicrobial resistance was higher in bacteria from exposed farm families than in neighbors. In another study of poultry farmers in the U.S. a randomized controlled trial design was combined with a case-control study design [101]. In the randomized, controlled part of the study, groups of 50 chicken were exposed to tetracycline in feed while controls did not receive any antimicrobial drugs. The emergence of resistance in the commensal bacteria on the chicken was tracked. At the same time, the commensal bacteria of farm families in contact with the chicken was tested for the emergence of resistance, and this was compared to the commensal bacteria from other farm families in the proximity, and to commensal bacteria from medical students. The study clearly demonstrated that antimicrobial resistance emerged in exposed chicken and the farm family contacts. Similarly, in a study of 47 turkey, 51 broiler and 25 layer farmers and their flocks as well as 46 poultry slaughterers in the Netherlands, the prevalence and degree of resistance in *E. coli* populations was analyzed and antibiotic use on the farms was recorded [104]. The prevalence of resistance was significantly higher in *E. coli* samples from turkey and broiler flocks than in those from laying hens, which was correlated with antibiotic use practices. The prevalence of resistance was also higher in bacteria from turkey and broiler farmers and slaughterers than in laying hen farmers. Individual isolates from farmers or slaughterers and birds or their meat seemed to match, despite some variability across farms. In another cross-sectional study, the prevalence of resistance in *E. coli* isolates from 290 pig farmers and 316 abattoir workers in the Netherlands was compared to that of 160 urban or suburban residents [103]. Fecal *E. coli* from the three human groups were tested for resistance to multiple antimicrobial drugs. The highest percentage of resistant *E. coli* was found in pig farmers, while urban/suburban residents had the lowest prevalence. In another very complex study design, the colonization of poultry workers with a specifically marked *E. coli* strain was evaluated [100]. Birds were experimentally inoculated with a challenge strain of *E. coli* (36 birds on a university farm, and 16 on a commercial farm). Poultry workers in direct contact with the challenged birds were sampled for colonization with the challenge strain. The results were compared to control workers with or without direct contact to control birds, and to samples collected from the exposed workers prior to exposure. In addition, the birds were sampled for colonization. The study clearly showed that after birds were challenged, the poultry workers in direct contact with the challenged birds were colonized; results were similar on the university and commercial farm.

Evidence for a transmission risk from farm animals to humans is also provided by other study types. For instance, a number of studies lack proper negative controls and apply complex study designs but, despite these limitations, provide evidence in support of a transmission risk. For instance, one study performed in the U.S. evaluated the spread of resistant *E. coli* to livestock, farmers and the environment [105]. In separate experiments, one pig and one cow were experimentally inoculated with a specific *E. coli* strain that carried a particular resistance to make it easier to detect. Animals in contact with the inoculated animals (pigs or cows and mice) were sampled for the *E. coli* strain, as were human caretakers and the environment. Contact animals, mice, flies and caretakers were found to excrete the challenge strain of *E. coli*. The length of colonization varied, but in several cases exceeded 4 weeks. The *E. coli* strain was also found in the environment and housing system and this finding impacted the dynamics of spread. Exposure to chlortetracycline use in the experiments led to increased resistance, even though transfer of resistance plasmid to other bacteria was not detected. The number of animals in this experiment was low (Table 6) and only the cattle experiment was repeated once, with one 'replicate' in indoor and one in outdoor settings. Nonetheless, the experiments provide evidence that transmission of resistant bacteria from livestock to human contacts can and does occur. In another uncontrolled transmission study, also conducted in the U.S., the spread of resistant *E. coli* from calves to human contacts was evaluated, and the impact of tetracycline exposure on the risk was assessed [113]. In this case, the experiment was repeated three times. Calves were inoculated with a rare *E. coli* strain carrying resistance genes and human volunteers in contact with the calves were sampled for carriage of the challenge strain. The study provided evidence that challenge bacteria were transferred from calves to human contacts. However, no statistically significant impact of tetracycline exposure on the transmission risk was detected. The exposure of calves to tetracycline did not result in a statistically significant difference in resistance levels of bacteria in the human volunteers. In yet another uncontrolled study, the transmission risk associated with consumer handling of contaminated carcasses was assessed [106]. An *E. coli* strain with an antimicrobial resistance marker was used to inoculate a chicken carcass, and the volunteer handling the carcass was evaluated for carriage of the marked strain. The study clearly showed that the *E. coli* strain was transferred from the chicken carcass to the volunteer handling it. Even though this study also lacked controls and replicates it does provide evidence that bacteria can be transferred to consumers through the handling of contaminated meat or poultry products.

Results from correlation studies, which compare bacterial populations in food producing animals and human contacts, also support a transmission risk even though the evidence is less-well controlled and less rigorous. In one study in Norway, for instance, 13 cattle, and 3 family members in contact with the cattle as well as the veterinarian, were evaluated for the presence of antimicrobial-resistant *E. coli*, and the sampling of human volunteers was repeated after one year, at which point samples from 4 other veterinarians were added [114]. The study found concurrent strains of multi-drug resistant *E. coli* in the animals and human contacts. In another Norwegian study, poultry farmers and their birds were sampled for vancomycin-resistant *Enterococcus faecium* and the genetic relatedness among the bacterial isolates was assessed [115]. On one of the farms, human and animal bacteria were genetically closely related. Notably, even genetically unrelated strains shared related vancomycin resistance genes, suggesting HGT. In another study in the U.S., 14 farm families in Missouri and their livestock (i.e., cattle or swine) were sampled for *E.coli* and the genetic relatedness among the human and animal isolates was assessed [116]. The frequency of animal contact was recorded and its potential impact on the genetic relatedness among the isolates was assessed. Notably, the frequency of animal contact was not significantly associated with the genetic relatedness among human and animal isolates. However, consumption of home-raised beef appeared to be associated with concordance between human and animal isolates.

Taken together, the data clearly support the notion that antimicrobial-resistant commensal bacteria that emerged in food-producing animals can be and are transferred to humans. This may occur through direct contact with the animals, or indirectly, for instance through handling of contaminated carcasses. Notably, in cases of transmission through direct contact directionality may not always be clear and in some instances bacteria may also be transmitted from humans to the animals they are in contact with. Nonetheless, the fact that commensal bacteria can be transferred to humans from food-producing animals is undoubtable.

Risk of resistance gene transfer from food-animal associated commensal bacteria to human pathogens

Resistance that emerged in commensal bacteria on farms or feedlots poses a human health risk if it can be transferred to human pathogens. This transfer may occur in the human gut, in the environment, or in the food-producing animals. The ability of human commensals to transfer their resistance genes to human pathogens has been extensively studied and is clearly possible, even though certain transfers are clearly more likely than others (see [117] for a review). Therefore this study focuses on evidence for a transfer of resistance genes between bacteria of human and animal origin regardless of the human-pathogenic potential of the human-associated recipient strain.

A number of in-vivo and in-vitro studies have investigated the ability of commensal bacteria of animal and human origin to transfer their resistance genes. In one study of six human volunteers, for instance, the transfer of resistance genes between *Enterococcus faecium* strains of chicken and human origin was investigated [108]. Resistance genes were readily transferred from chicken to human isolates in the gut of the human volunteers. Notably, in one volunteer, additional resistance genes were also transferred. In another study, transfer of vancomycin resistance between *Enterococcus faecium* isolates of human and swine origin was investigated in the gut of gnotobiotic mice (i.e., mice reared under conditions so that colonization with bacteria is fully known) [106]. Vancomycin resistance was readily transferred from porcine to human isolates in the gut of the mice. Notably, tylosin exposure through drinking water favored colonization with strains that had undergone conjugation. Similar results were observed in another study, which evaluated the transfer of vancomycin resistance between *Enterococci faecium* strains of human and animal origin in the environment and in the gut of germ-free mice [107]. Vancomycin resistance was readily transferred among *Enterococci* of different origin. Notably, the frequency of conjugation was higher in the mouse gut than in the environment. In most cases, resistance disappeared within 3 days but one of the bacterial strains persisted for more than 20 days in the absence of antimicrobial exposure.

Exchange of resistance genes between isolates of animal and human origin has also been demonstrated for other bacteria [118]. In one study, for instance, the transfer of resistance genes from a multi-drug resistant *Klebsiella* strain isolated from a human pneumonia patient to a mouse-adapted *E. coli* strain was investigated in the mouse intestine and under in-vitro conditions [112]. Some of the mice were exposed to antimicrobial drugs during the study. Resistance genes were readily transferred in vitro and in vivo. Antimicrobial exposure selected for resistant strains, which rapidly disappeared in the guts of mice not exposed to antibiotics. Even though transfer in this case occurred from human to animal –associated bacteria it clearly demonstrates that the exchange of genetic material is possible. In another study, the transfer of resistance genes between commensal *E. coli* and two pathogens (*E. coli* O157 and *Salmonella)*, all of porcine origin, was investigated in an in-vitro model of the porcine gut [108]. Antimicrobial resistance genes were readily transferred between the bacteria and in one example persisted throughout the duration of the study. In yet another study, the transfer of resistance genes among *E.coli*, *Vibrio* and *Aeromonas* was investigated in a number of environments (e.g., meat, seawater, hand towel) [107]. Plasmids were readily transferred from one bacterium to another, across bacterial species and in a number of different environments. Similar findings have also been reported for MRSA. In one study, for instance, gnotobiotic piglets were co-colonized with human- and pig-associated variants of MRSA ST 398 and the bacterial populations were followed for 16 days and analyzed by whole-genome sequencing [119]. Transfer of mobile genetic elements from the pig to the human isolates was detected as early as 4 h after co-colonization. Plasmids and bacteriophages were extensively and repeatedly transferred among the isolates, indicating a very high frequency of horizontal gene transfer. Interestingly, bacterial populations differed considerably across pigs, implying limited transfer among the pigs in this study. In another study, nine human volunteers ingested an *E. coli* strain of human origin that carried resistance to rifampicin but was susceptible to sulfonamides. This was followed three hours later by ingestion of another *E. coli* strain, of pig origin and carrying sulfonamide resistance. Stool samples from the volunteers were collected 24 h prior to the challenge, and on days 1 to 7 as well as 14 and 35 after. Conjugation was detected on day 2 in one of the volunteers, mediated through the exchange of a plasmid containing the sulfonamide resistance gene *sul2*, and co-transfer of ampicillin resistance was also demonstrated. Notably, however, the *sul2* resistance gene was identical to one carried by commensal bacteria present in the gut of the volunteer before the experiment but differed from that carried by the pig strain, demonstrating the complexity of these types of investigations, in particular if the resident bacterial populations are not fully known or controlled. A number of other studies have also investigated the transfer of various resistance genes among a diverse group of bacteria in the guts of various animals and other environments and found ample evidence that resistance genes are readily transferred (see [117] for a review). In addition, phylogenetic studies provide further support for horizontal gene transfer of resistance by identifying virtually identical resistance genes in distantly related bacterial species from varying geographic regions [120].

Taken together, there is considerable evidence that resistant animal-associated commensals can and do, at least transiently, colonize humans that are in contact with the animals or, in some cases, their food and that these commensals can transfer resistance genes to human-associated commensals and to human pathogens. Notably, antimicrobial exposure seems to favor the selection and maintenance of conjugates with newly-acquired antimicrobial resistance genes, even though this selection pressure does not seem to be necessary in all cases. There is also strong evidence that the same resistance genes are present in bacteria from animals and humans. What has so far remained less clear is how frequently this transfer occurs under real-world conditions, what other factors such as management practices or antibiotic exposures favor or limit this transfer, exactly when, where and how the transfers occur, and what fraction of resistance genes present in populations of human pathogens originated in commensals on farms.

Excess morbidity and mortality caused by antimicrobial resistance traits that emerged on farms

To fully evaluate the impact of antimicrobial resistance as a public health burden, it is important to quantify the excess morbidity and mortality caused by the fact that a certain pathogen is resistant to antimicrobial drugs. This section focuses on antimicrobial resistant zoonotic and foodborne pathogens. However, the origin of resistance genes is complex and it is not clear that the resistance genes carried by these foodborne or zoonotic pathogens necessarily emerged in animal agriculture rather than other settings such as human healthcare. Regardless of the origin of the resistance genes, the studies are relevant to the question of whether infections with antimicrobial-resistant bacteria pose an increased public health risk.

For ethical reasons, RCTs comparing health outcomes associated with resistant as compared to susceptible human pathogens are not feasible. However, observational studies as well as other study types such as outbreak analyses are available. Observational studies typically compare outcomes such as hospitalizations or deaths among patients infected with resistant or susceptible strains.

A number of observational studies have compared health outcomes for patients infected with susceptible versus resistant strains of foodborne or zoonotic pathogens such as *Salmonella*, *Campylobacter* or *Staphylococcus aureus* (Table 7). One study in the U.S., for instance, compared the frequency of hospitalization and bloodstream infections in patients with resistant and susceptible *Salmonella* strains [121]. Resistant isolates were significantly more likely to be associated with bloodstream infections than susceptible isolates. For example, for serotype Typhimurium, 3% of patients infected with susceptible isolates had bloodstream infections, compared to 6% of patients infected with resistant strains. Patients infected with resistant isolates also were more likely to be hospitalized because of bloodstream infection than those infected with susceptible isolates. Among the hospitalized patients, those infected with resistant isolates had longer stays than those infected with susceptible isolates. Similar results were obtained in another U.S. based study of 875 patients with gastro-intestinal and bloodstream infections due to *Salmonella* [122]. Bloodstream infections and hospitalizations were significantly more likely among patients with resistant compared to susceptible *Salmonella* isolates. Results from yet another U.S. based study of patients infected with *Salmonella* further support this finding [123]. Patients with resistant infections were significantly more likely to be hospitalized than those with susceptible infections. Notably, recent antimicrobial treatment as well as age and race were significant predictors of resistance.

Another observational study, conducted in Canada to compare the risk of hospitalization in response to infection with resistant *Salmonella* Typhimurium strains found similar results [124]. Hospitalization was significantly more likely in patients infected with resistant compared to susceptible strains. In fact, an estimated 57–72% of hospitalizations were attributable to the resistance patterns. A Danish study of patients infected with *Salmonella* Typhimurium infections that occurred between 1995 and 1999 evaluated death rates in patients infected with *Salmonella* Typhimurium strains carrying various antimicrobial resistance genes [125]. For every patient enrolled in the study, 10 random controls were found, matched by age, sex and county of residence. Subjects were followed for up to 2 years. Patients with susceptible *Salmonella* Typhimurium infection were 2.3 times (95% CI 1.5 to 3.5) more likely to die during the study period than the general population. By comparison, patients infected with the most resistant strains were 4.8 times (95% CI: 2.2–10.2) more likely, and patients infected with quinolone-resistant isolates were 10.3 times (95% CI 2.8-37.8) more likely to die than the general population.

Similar results have also been obtained for other bacteria. One Danish study of *Campylobacter* infections, for instance, compared the risk of invasive illness and death within up to 90 days of sample collection in 3471 patients infected with quinolone and erythromycin resistant or susceptible strains [126]. Patients infected with quinolone-resistant *Campylobacter* strains had a 6-fold increased risk of invasive illness or death within 30 days of sample collection compared with patients infected with susceptible isolates. Similarly, infection with erythromycin-resistant *Campylobacter* strains was associated with more than a 5-fold higher risk within 90 days compared to infections with susceptible strains. A meta-analysis of cohort studies focused on patients with bloodstream infections due to *Staphylococcus aureus* in multiple countries found similar results [127]. Data from a total of 3963 patients from 31 individual studies were analyzed, comparing mortality rates due to infections with methicillin susceptible and resistant strains. A significantly increased mortality rate was associated with MRSA infections compared to methicillin –susceptible strains (OR: 1.93; 95% CI – 1.52 – 2.42). Data from outbreaks further support worse health outcomes for infections with resistant compared to susceptible strains (see for instance [128]), even though potential confounding effects such as virulence differences among strains or differences in exposed populations have to be considered.

Taken together, there is unequivocal evidence, from epidemiological studies, meta-analyses, and the analysis of outbreaks, that infections with antimicrobial resistant bacteria tend to be associated with worse public health outcomes than infections with susceptible strains. Notably, the impact appears to differ by pathogen as well as resistance involved [121, 126]. The underlying reasons may not always be clear, but can include delayed treatment onset, the need to choose less-desirable treatment options, and, at least in some cases, increased virulence of antimicrobial drug resistant strains because of co-selection for resistance and virulence genes. Regardless of what drives the increased public health cost, infections with antimicrobial resistant bacteria are a public health threat that needs to be addressed.

Conclusions

The review clearly demonstrates that there is ample scientific support, based on observational studies, a variety of

Table 7 Examples of study types evaluating the health impacts associated with human infections due to resistant as compared to susceptible bacterial strains

Reference	Study									Key findings relevant to antimicrobial resistance
	Type[a]	subjects	country	time period	bacterial target	relevant study outcomes	sample size	controls	comments	
GRADE level: Controlled trial										
n/a										
GRADE level: observational trial										
[121]	Cohort	Patients with *Salmonella* infections	US	1996–2001	*Salmonella*	Frequency of hospitalization and bloodstream infection	*n* = 1415 patients (FoodNet) and *n* = 7370 isolates (NARMS)	Patients infected with susceptible *Salmonella* strains	Two analyses were performed, one of *Salmonella* isolates collected through NARMS, and one of patients with NARMS *Salmonella* isolates and corresponding FoodNet interviews	Resistant isolates were more likely associated with bloodstream infections than susceptible isolates (for example, for serotype Typhimurium, 3% of patients infected with susceptible isolates had bloodstream infections, compared to 6% of patients infected with resistant strains); patients infected with resistant isolates were more likely to be hospitalized because of bloodstream infection than those infected with susceptible isolates; among hospitalized patients, those infected with resistant isolates had longer stays than those infected with susceptible isolates;
[122]	Cohort	Patients with *Salmonella* infections (bloodstream and GI infection)	US	2006–2008	*Salmonella*	Clinical outcomes	*n* = 875 patients	Patients infected with susceptible *Salmonella* strains		Bloodstream infections and hospitalizations more likely among patients with resistant than susceptible isolates
[123]	Cohort	Patients infected with *Salmonella*	US	1989–1990	*Salmonella*	Infection and hospitalization		Patients infected with susceptible *Salmonella* strains	Results were compared to similar study conducted in 1979–1980	Patients with resistant infections were more likely to be hospitalized than those with susceptible infections; recent antimicrobial treatment as well as age and race were significant predictors of resistance
[124]	Cohort	Patients with *Salmonella* infections	Canada	1999–2000	*Salmonella Typhimurium*	Risk of hospitalization	*n* = 440 patients	Patients infected with susceptible *Salmonella* strains		Hospitalization was more likely in patients infected with resistant than susceptible strains; an estimated 57–72% of hospitalizations were attributable to resistance patterns

Table 7 Examples of study types evaluating the health impacts associated with human infections due to resistant as compared to susceptible bacterial strains *(Continued)*

[125]	Cohort	Patients infected with *Salmonella* Typhimurium	Denmark	1995–1999	*Salmonella Typhimurium*	Death rates	N = 2047	10 random controls (matched by age, sex and county of residence); comparison between susceptible and resistant infections	Subjects were followed for up to 2 years after entering the study	Patients with susceptible *Salmonella* Typhimurium infection were 2.3 times more likely to die during the study period than the general population; patients with most resistant strains were 4.8 times (95% CI: 2.2–10.2) more likely; patients infected with quinolone-resistant isolates were 10.3 times more likely to die than the general population.
[126]	Cohort	Patients with *Campylobacter* infections	Denmark		*Campylobacter (quinolone and erythromycin-resistant)*	Risk of invasive illness and death within up to 90 days of sample receipt	n = 3471 patients	Patients infected with susceptible *Campylobacter* isolates		Patients infected with quinolone-resistant *Campylobacter* strains had a 6-fold increased risk of invasive illness or death within 30 days of sample collection compared with patients infected with susceptible isolates; infection with erythromycin-resistant *Campylobacter* strains was associated with >5-fold higher risk within 90 days compared to infections with susceptible strains
[127]	Meta-analysis of cohort studies	Studies of patients with bloodstream infection due to *Staph. aureus*	multiple countries	1980–2000	*Staphylococcus aureus, MRSA*	Mortality rates due to infections with methicillin susceptible and resistant *Staphylococcus aureus*	n = 3963 patients in n = 31 studies	Patients infected with methicillin susceptible strain	Results pooled with random effects model	Increased mortality associated with MRSA infections compared to methicillin –susceptible strains (OR: 1.93; 95% CI – 1.52 – 2.42)
GRADE level: other										
[128]	Outbreak analysis	Outbreaks of patients infected with *Salmonella*	US	1984–2002	*Salmonella*	Hospitalization due to infection with susceptible or resistant *Salmonella* strains	n = 23,206 patients in n = 32 outbreaks	Outbreaks with susceptible *Salmonella* strains		The median proportion hospitalized for each type of outbreak caused by resistant strains was 26%, 2.5 times higher than the median proportion hospitalized for outbreaks caused by pan-susceptible strains

[a] *CC* case-control study (or case-case study where controls are cases of infection with other strains), *CS* cross-sectional study

other relevant scientific evidence, and, where ethically feasible, also RCTs to support each step in the causal pathway from antimicrobial use on farms to the public health burden caused by antimicrobial resistant infections in humans. These studies reach across the major food-producing species and a variety of bacterial species including *Salmonella*, *Campylobacter*, *E. coli* and *Enterococci* even though there seem to be some important differences among the bacterial species and data are not readily available for all bacterial species and antimicrobial drugs of interest. Yet, taken together, the data support what the scientific community, national governments, and international organizations such as the World Health Organization, the Food and Agricultural Organization of the United Nations, and the World Organization for the Health of Animals (OIE) have long recognized: antimicrobial use on farms clearly contributes to the emergence of resistance and poses a human public health risk.

Because the molecular and evolutionary determinants of antimicrobial resistance are complex, resistance does not strictly follow a simple epidemiological model of causation; rather, a more sophisticated model typically used for chronic diseases applies. For example, antimicrobial use may not in all cases lead to the immediate emergence of resistance, and its discontinuation may not lead to an immediate drop in resistance. The antimicrobial drug and treatment regimen as well as external factors such as the feed type used on a given operation can have significant impacts on resistance, and rates of resistance emergence may be markedly different across bacterial species or even strains.

Bacterial resistance genes can be readily shared across bacteria, and some may be pre-existing or persist in environmental reservoirs such as soils. Tracing their origin back across bacterial backgrounds is challenging, even though technological advances such as whole-genome sequencing and more advanced phylogenetic and population genetic models make their trace-back increasingly feasible. Currently, it may be impossible to exactly quantify the contribution of animal agriculture to the overall burden of resistance, but this goal is becoming increasingly feasible.

Importantly, even if some data gaps remain to be filled, there is no doubt that antimicrobial use on farms or feedlots contributes to the problem of antimicrobial resistance. It is therefore important to take action now to ensure antimicrobial drugs are used judiciously, and only when needed to ensure animal health and well-being. Almost 50 years have passed since the Swann report called for the discontinuation of growth promotion uses for medically important antibiotics, and the practice has just now been phased out in the U.S. Many of the studies reviewed here are not new – in fact, many well-designed, compelling studies were published more than 20 or 30 years ago. Time is running out on curtailing antimicrobial resistance. Antimicrobial use on farms contributes to the burden of antimicrobial resistance. Science has shown it, many times over, and stakeholders around the world have come to accept it. It is time to move the public debate away from the problem to its potential solutions.

Abbreviations

GRADE: Grades of recommendations assessment, development and evaluation; HGT: Horizontal gene transfer; JETACAR: Joint expert technical advisory committee on antibiotic resistance; MIC: Minimum inhibitory concentration; MRSA: Methicillin resistant *Staphylococcus aureus*; OIE: World Organization for Animal Health; RCT: Randomized controlled trial; VRE: Vancomycin resistant *Enterococci*

Acknowledgements

Not applicable.

Authors' contributions

KH, KT, EJ and AC conceived the study. KH, NW and JT provided analysis for the manuscript. KH drafted the manuscript. KT, EJ and AC critically and substantially revised the manuscript. All authors approved the manuscript.

Competing interests

The authors declare that they have no competing interests.

References

1. U.S. Centers for Disease Control and Prevention. Antibiotic Resistance Threats in the United States, 2013. Atlanta: U.S. Department of Health and Human Services. 2013. https://www.cdc.gov/drugresistance/pdf/ar-threats-2013-508.pdf.
2. McEwen SA, Fedorka-Cray PJ. Antimicrobial use and resistance in animals. Clin Infect Dis. 2002;34(Supplement 3):S93–S106.
3. Marshall BM, Levy SB. Food animals and antimicrobials: impacts on human health. Clin Microbiol Rev. 2011;24(4):718–33.
4. Codex Alimentarius. Code of Practice to Minimize and Contain Antimicrobial Resistance. List of Standards- FAO. CAC/RCP 61–2005. www.fao.org/input/download/standards/10213/CXP_061e.pdf. Accessed 10 Apr 2017.
5. Casewell M, Friis C, Marco E, McMullin P, Phillips I. The European ban on growth-promoting antibiotics and emerging consequences for human and animal health. J Antimicrob Chemother. 2003;52(2):159–61.
6. World Health Organization. Critically important antimicrobials for human medicine. 4th revision. 2016. p. 1–31.
7. European Commission. Ban on antibiotics as growth promoters in animal feed enters into effect. European Commission. 2005. http://europa.eu/rapid/press-release_IP-05-1687_en.htm. Accessed 28 June 2017.
8. Food and Drug Administration. Guidance for Industry #152. Center for Veterinary Medicine. 2003. p. 1–35. https://www.fda.gov/downloads/AnimalVeterinary/GuidanceComplianceEnforcement/GuidanceforIndustry/UCM052519.pdf.
9. Moulin G, Góchez, D, Lasley J, Erlacher-Vindel E. OIE Annual report on the use of antimicrobial agents in animals. OIE. 2016. p. 1–65. http://www.oie.int/fileadmin/Home/fr/Our_scientific_expertise/docs/pdf/AMR/Survey_on_monitoring_antimicrobial_agents_Dec2016.pdf.
10. Food and Drug Administration. FDA's CVM Key Initiatives for Antimicrobial Stewardship. https://www.fda.gov/AnimalVeterinary/SafetyHealth/

AntimicrobialResistance/JudiciousUseofAntimicrobials/ucm535158.htm. Accessed 11 April 2017.
11. MacGowan AP. Clinical implications of antimicrobial resistance for therapy. J Antimicrob Chemother. 2008;62(suppl 2):ii105–14.
12. Levy SB, Marshall B. Antibacterial resistance worldwide: causes, challenges and responses. Nat Med. 2004;
13. Parascandola M, Weed DL. Causation in epidemiology. J Epidemiol Community Health. 2001;55(12):905–12.
14. Davies J, Davies D. Origins and evolution of antibiotic resistance. Microbiol Mol Biol Rev. 2010;74(3):417–33.
15. Tavares LS, Silva CS, de Souza VC, da Silva VL, Diniz CG, Santos MO. Strategies and molecular tools to fight antimicrobial resistance: resistome, transcriptome, and antimicrobial peptides. Front Microbiol. 2013;4:412.
16. Rothman KJ. Causal inference in epidemiology. Modern Epidemiology. Boston: Little, Brown and Company. 1986;7–21.
17. Tlaskalová-Hogenová H, Štěpánková R, Hudcovic T, Tučková L, Cukrowska B, Lodinová-Zádníková R, et al. Commensal bacteria (normal microflora), mucosal immunity and chronic inflammatory and autoimmune diseases. Immunol Lett. 2004;93(2–3):97–108.
18. Huddleston JR. Horizontal gene transfer in the human gastrointestinal tract: potential spread of antibiotic resistance genes. Infect Drug Resist. 2014;7:167–76.
19. Casey JA, Curriero FC, Cosgrove SE, Nachman KE, Schwartz BS. High-density livestock operations, crop field application of manure, and risk of community-associated methicillin-resistant *Staphylococcus aureus* infection in Pennsylvania. JAMA Intern Med. 2013;173(21):1980–90.
20. Rule AM, Evans SL, Silbergeld EK. Food animal transport: a potential source of community exposures to health hazards from industrial farming (CAFOs). J Infect Public Health. 2008;1(1):33–9.
21. McEachran AD, Blackwell BR, Hanson JD, Wooten KJ, Mayer GD, Cox SB, Smith PN. Antibiotics, bacteria, and antibiotic resistance genes: aerial transport from cattle feed yards via particulate matter. Environmental Health Perspectives. 2015;123(4):337.
22. Ward MJ, Gibbons CL, McAdam PR, Van Bunnik BAD, Girvan EK, Edwards GF, et al. Time-scaled evolutionary analysis of the transmission and antibiotic resistance dynamics of *Staphylococcus aureus* clonal complex 398. Appl Environ Microbiol. 2014;80(23):7275–82.
23. Pantosti A. Methicillin-resistant Staphylococcus aureus associated with animals and its relevance to human health. Frontiers in Microbiology. 2012; 3:127.
24. van Rijen MML, Bosch T, Verkade EJM, Schouls L, Kluytmans JAJW. On behalf of the CAMSG. Livestock-associated MRSA carriage in patients without direct contact with livestock. PLoS One. 2014;9(6):e100294.
25. Barza M. Potential mechanisms of increased disease in humans from antimicrobial resistance in food animals. Clin Infect Dis. 2002;34(Supplement 3):S123–5.
26. Eliopoulos GM, Cosgrove SE, Carmeli Y. The impact of antimicrobial resistance on health and economic outcomes. Clin Infect Dis. 2003;36(11): 1433–7.
27. Travers K, Michael B. Morbidity of infections caused by antimicrobial-resistant bacteria. Clin Infect Dis. 2002;34(Supplement 3):S131–4.
28. Kaye KS, Engemann JJ, Mozaffari E, Carmeli Y. Reference group choice and antibiotic resistance outcomes. Emerg Infect Dis. 2004;10(6):1125–8.
29. Jones TF, Ingram LA, Cieslak PR, Vugia DJ, Tobin-D'Angelo M, Hurd S, et al. Salmonellosis outcomes differ substantially by serotype. J Infect Dis. 2008; 198(1):109–14.
30. Oxman AD, Group GW. Grading quality of evidence and strength of recommendations. BMJ. 2004;328(19):1490–4.
31. GRADE Working Group. http://www.gradeworkinggroup.org/. Accessed 12 July 2016.
32. Ferguson JK, Dalton CB, McGettigan P, Hill S. Antimicrobial resistance in animal enteric bacteria and human disease—a review of the scientific literature. Commissioned Report Jt Expert Tech Advis Comm Antibiot Resist (JETACAR) Canberra. 1998;
33. Australian Government Department of Health. The Use of Antibiotics in Food-Producing Animals: Antibiotic-Resistant Bacteria in Animals and Humans. Commonwealth of Australia. 2014. http://www.health.gov.au/internet/main/publishing.nsf/content/health-pubs-jetacar-cnt.htm. Accessed 28 June 2017.
34. Andreoletti O, Budka H, Buncic S, Colin P, Collins JD, De Koeijer A, Griffin J, Havelaar A, Hope J, Klein G, Kruse H. Foodborne antimicrobial resistance as a biological hazard. EFSA J. 2008;765:2–87.
35. Chauvin C, Querrec M, Perot A, Guillemot D, Sanders P. Impact of antimicrobial drug usage measures on the identification of heavy users, patterns of usage of the different antimicrobial classes and time-trends evolution. J Vet Pharmacol Ther. 2008;31(4):301–11.
36. Jensen VF, Jacobsen E, Bager F. Veterinary antimicrobial-usage statistics based on standardized measures of dosage. Prev Vet Med. 2004;64(2–4):201–15.
37. Timmerman T, Dewulf J, Catry B, Feyen B, Opsomer G. Kruif ad, Maes D. Quantification and evaluation of antimicrobial drug use in group treatments for fattening pigs in Belgium. Prev Vet Med. 2006;74(4):251–63.
38. Gow SP, Waldner CL. Antimicrobial drug use and reason for treatment in 203 western Canadian cow-calf herds during calving season. Prev Vet Med. 2009;90(1–2):55–65.
39. Merle R, Mollenhauer Y, Hajek P, Robanus M, Hegger-Gravenhorst C, Honscha W, et al. Monitoring of antibiotic consumption in cattle on agricultural farms. Berliner und Munchener tierarztliche Wochenschrift. 2013; 126(7–8):318–25.
40. Thomson K, Rantala M, Hautala M, Pyörälä S, Kaartinen L. Cross-sectional prospective survey to study indication-based usage of antimicrobials in animals: results of use in cattle. BMC Vet Res. 2008;4(1):1.
41. Zwald AG, Ruegg PL, Kaneene JB, Warnick LD, Wells SJ, Fossler C, et al. Management practices and reported antimicrobial usage on conventional and organic dairy farms. J Dairy Sci. 2004;87(1):191–201.
42. Carrique-Mas JJ, Trung NV, Hoa NT, Mai HH, Thanh TH, Campbell JI, et al. Antimicrobial usage in chicken production in the Mekong Delta of Vietnam. Zoonoses Public Health. 2015;62:70–8.
43. National Animal Health Monitoring System (NAHMS). https://www.aphis.usda.gov/aphis/ourfocus/animalhealth/monitoring-and-surveillance/nahms. Accessed 12 July 2016.
44. Kim DP, Saegerman C, Douny C, Dinh TV, Xuan BH, Vu BD, et al. First survey on the use of antibiotics in pig and poultry production in the Red River Delta region of Vietnam. Food Public Health. 2013;3(5):247–56.
45. Agricultural Resource Management Survey (ARMS). http://www.ers.usda.gov/data-products/arms-farm-financial-and-crop-production-practices/arms-data.aspx. Accessed 12 July 2016.
46. McDermott PF, Bodeis SM, English LL, White DG, Walker RD, Zhao S, et al. Ciprofloxacin resistance in campylobacter jejuni evolves rapidly in chickens treated with fluoroquinolones. J Infect Dis. 2002;185(6):837–40.
47. Delsol AA, Anjum M, Woodward MJ, Sunderland J, Roe JM. The effect of chlortetracycline treatment and its subsequent withdrawal on multi-resistant salmonella enterica serovar Typhimurium DT104 and commensal *Escherichia coli* in the pig. J Appl Microbiol. 2003;95(6):1226–34.
48. Mathew AG, Jackson F, Saxton AM. Effects of antibiotic regimens on resistance of *Escherichia coli* and salmonella serovar Typhimurium in swine. J Swine Health Prod. 2002;10(1):7–14.
49. Jacobs-Reitsma WF, Kan CA, Bolder NM. The induction of quinolone resistance in campylobacter bacteria in broilers by quinolone treatment. Lett Appl Microbiol. 1994;19(4):228–31.
50. Inglis GD, McAllister TA, Busz HW, Yanke LJ, Morck DW, Olson ME, et al. Effects of subtherapeutic administration of antimicrobial agents to beef cattle on the prevalence of antimicrobial resistance in campylobacter jejuni and campylobacter hyointestinalis. Appl Environ Microbiol. 2005; 71(7):3872–81.
51. Mathew AG, Garner KN, Ebner PD, Saxton AM, Clift RE, Liamthong S. Effects of antibiotic use in sows on resistance of *E. coli* and salmonella enterica Typhimurium in their offspring. Foodborne Pathog Dis. 2005;2(3):212–20.
52. Delsol AA, Sunderland J, Woodward MJ, Pumbwe L, Piddock LJ, Roe JM. Emergence of fluoroquinolone resistance in the native campylobacter coli population of pigs exposed to enrofloxacin. J Antimicrob Chemother. 2004 May 1;53(5):872–4.
53. Ebner PD, Mathew AG. Effects of antibiotic regimens on the fecal shedding patterns of pigs infected with salmonella Typhimurium. J Food Prot. 2000 Jun;63(6):709–14.
54. Ray KA, Warnick LD, Mitchell RM, Kaneene JB, Ruegg PL, Wells SJ, et al. Antimicrobial susceptibility of salmonella from organic and conventional dairy farms. J Dairy Sci. 2006;89(6):2038–50.
55. Sato K, Bartlett PC, Kaneene JB, Downes FP. Comparison of prevalence and antimicrobial susceptibilities of campylobacter spp. isolates from organic and conventional dairy herds in Wisconsin. Appl Environ Microbiol. 2004; 70(3):1442–7.
56. Luangtongkum T, Morishita TY, Ison AJ, Huang S, McDermott PF, Zhang Q. Effect of conventional and organic production practices on the prevalence

and antimicrobial resistance of campylobacter spp. in poultry. Appl Environ Microbiol. 2006;72(5):3600–7.

57. Griggs DJ, Johnson MM, Frost JA, Humphrey T, Jørgensen F, Piddock LJV. Incidence and mechanism of ciprofloxacin resistance in campylobacter spp. isolated from commercial poultry flocks in the United Kingdom before, during, and after fluoroquinolone treatment. Antimicrob Agents Chemother. 2005;49(2):699–707.
58. Avrain L, Humbert F, L'Hospitalier R, Sanders P, Vernozy-Rozand C, Kempf I. Antimicrobial resistance in campylobacter from broilers: association with production type and antimicrobial use. Vet Microbiol. 2003;96(3):267–76.
59. Price LB, Leila GL, Vailes R, Silbergeld E. The persistence of Fluoroquinolone-resistant campylobacter in poultry production. Environ Health Perspect. 2007;115(7):1035–9.
60. Klare I, Badstübner D, Konstabel C, Böhme G, Claus H, Witte W. Decreased incidence of VanA-type vancomycin-resistant enterococci isolated from poultry meat and from fecal samples of humans in the community after discontinuation of avoparcin usage in animal husbandry. Microb Drug Resist. 1999;5(1):45–52.
61. Endtz HP, Ruijs GJ, van Klingeren B, Jansen WH, van der Reyden T, Mouton RP. Quinolone resistance in campylobacter isolated from man and poultry following the introduction of fluoroquinolones in veterinary medicine. J Antimicrob Chemother. 1991;27(2):199–208.
62. Desmonts M-H, Dufour-Gesbert F, Avrain L, Kempf I. Antimicrobial resistance in campylobacter strains isolated from French broilers before and after antimicrobial growth promoter bans. J Antimicrob Chemother. 2004;54(6):1025–30.
63. Dutil L. Ceftiofur Resistance in Salmonella enterica Serovar Heidelberg from Chicken Meat and Humans, Canada-Volume 16, Number 1—January 2010-Emerging Infectious Disease journal-CDC.
64. Boerlin P, Wissing A, Aarestrup FM, Frey J, Nicolet J. Antimicrobial growth promoter ban and resistance to Macrolides and Vancomycin in Enterococci from pigs. J Clin Microbiol. 2001;39(11):4193–5.
65. Alexander TW, Yanke LJ, Topp E, Olson ME, Read RR, Morck DW, et al. Effect of subtherapeutic administration of antibiotics on the prevalence of antibiotic-resistant *Escherichia coli* bacteria in feedlot cattle. Appl Environ Microbiol. 2008;74(14):4405–16.
66. Berge ACB, Epperson WB, Pritchard RH. Assessing the effect of a single dose florfenicol treatment in feedlot cattle on the antimicrobial resistance patterns in faecal *Escherichia coli*. Vet Res. 2005;36(5–6):723–34.
67. Kanwar N, Scott HM, Norby B, Loneragan GH, Vinasco-Torres J, Cottell JL, et al. Impact of treatment strategies on cephalosporin and tetracycline resistance gene quantities in the bovine fecal metagenome. Sci Rep. 2014 Jul 23;4(Article number: 5100):1–0.
68. Aarestrup FM, Carstensen B. Effect of tylosin used as a growth promoter on the occurrence of macrolide-resistant enterococci and staphylococci in pigs. Microb Drug Resist. 1998;4(4):307–12.
69. Linton AH, Hedges AJ, Bennett PM. Monitoring for the development of antimicrobial resistance during the use of olaquindox as a feed additive on commercial pig farms. J Appl Bacteriol. 1988;64(4):311–27.
70. Dunlop RH, McEwen SA, Meek AH, Clarke RC, Black WD, Friendship RM. Associations among antimicrobial drug treatments and antimicrobial resistance of fecal *Escherichia coli* of swine on 34 farrow-to-finish farms in Ontario, Canada. Prev Vet Med. 1998;34(4):283–305.
71. Akwar HT, Poppe C, Wilson J, Reid-Smith RJ, Dyck M, Waddington J, et al. Associations of antimicrobial uses with antimicrobial resistance of fecal *Escherichia coli* from pigs on 47 farrow-to-finish farms in Ontario and British Columbia. Canadian J Vet Res = Revue Canadienne De Recherche Veterinaire. 2008;72(2):202–10.
72. Chantziaras I, Boyen F, Callens B, Dewulf J. Correlation between veterinary antimicrobial use and antimicrobial resistance in food-producing animals: a report on seven countries. J Antimicrob Chemother. 2014;69(3):827–34.
73. Pantosti A, Del Grosso M, Tagliabue S, Macri A, Caprioli A. Decrease of vancomycin-resistant enterococci in poultry meat after avoparcin ban. Lancet. 1999;354(9180):741–2.
74. Zilberberg MD, Chen J, Mody SH, Ramsey AM, Shorr AF. Imipenem resistance of pseudomonas in pneumonia: a systematic literature review. BMC Pulm Med. 2010;10:45.72.
75. Bliziotis IA, Samonis G, Vardakas KZ, Chrysanthopoulou S, Falagas ME. Effect of aminoglycoside and β-lactam combination therapy versus β-lactam monotherapy on the emergence of antimicrobial resistance: a meta-analysis of randomized, controlled trials. Clin Infect Dis. 2005;41(2):149–58.
76. Costelloe C, Metcalfe C, Lovering A, Mant D, Hay AD. Effect of antibiotic prescribing in primary care on antimicrobial resistance in individual patients: systematic review and meta-analysis. BMJ. 2010;340
77. Carmeli Y, Troillet N, Eliopoulos GM, Samore MH. Emergence of antibiotic-resistant Pseudomonas Aeruginosa: comparison of risks associated with different antipseudomonal agents. Antimicrob Agents Chemother. 1999; 43(6):1379–82.
78. Harbarth S, Samore MH, Lichtenberg D, Carmeli Y. Prolonged antibiotic prophylaxis after cardiovascular surgery and its effect on surgical site infections and antimicrobial resistance. Circulation. 2000;101(25):2916–21.
79. El Amari EB, Chamot E, Auckenthaler R, Pechère JC, Van Delden C. Influence of previous exposure to antibiotic therapy on the susceptibility pattern of Pseudomonas Aeruginosa Bacteremic isolates. Clin Infect Dis. 2001;33(11):1859–64.
80. Pechere JC, Marchou B, Michea-Hamzehpour M, Auckenthaler R. Emergence of resistance after therapy with antibiotics used alone or combined in a marine model. J Antimicrob Chemother. 1986;17(suppl A):11–8.
81. Tan C-H, Li J, Nation RL. Activity of colistin against heteroresistant Acinetobacter Baumannii and emergence of resistance in an in vitro pharmacokinetic/pharmacodynamic model. Antimicrob Agents Chemother. 2007;51(9):3413–5.
82. Goossens H, Ferech M, Vander Stichele R, Elseviers M. Outpatient antibiotic use in Europe and association with resistance: a cross-national database study. Lancet. 365(9459):579–87.
83. Olofsson SK, Cars O. Optimizing drug exposure to minimize selection of antibiotic resistance. Clin Infect Dis. 2007;45(Supplement 2):S129–36.
84. Melnyk AH, Wong A, Kassen R. The fitness costs of antibiotic resistance mutations. Evol Appl. 2015;8(3):273–83.
85. Cometta A, Baumgartner JD, Lew D, Zimmerli W, Pittet D, Chopart P, et al. Prospective randomized comparison of imipenem monotherapy with imipenem plus netilmicin for treatment of severe infections in nonneutropenic patients. Antimicrob Agents Chemother. 1994;38(6):1309–1313.83.
86. Geli P, Laxminarayan R, Dunne M, Smith DL. "one-size-fits-all"? Optimizing treatment duration for bacterial infections. PLoS One. 2012;7(1):e29838.
87. Gupta A, Fontana J, Crowe C, Bolstorff B, Stout A, Duyne SV, et al. Emergence of multidrug-resistant salmonella enterica serotype Newport infections resistant to expanded-Spectrum Cephalosporins in the United States. J Infect Dis. 2003;188(11):1707–1716.85.
88. Varma JK, Marcus R, Stenzel SA, Hanna SS, Gettner S, Anderson BJ, et al. Highly resistant salmonella Newport-MDRAmpC transmitted through the domestic US food supply: a FoodNet case-control study of sporadic salmonella Newport infections, 2002–2003. J Infect Dis. 2006;194(2):222–30.
89. Karon AE, Archer JR, Sotir MJ, Monson TA, Kazmierczak JJ. Human multidrug-resistant salmonella Newport infections, Wisconsin, 2003-2005. Emerg Infect Dis. 2007;13(11):1777.87.
90. Spika JS, Waterman SH, Hoo GWS, St. Louis ME, Pacer RE, James SM, et al. Chloramphenicol-resistant salmonella newport traced through hamburger to dairy farms. N Engl J Med. 1987;316(10):565–570.88.
91. van Loo I, Huijsdens X, Tiemersma E, de Neeling A, van de Sande-Bruinsma N, Beaujean D, et al. Emergence of methicillin-resistant *Staphylococcus aureus* of animal origin in humans. Emerg Infect Dis. 2007;13(12):1834–9.
92. Graveland H, Wagenaar JA, Heesterbeek H, Mevius D, van Duijkeren E, Heederik D. Methicillin resistant *Staphylococcus aureus* ST398 in veal calf farming: human MRSA carriage related with animal antimicrobial usage and farm hygiene. PLoS One. 2010;5(6):e10990.
93. Denis O, Suetens C, Hallin M, Catry B, Ramboer I, Dispas M, et al. Methicillin-resistant *Staphylococcus aureus* ST398 in swine farm personnel, Belgium. Emerg Infect Dis. 2009;15(7):1098–101.
94. Mølbak K, Baggesen DL, Aarestrup FM, Ebbesen JM, Engberg J, Frydendahl K, et al. An outbreak of multidrug-resistant, Quinolone-resistant salmonella enterica serotype Typhimurium DT104. N Engl J Med. 1999;341(19):1420–5.
95. Holmberg SD, Osterholm MT, Senger KA, Cohen ML. Drug-resistant salmonella from animals fed antimicrobials. N Engl J Med. 1984;311(10):617–22.
96. Fey PD, Safranek TJ, Rupp ME, Dunne EF, Ribot E, Iwen PC, et al. Ceftriaxone-resistant salmonella infection acquired by a child from cattle. N Engl J Med. 2000;342(17):1242–9.

97. Huijsdens XW, van Dijke BJ, Spalburg E, van Santen-Verheuvel MG, Heck ME, Pluister GN, et al. Community-acquired MRSA and pig-farming. Ann Clin Microbiol Antimicrob. 2006;5(1):1–4.
98. Smith TC, Male MJ, Harper AL, Kroeger JS, Tinkler GP, Moritz ED, et al. Methicillin-resistant *Staphylococcus aureus* (MRSA) strain ST398 is present in Midwestern U.S. swine and swine workers. PLoS One. 2009;4(1):e4258.
99. Juhasz-Kaszanyitzky E, Janosi S, Somogyi P, Dan A, van der Graaf-van Bloois L, van Duijkeren E, et al. MRSA transmission between cows and humans. Emerg Infect Dis. 2007;13(4):630–2.
100. Ojeniyi AA. Direct transmission of *Escherichia coli* from poultry to humans. Epidemiol Infect. 1989;103(03):513–22.
101. Levy SB. Emergence of antibiotic-resistant bacteria in the intestinal Flora of farm inhabitants. J Infect Dis. 1978;137(5):688–90.
102. Levy SB, FitzGerald GB, Macone AB. Changes in intestinal Flora of farm personnel after introduction of a tetracycline-supplemented feed on a farm. N Engl J Med. 1976;295(11):583–8.
103. Nijsten R, London N, Bogaard AVD, Stobberingh E. Resistance in faecal *Escherichia coli* isolated from pigfarmers and abattoir workers. Epidemiol Infect. 1994;113(01):45–52.
104. Van den Bogaard AE, London N, Driessen C, Stobberingh EE. Antibiotic resistance of faecal *Escherichia coli* in poultry, poultry farmers and poultry slaughterers. J Antimicrob Chemother. 2001;47(6):763–71.
105. Marshall B, Petrowski D, Levy SB. Inter- and Intraspecies spread of *Escherichia coli* in a farm environment in the absence of antibiotic usage. Proc Natl Acad Sci U S A. 1990;87(17):6609–13.
106. Linton AH, Howe K, Bennett PM, Richmond MH, Whiteside EJ. The colonization of the human gut by antibiotic resistant *Escherichia coli* from chickens. J Appl Bacteriol. 1977;43(3):465–9.
107. Kruse H, Sørum H. Transfer of multiple drug resistance plasmids between bacteria of diverse origins in natural microenvironments. Appl Environ Microbiol. 1994;60(11):4015–21.
108. Blake DP, Hillman K, Fenlon DR, Low JC. Transfer of antibiotic resistance between commensal and pathogenic members of the Enterobacteriaceae under ileal conditions. J Appl Microbiol. 2003;95(3):428–36.
109. Moubareck C, Bourgeois N, Courvalin P, Doucet-Populaire F. Multiple antibiotic resistance gene transfer from animal to human enterococci in the digestive tract of gnotobiotic mice. Antimicrob Agents Chemother. 2003; 47(9):2993–6.
110. Dahl KH, Mater DDG, Flores MJ, Johnsen PJ, Midtvedt T, Corthier G, et al. Transfer of plasmid and chromosomal glycopeptide resistance determinants occurs more readily in the digestive tract of mice than in vitro and exconjugants can persist stably in vivo in the absence of glycopeptide selection. J Antimicrob Chemother. 2007;59(3):478–86.
111. Lester CH, Frimodt-Møller N, Sørensen TL, Monnet DL, Hammerum AM. In vivo transfer of the vanA resistance gene from an Enterococcus faecium isolate of animal origin to an E. Faecium isolate of human origin in the intestines of human volunteers. Antimicrob Agents Chemother. 2006;50(2):596–9.
112. Schjørring S, Struve C, Krogfelt KA. Transfer of antimicrobial resistance plasmids from *Klebsiella pneumoniae* to *Escherichia coli* in the mouse intestine. J Antimicrob Chemother. 2008;62(5):1086–93.
113. Hirsh DC, Wiger N. The effect of tetracycline upon the spread of bacterial resistance from calves to man. J Anim Sci. 1978;46(5):1437–46.
114. Oppegaard H, Steinum TM, Wasteson Y. Horizontal transfer of a multi-drug resistance plasmid between coliform bacteria of human and bovine origin in a farm environment. Appl Environ Microbiol. 2001;67(8):3732–4.
115. Simonsen GS, Haaheim H, Dahl KH, Kruse H, Løvseth A, Olsvik Ø, et al. Transmission of VanA-type vancomycin-resistant enterococci and vanA resistance elements between chicken and humans at avoparcin-exposed farms. Microb Drug Resist. 1998;4(4):313–8.
116. Dorn CR, Tsutakawa RK, Fein D, Burton GC, Blenden DC. Antibiotic resistance patterns of *Escherichia coli* isolated from farm families consuming home-raised meat. Am J Epidemiol. 1975;102(4):319–26.
117. Huddleston JR. Horizontal gene transfer in the human gastrointestinal tract: potential spread of antibiotic resistance genes. Infect Drug Resist. 2014 Jun 20;7:167–76.
118. Trobos M, Lester CH, Olsen JE, Frimodt-Møller N, Hammerum AM. Natural transfer of sulphonamide and ampicillin resistance between *Escherichia coli* residing in the human intestine. J Antimicrob Chemother. 2009 Jan 1;63(1):80–6.
119. McCarthy AJ, Loeffler A, Witney AA, Gould KA Lloyd DH, Lindsay JA. Extensive horizontal gene transfer during *Staphylococcus aureus* co-colonization in vivo. Genome Biol Evol. 2014 Oct 1;6(10):2697–708.
120. Nikolich MP, Hong G, Shoemaker NB, Salyers AA. Evidence for natural horizontal transfer of tetQ between bacteria that normally colonize humans and bacteria that normally colonize livestock. Appl Environ Microbiol. 1994; 60(9):3255–60.
121. Varma JK, Mølbak K, Barrett TJ, Beebe JL, Jones TF, Rabatsky-Ehr T, et al. Antimicrobial-resistant nontyphoidal salmonella is associated with excess bloodstream infections and hospitalizations. J Infect Dis. 2005;191(4):554–61.
122. Krueger AL, Greene SA, Barzilay EJ, Henao O, Vugia D, Hanna S, et al. Clinical outcomes of Nalidixic acid, Ceftriaxone, and multidrug-resistant Nontyphoidal salmonella infections compared with Pansusceptible infections in FoodNet sites, 2006–2008. Foodborne Pathog Dis. 2014l;11(5):335–41.
123. Lee LA, Puhr ND, Maloney EK, Bean NH, Tauxe RV. Increase in antimicrobial-resistant salmonella infections in the United States, 1989–1990. J Infect Dis. 1994;170(1):128–34.
124. Martin LJ, Fyfe M, Doré K, Buxton JA, Pollari F, Henry B, et al. Increased burden of illness associated with antimicrobial-resistant salmonella enterica serotype Typhimurium infections. J Infect Dis. 2004;189(3):377–84.
125. Helms M, Vastrup P, Gerner-Smidt P, Molbak K. Excess mortality associated with antimicrobial drug-resistant salmonella typhimurium. Emerg Infect Dis. 2002;8(5):490–5.
126. Helms M, Simonsen J, Olsen KEP, Mølbak K. Adverse health events associated with antimicrobial drug resistance in campylobacter species: a registry-based cohort study. J Infect Dis. 2005;191(7):1050–5.
127. Cosgrove SE, Sakoulas G, Perencevich EN, Schwaber MJ, Karchmer AW, Carmeli Y. Comparison of mortality associated with methicillin-resistant and methicillin-susceptible *Staphylococcus aureus* bacteremia: a meta-analysis. Clin Infect Dis. 2003;36(1):53–9.
128. Jay KV, Katherine DG, Jessa O, Timothy JB, Felicita M, Frederick JA. Hospitalization and Antimicrobial Resistance in Salmonella Outbreaks, 1984–2002. Emerg Infect Dis J. 2005;11(6):943.
129. ADUFA Reports. http://www.fda.gov/ForIndustry/UserFees/AnimalDrugUserFeeActADUFA/ucm042896.htm. Accessed 12 July 2016.
130. Funk JA, Lejeune JT, Wittum TE, Rajala-Schultz PJ. The effect of subtherapeutic chlortetracycline on antimicrobial resistance in the fecal flora of swine. Microb Drug Resist. 2006;12(3):210–8.

9

Elimination kinetics of eugenol in grass carp in a simulated transportation setting

Dong-Hao Zhao[1,2,3,4†], Chang-Liang Ke[1,2,3,4†], Qi Liu[1,2,3,4], Xu-Feng Wang[1,2,3,4], Qiang Wang[1,2,3,4] and Liu-Dong Li[1,2,3,4*]

Abstract

Background: Fish are vulnerable to stress from over-crowding during transportation and eugenol is the most common sedative used to minimize fish injury. The ADI value of 2.5 mg/kg is recommended by the Joint FAO/WHO Expert Committee on Food Additives. The aim of this work was to study the elimination kinetics of eugenol following exposure of grass carp to a eugenol bath in a simulated transportation setting.

Results: Grass carp, *Ctenopharyngodon idella* (120 fish) were exposed for 24 h to a 10 mg/L eugenol bath. Sampling was performed during a 96 h period after the 24 h bath. Eight fish were sampled at each time point and muscle, plasma and liver concentrations of the drug were determined by ultra-performance liquid chromatography-tandem mass spectrometry. The concentration-time data of eugenol in each tissue were analyzed using non-compartmental methods. The peak concentrations (C_{max}) in plasma, muscle and liver were 7.68, 5.30 and 24.63 mg/kg and the elimination half-lives ($t_{1/2\beta}$) were 19.79, 10.27 and 55.28 h, respectively. The clearance (CL) values were 0.10, 0.44 and 0.04 L/h/kg and the areas under the concentration-time curve ($AUC_{0\text{-}96h}$) were 91.54, 22.44, and 214.12 mg·h/L in plasma, muscle and liver, respectively. After a eugenol exposure bath, drug concentrations in muscle tissue of grass carp were below 1 mg/kg at 8 h and 0.1 mg/kg at 24 h.

Conclusions: The drug concentrations in muscle tissue at 8 h were lower than the recommended ADI value.

Keywords: *Ctenopharyngodon idella*, Clove oil, Anesthetic, Food safety risk, Drug elimination

Background

Eugenol (2-Methoxy-4-(2-propen-1-yl) phenol) and its derivatives isoeugenol and methyleugenol (Fig. 1) are volatile oils extracted from flower buds, leaves and stems of clove, nutmeg, cinnamon, basil and myrcia [1, 2]. The yellowish or colorless liquid has an intense aromatic odor of cloves, is approved as a food additive, and is a Generally Recognized as Safe (GRAS) compound in the United States and European Union [3, 4]. In addition, eugenol has been widely used in dentistry due to its anesthetic and disinfection functions that are active against the bacteria causing gingivitis and dental plaque [5]. Eugenol is also used as a fish sedative because of its fast, stable anesthetic effect and shorter recovery time for freshwater and saltwater fish, although it is not universally approved for this purpose [6].

Fish are vulnerable to stress from over-crowding during long distance transportation and anesthetics can diminish mortality and decrease metabolism [7]. Eugenol is an inexpensive and plentiful anesthetic for fish and is often used to sedate or anesthetize fish in China. However, the use of eugenol and isoeugenol as an anaesthetic for edible fish is controversial.

Australia allows the use of isoeugenol but not eugenol as a fish anaesthetic and the maximum residue limit (MRL) is 100 mg/kg in aquatic products [8]. The relatively new anesthetic Aqui-S that contains approximately 50% isoeugenol is also approved in EU and Norway.

In New Zealand, the MRL of eugenol was 0.1 mg/kg in 2005 but this limit was revoked in 2013 [9, 10]. Eugenol is approved for aquatic medicine as an anaesthetic with an MRL of 0.05 mg/kg in Japan [11]. The acceptable daily intake (ADI) of eugenol at 2.5 mg/kg was recommended by the Joint FAO/WHO Expert

* Correspondence: dhao1[illegible]8@126.com
†Equal contributors
[1]Key Laboratory of Aquatic Product Processing, Ministry of Agriculture, Guangzhou 510300, People's Republic of China
[2]Laboratiry of Quality & Safety Risk Assessment for Aquatic Product on Storage and Preservation, Guangzhou 510300, People's Republic of China
Full list of author information is available at the end of the article

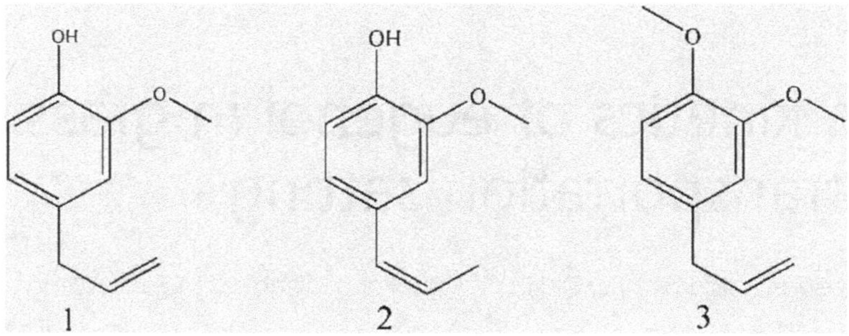

Fig. 1 Chemical structures of (1) eugenol (2) isoeugenol and (3) methyleugenol

Committee on Food Additives (JECFA) [12]. Although the United States FDA lists eugenol as a GRAS additive, they do not consider eugenol to be safe as a fish anaesthetic [13]. The Canadian Council on Animal Care approved eugenol for fish euthanasia but not as an anaesthetic [14].

There are numerous studies focusing on the anesthetic action of eugenol in zebrafish, spotted maigre, *Cynoglossus semilaevis, Salmo salar* (Atlantic salmon), rainbow trout, common carp, channel catfish and striped bass [7, 15]. The objective of the current work was to establish the elimination kinetics of eugenol following an exposure bath in grass carp. We wanted to assess the residue risk by simulating eugenol anesthesia during the transportation of live fish.

Methods

Animals and reagents

One hundred and twenty grass carp (*Ctenopharyngodon idella*, 1.5 ± 0.1 kg) were purchased from Huanqiu Aquatic Products Market (Foshan, China) and were used in the elimination kinetics experiment. The fish were transported to the lab in a specialized truck and housed in a fiber reinforced plastic tank. Prior to drug exposure, the grass carp were acclimatized and fasted for one week with a continuous flow of aerated tap water. The water temperature was sustained at 25 ± 2 °C and the pH, temperature, ammonia and dissolved oxygen levels were monitored every day during the experimental period.

Eugenol (99.5%) was purchased from Xiashan Aquatic Products Market in Zhanjiang, China. Deuterated eugenol (97.2%) was obtained from Accustandard (USA). The oily liquid was dissolved in aqueous alcohol (analytical grade, 1:10 *v*/v) for use as a tank additive.

Anesthetic effect of eugenol on grass carp at different concentrations

To acquire a satisfactory anesthetic or sedative effect to study elimination kinetics, we determined the anesthetic activity of eugenol on grass carp at different concentrations. Another thirty grass carp were divided equally into six groups. The fish were medicated with concentrations of eugenol at 5, 10, 15, 20, 30 and 40 mg/L for 8 h and physiological characteristics of breathing rate, body balance and response to stimulation were closely observed. Fish survival was also assessed and the minimum eugenol concentration that kept the fish in deep sedation without mortality was used for the remaining experiments.

Sample collection

The fish were randomly divided into 15 groups and 8 fish were sampled at each time point. After 24 h exposure bath of eugenol, grass carp were transferred to drug-free water with a net, sacrificed with a blow to the head, and blood, liver and muscle samples were collected at 0, 0.25, 0.5, 1, 2, 4, 8, 12, 16, 24, 36, 48, 72 and 96 h. Blank samples without anesthetic from the fifteenth group were simultaneously collected. Blood samples were collected with anticoagulants and centrifuged immediately at 2000 g for 10 min. Plasma was separated and stored at 4 °C. After rinsing with deionized water to eliminate blood, the tissue samples were wiped with disposable tissues and frozen at −20 °C until analysis.

Sample preparation

An aliquot of 0.5 mL plasma sample was transferred into a capped 1.5 mL centrifuge tube and mixed with 0.5 mL of acetonitrile. A 0.1 mL aliquot of deuterated eugenol (eugenol-d3) internal standard solution (100 ng/mL) was added and the mixture was vortexed for 30 s and then centrifuged at 12,000 g for 10 min. The supernatant was collected for solid-phase extraction (SPE).

Muscle and liver tissues were homogenized and a 2.00 g sample transferred to a 15 mL polypropylene centrifuge tube and was spiked with 10 ng of eugenol-d3 internal standard solution. After 30 min incubation by standing at room temperature, 5 mL n-hexane was added and the tube was vortexed and then shaken for 5 min. The tube was centrifuged at 5000 *g* for 5 min and the supernatant was transferred into a 10 mL glass-tube. The extraction procedure was repeated and the combined supernatants were evaporated to dryness under a gentle nitrogen stream at 40 °C. The residue was dissolved in 3 mL a 60% methanol–water solution.

The dissolved residue was loaded onto an HLB cartridge (60 mg/3 cm^3, Waters, Milford, MA) that had been activated with 3 mL methanol and 3 mL water successively. The cartridge was washed with 3 mL 60% methanol–water and eluted with 4 mL methanol. The eluate was concentrated to less than 0.5 mL with a nitrogen stream and adjusted to 1 mL with deionized water. The solution was filtered using a 0.22 μm syringe filter for LC-MS/MS determination.

LC-MS-MS analysis

The concentrations of eugenol in the plasma, muscle and liver samples were determined by LC-MS/MS. The instrument system was a Waters Acquity Series UPLC equipped with an autosampler, a column heater, a binary pump coupled to a Xevo TQ-S triple-quadrupole mass spectrometer with an electrospray ionization source (Waters, Milford, MA). MassLynx software was used for instrument control and data processing. Gradient elution for LC separation was performed at 35 °C using a BEH C_{18} column (50 mm × 2.1 mm i.d., 1.7 μm particle size) by employing a mobile phase consisting of methanol and water with a flow rate of 0.35 mL/min (Table 1). The injection volume was 10 μL.

The electrospray ionization source was used in negative mode with the following mass operating conditions: capillary voltage, 2 kV, desolvation temperature at 350 °C with a N_2 gas flow rate of 700 L/h, cone voltage, 20 V, cone gas flow rate 30 L/h. Qualitative and quantitative analysis of eugenol were carried out using the multiple reaction monitoring (MRM) mode. The protonated molecular ion $[M-H]^-$ of 163 was selected as parent ion due to its high abundance in full scan mode. Two characteristic fragment ions of 148 and 121 were identified as daughter ions with appropriate collision energy in product ion scan mode. The ion transitions of 163 → 148 and 163 → 121 were employed in the MRM experiment. The distinctive transition of 166 → 148 for eugenol-d3 that specified the internal standard compound was used for quantitation.

Elimination kinetics analysis

The concentration-time data of eugenol in plasma, muscle and liver were analyzed using a non-compartmental method using WinNonlin, Version 6.3 software (Pharsight, CA, USA). The area under the plasma, muscle or liver concentration-time curves (AUC) and mean residence time (MRT) were evaluated using the trapezoidal rule with extrapolation to infinity. The elimination or terminal half-life ($t_{1/2\beta}$) was calculated by dividing 0.693 by λ_z, where 0.693 is the natural logarithm of 2 and λ_z was estimated from the slope of the terminal phase [16]. Clearance (CL) was derived from dose/AUC [17] and volume of distribution in the terminal phase (Vz) was calculated by the equation: $Vz = Dose/(\lambda_z \times AUC)$ [18].

Table 1 Linear gradient elution program

Time (min)	0	0.5	1.5	2.5	3	4
Methanol (%)	25	25	95	95	25	25
Water (%)	75	75	5	5	75	75

Results

Physiological characteristics of grass carp in the exposure bath

Eugenol induced grass carp anesthesia rapidly with little apparent stress after 10 min exposure to a concentration of 10 mg/L (Table 2). Conversely, mortality was as high as 100% if grass carp were exposed to eugenol levels greater than 40 mg/L (Fig. 2).

We obtained a state of deep sedation when the fish were exposed to a medicated bath containing eugenol at 10 mg/L. The fish could keep their balance with gentle breathing, little activity and no response to touch stimuli. After 8 h exposure bath, they would return to a normal state in several minutes with zero mortality when they were transferred to anesthetic free water. However, five fish died in the elimination kinetics study, and mortality after 24 h was below 5%. Therefore, the ideal anesthetic concentration of 10 mg/L was the optimal dosage and was employed in the following experiments.

LC-MS-MS analysis

The coefficient of determination (R^2) for the determination of eugenol levels was above 0.99 in the linear range of 1–500 μg/L. Plasma, muscle and liver samples that were fortified with eugenol at three concentrations of 5, 25, and 100 μg/L (or μg/kg) had recoveries ranging from 89.2% to 96.5%. The limit of quantitation (LOQ) was 0.5 μg/L in plasma and 0.25 μg/kg in muscle or liver sample, respectively.

Elimination kinetics of eugenol following exposure bath in grass carp

No conspicuous paradoxical reactions were observed in grass carp after drug exposure in the bath format. The semi-logarithmic concentration-time plots of plasma, muscle and liver indicated that after a 24 h exposure to 10 mg/L eugenol, the C_{max} were 7.68, 5.30, and 24.63 mg/kg in plasma, muscle and liver, respectively (Fig. 3).

The elimination kinetics were simulated using a non-compartmental model. Compared with plasma and muscle, the drug residue level in liver was noticeably higher. The $t_{1/2\beta}$ of plasma, muscle and liver were 19.79, 10.27 and 55.28 h, respectively. The CL of plasma (0.10 L/h/kg) and muscle (0.44 L/h/kg) were large

Table 2 Physiological characteristics of grass carp exposed to eugenol for 10 min at 25 °C

Eugenol (mg/L)	*Physiological characteristics*				*Mortality (%)*	*Condition*
	Breathing	Motion	Equilibrium	Response		
0	Normal	Normal	Normal	Normal	0	Normal
5	Accelerated	Reduced	Normal	Delayed reaction to touch stimuli	0	Sedation
10	Reduced	Stop	Normal	No reaction to touch stimuli	0	Deep sedation
15	Reduced	Stop	Partial loss of equilibrium	No reaction to touch stimuli	10	Deep sedation
20	Reduced	Stop	Total loss of equilibrium	No reaction to touch stimuli	30	Anesthesia
30	Reduced	Stop	Total loss of equilibrium	No reaction to touch stimuli	60	Deep anesthesia
40	Stop	Stop	Total loss of equilibrium	No reaction to touch stimuli	100	Death

Ten min observation time

compared with the liver (0.04 L/h/kg). The $AUC_{0\text{-}96h}$ were 91.54, 22.44, and 214.12 mg·h/L for plasma, muscle and liver, respectively. The $AUC_{0\text{-}96h}$ for muscle was only a quarter of that in plasma and one-tenth of that in liver. The mean residence times (MRT) for plasma and liver were 24.25 h and 24.65 h, significantly higher than the 8.50 h for muscle (Table 3).

Discussion

We determined that the appropriate anesthetic dose of eugenol that produced deep sedation sufficient to transport grass carp was 10 mg/L. However, different fish have a different sensitivity to eugenol. The effective dosages of clove oil for Atlantic salmon, rainbow trout, common carp, channel catfish and striped bass were 10–50 mg/L, 40–120 mg/L, 40–100 mg/L, 100 mg/L and 60 mg/L, respectively [19]. Compared to these fish, grass carp have a high sensitivity to eugenol. The mortality reached 10% if the concentration of eugenol was 15 mg/L (Fig. 2). Therefore, the administered dose of eugenol should be precisely prepared for the exposure bath experiment to avoid producing unsatisfactory anesthetic effects or death.

Drug levels in blood are normally higher than liver or muscle tissues in the absorption and distribution phases. However, in this study we simulated a practical situation in which grass carp were exposed to the drug for an extended period. The drug concentration in the fish body had already reached the steady state by the end of the 24-h exposure. Therefore, the concentration-time data in this experiment actually described the disposition process of metabolism and elimination, even at the first sampling time point. Correspondingly, the concentration of eugenol in liver was higher than blood at 0 h after the 24-h medicated bath. During the 96-h elimination kinetics experimental period, the drug level in liver was always higher than blood, and muscle remained at the lowest drug concentration. These data suggest that the liver is the main organ for eugenol metabolism.

The concentration-time curves of eugenol in plasma, liver and muscle exhibited a monophasic decline, so a non-compartmental model fit the elimination kinetics data well (Fig. 3). Within the first day, levels of eugenol declined quickly in the three sample types. The trend of rapid elimination lasted to the second day for plasma and muscle. However, the elimination rate of eugenol slowed down in each tissue from 48 to 96 h. After drug exposure, eugenol decreased rapidly in liver, from 24.63 ± 4.67 mg/kg to approximately 2 mg/kg at

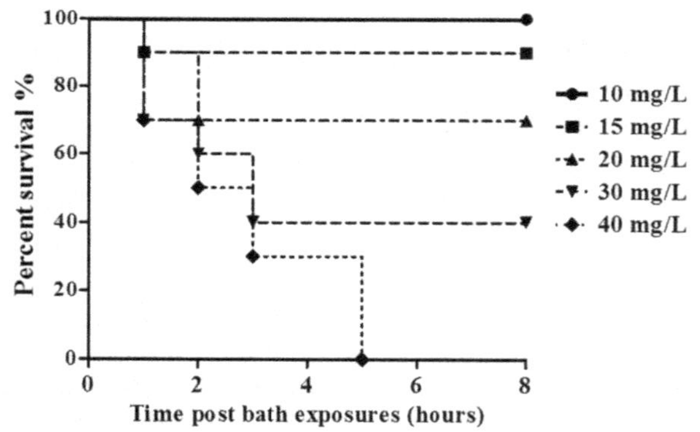

Fig. 2 Survival curves for grass carp at various concentrations of eugenol during bath exposure over an 8 h period. Curves were plotted from single experiments using 8 fish at each timepoint

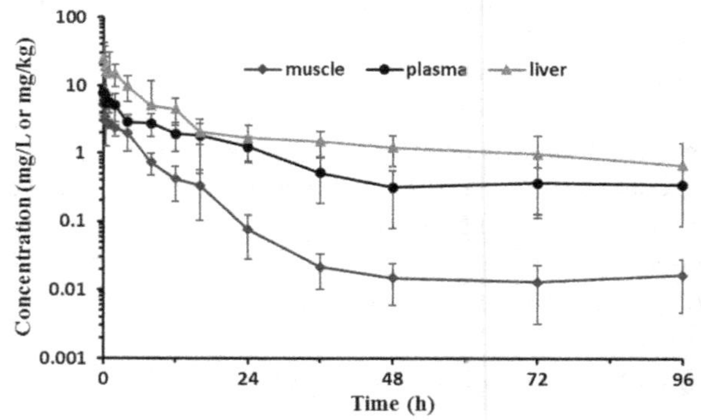

Fig. 3 Plasma, muscle and liver concentration-time semilogarithmic profile of eugenol following medicated bath administration for 24 h at a single dose of 10 mg/L ($n = 8$)

Table 3 Elimination kinetics of eugenol in grass carp following exposure for 24 h at 10 mg/L ($n = 8$)

Parameters	Plasma (mean ± SD)	Muscle (mean ± SD)	Liver (mean ± SD)
C_{max} (mg/L or mg/kg)	7.68 ± 0.31	5.30 ± 0.44	24.63 ± 4.67
AUC_{last} (mg·h/L)	91.54	22.44	214.12
$AUC_{0-\infty}$ (mg·h/L)	101.35	22.68	267.29
MRT (h)	24.25	8.50	24.65
CL (L/h/kg)	0.10	0.44	0.04
V_z (L/kg)	2.82	6.53	2.98
$t_{1/2\beta}$ (h)	19.79	10.27	55.28

about 12 h, again confirming eugenol is primarily metabolized in the liver.

The C_{max} in muscle tissue was 5.30 ± 0.44 mg/kg, which was one tenth of the C_{max} in rainbow trout after a 100 mg/L exposure for 240 min [20]. The $t_{1/2\beta}$ of eugenol in muscle tissue was 10.27 h, shorter than in blood and liver. In a previous report, mean concentrations of eugenol decreased from approximately 16 mg/kg to 3 mg/kg within 6 h, and the clearance rate was similar to this work [21]. For liver, a $t_{1/2\beta}$ of 55.28 h was noticeably different from the methyl eugenol $t_{1/2\beta}$ of 67.66 min in rats [22]. The species type may have a significant influence on the metabolism and elimination of eugenol. In comparison with mammals, the metabolism velocity of the drug in many fish was slower due to their lower body temperature.

Biotransformation of eugenol leads to the formation of multiple metabolites, such as isoeugenol and methyl eugenol [23]. Their concentrations were determined in another study (Li et al., unpublished data). Methyl eugenol was not detected 30 min after drug exposure. Subsequently, its concentrations in blood, muscle or liver were less than 0.01 mg/kg or mg/L. These residue levels indicated only a small transformation of eugenol methyl eugenol in the grass carp.

On the other hand, the concentrations of isoeugenol were high in grass carp after the medicated bath. However, this metabolite was eliminated rapidly. The residue levels of isoeugenol dropped sharply from the original 5 mg/kg to 0.02 mg/kg in muscle during which time the grass carp recovered from anesthesia (1 h). The compound was not detected at 8 h. On the contrary, the maximum isoeugenol concentrations in blood and liver samples were below 0.5 mg/L or mg/kg, but the residence times was longer. Isoeugenol could not be detected at 72 h in blood and 96 h in liver after recovery from exposure in the eugenol bath. Depletion of isoeugenol from muscle tissue in rainbow trout has been reported but the medicated bath consisted of primarily isoeugenol [24]. Therefore, the residual level of isoeugenol should be also monitored when grass carp are exposed to eugenol.

The JECFA recommended an ADI for eugenol of 2.5 mg/kg. This means that a 70 kg adult ingests less than 175 mg from grass carp if 1 kg is eaten. Fish muscle is the primary edible part of the grass carp and most fish. In the current work, we determined that the concentration of eugenol in muscle at 8 h was below 1 mg/kg. However, due to lack of accurate MRL data, it is not appropriate to declare that aquatic products are safe when fish are anesthetized with eugenol during transportation merely based on this single study. Metabolism and elimination of eugenol in other fish may be significantly different. In addition, we used fasting conditions before eugenol exposure because of the buildup of excrement resulted in turbid water. However, since this might change fat/muscle stores or increase stress to the fish, additional studies are needed to address this issue. The crowding and actual stress of transport were not evaluated, and the safety margin of the drug might be quite different in that setting.

Conclusions

This work simulated the practical situation of eugenol anesthesia according to the actual usage of this drug during fish transportation procedures. A medicated bath of 10 mg/L eugenol lasting 24 h produced drug concentrations in grass carp muscle that were below 1 mg/kg at 8 h and 0.1 mg/kg at 24 h, it was less than the ADI value recommended by the JECFA.

Abbreviations

ADI: Acceptable daily intake; AUC: Areas under the concentration-time curve; CL: Clearance; C_{max}: Peak concentrations; EFSA: European Food Safety Authority; FEMA: Flavor and Extract Manufacturers Association; GRAS: Generally Recognized as Safe; JECFA: Joint FAO/WHO Expert Committee on Food Additives; MRL: Maximum residue limit; MRT: Mean residence times; $t_{1/2\beta}$: Elimination half-lives; UPLC-MS/MS: Ultra-performance liquid chromatography-tandem mass spectrometry; Vz: Volume of distribution in the terminal phase

Acknowledgements

None.

Funding

This work was supported by the National Key Project for Agro-product Quality & Safety Risk Assessment, PRC (No. GJFP201501003).

Authors' contributions

LDL conceived of the study and participated in its design and coordination. DHZ and CLK design the experiment. QL, XFW and QW participated in the elimination kinetics experiment and analyzed the resulting data. DHZ drafted the manuscript. All authors read, revised and approved the final manuscript.

Consent for publication

Not applicable.

Competing interests

The authors declare that there are no competing interest.

Author details

[1]Key Laboratory of Aquatic Product Processing, Ministry of Agriculture, Guangzhou 510300, People's Republic of China. [2]Laboratiry of Quality & Safety Risk Assessment for Aquatic Product on Storage and Preservation, Guangzhou 510300, People's Republic of China. [3]Fishery Environments and Aquatic Products Quality Inspection & Testing Center of the Ministry of Agriculture, Guangzhou 510300, People's Republic of China. [4]South China Sea Fisheries Research Institute, Chinese Academy of Fishery Sciences, Guangzhou 510300, People's Republic of China.

References

1. Razafimamonjison G, Jahiel M, Duclos T, Ramanoelina P, Fawbush F, Danthu P. Bud, leaf and stem essential oil composition of Syzygium Aromaticum from Madagascar, Indonesia and Zanzibar. Int J Basic Appl Sci. 2014;3(3):224.
2. Authority E. Conclusion on the peer review of the pesticide risk assessment of the active substance eugenol. EFSA J. 2012;10(11):9–14.
3. Library FFI: The Flavor and Extract Manufacturers Association of the United States. https://www.femaflavor.org/flavor-library/eugenol.
4. (EFSA) EFSA: Database of flavouring substances - European Commission. 2016. http://www.efsa.europa.eu/en/topics/topic/flavourings.
5. Alma MH, Ertas M, Nitz S, Kollmannsberger H. Chemical composition and content of essential oil from the bud of cultivated Turkish clove (Syzygium Aromaticum L.). Bioresources. 2007;2(2):265–9.
6. Cooke SJ, Suski CD, Ostrand KG, Tufts BL, Wahl DH. Behavioral and physiological assessment of low concentrations of clove oil anaesthetic for handling and transporting largemouth bass (Micropterus Salmoides). Aquaculture. 2004;239(1):509–29.
7. Akbari S, Khoshnod MJ, Rajaian H, Afsharnasab M. The use of eugenol as an anesthetic in transportation of with Indian shrimp (Fenneropenaeus Indicus) post larvae. *Turkish.* J Fish Aquat Sci. 2010;10(3):423–9.
8. Food standard Australia and New Zealand: Standard 1.4.2 Maximum Residue Limits. (Australia only) volume 2. 2011. https://www.legislation.gov.au/Details/F2011C00786/Html/Volume_2.
9. Ministry for Primary Industries of New Zealand: (Maximum Residue Limits of Agricultural Compounds) Food Standards. 2013. http://www.foodsafety.govt.nz/elibrary/industry/news-views-feb-2014.pdf.
10. Ministry for Primary Industries of New Zealand: Food standard 2015 Maximum Residue Limits (MRLs) for Agricultural Compounds. 2015. http://www.foodsafety.govt.nz/elibrary/industry/register-list-mrl-agricultural-compounds.htm.
11. Foundation TJFCR: Revision of MRLs of agricultural chemicals, feed additives and veterinary drugs in foods. 2015. http://www.ffcr.or.jp/zaidan/ffcrhome.nsf/TrueMainE?OpenFrameSet.
12. Additives JFWECof. WHO technical report series 934: evaluation of certain food additives. Geneva: World Health Organization; 2006. p. 49–54. http://apps.who.int/iris/bitstream/10665/43408/1/WHO_TRS_934_eng.pdf.
13. FDA: Guidance for Industry: Concerns Related to the Use of Clove Oil as an Anesthetic for Fish, Guideline No. 150. US Food and Drug Administration Center for Veterninary Medicine. 2007. https://www.fda.gov/downloads/animalveterinary/guidancecomplianceenforcement/guidanceforindustry/ucm052520.pdf.
14. Canadian Council on Animal Care: Guidelines for additional information on effects of euthanasia methods on research results: clove oil (eugenol). 2016. http://www.ccac.ca/Documents/Standards/Guidelines/Add_PDFs/Fish_Anesthetics.pdf.
15. Iversen M, Finstad B, McKinley RS, Eliassen RA. The efficacy of metomidate, clove oil, Aqui-S™ and Benzoak® as anaesthetics in Atlantic salmon (Salmo Salar L.) smolts, and their potential stress-reducing capacity. Aquaculture. 2003;221(1):549–66.
16. Toutain PL, Bousquet-Melou A. Plasma terminal half-life. J Vet Pharmacol Ther. 2004;27(6):427–39.
17. Toutain PL, Bousquet-Melou A. Plasma clearance. J Vet Pharmacol Ther. 2004;27(6):415–25.
18. Toutain PL, Bousquet-Melou A. Volumes of distribution. J Vet Pharmacol Ther. 2004;27(6):441–53.
19. Coyle SD, Durborow RM, Tidwell JH. Anesthetics in aquaculture. In: Southern regional aquaculture center publication no. 3900. Stoneville; 2004.
20. Meinertz JR, Porcher ST, Smerud JR, Gaikowski M. Determination of the exposure parameters that maximise the concentrations of the anaesthetic/sedative eugenol in rainbow trout (Oncorhynchus Mykiss) skin-on fillet tissue. Food Addit Contam Part A. 2014;31(9):1522–8.
21. Kildea MA, Allan GL, Kearney RE. Accumulation and clearance of the anaesthetics clove oil and AQUI-S™ from the edible tissue of silver perch (Bidyanus Bidyanus). Aquaculture. 2004;232(1):265–77.
22. Meng X, Zhao X, Wang S, Jia P, Bai Y, Liao S, Zheng X: Simultaneous Determination of Volatile Constituents from Acorus tatarinowii Schott in Rat Plasma by Gas chromatography–mass spectrometry with Selective Ion Monitoring and Application in Pharmacokinetic Study. J Anal Methods Chem. 2013:949830. https://www.ncbi.nlm.nih.gov/pmc/articles/PMC3855985/pdf/JAMC2013-949830.pdf.
23. Ke C, Liu Q, Li L, Chen J, Wang X, Huang K. Simultaneous determination of eugenol, isoeugenol and methyleugenol in fish fillet using gas chromatography coupled to tandem mass spectrometry. J Chromatogr B Analyt Technol Biomed Life Sci. 2016;1031:189–94.
24. Meinertz JR, Schreier TM. Depletion of isoeugenol residues from the fillet tissue of AQUI-S™ exposed rainbow trout (Oncorhynchus Mykiss). Aquaculture. 2009;296(3):200–6.

10

National post-market surveillance assessment of veterinary medicines in Korea during the past decade

JeongWoo Kang, Hae-chul Park, Yang ho Jang, Md Akil Hossain, Kyunghun Jeong, Mi young Jeong, Seon-Jong Yun, Sung-won Park, Dae gyun Kim and Kwang-jick Lee*

Abstract

Background: Veterinary medicines have been widely used for the prevention and treatment of diseases, growth promotion, and to promote feeding efficacy in livestock. As the veterinary medicine industry has steadily grown, it is crucial to set up a baseline for the quality of medicine as well as the insufficiency or excessiveness of the active ingredients in drug products to ensure the compliance, safety and efficacy of these medicines. Thus, the 10 years data of post-marketing quality control study was summarized to determine the rate and extent of non-compliance of these medicines and to establish baseline data for future quality control measures of veterinary medicine.

Results: In this study, 1650 drugs for veterinary use were collected per year from each city and province in Korea and analysed for the quantity of active ingredients according to the "national post-market surveillance (NPMS) system" over the past decade. The NPMS assessment was performed using liquid and gas chromatography, titration, UV/Vis spectrophotometry, and bioassays. A total of 358 cases were deemed noncompliant, with the average noncompliance rate for all medicine types being 2.0%. The average noncompliance rates for antibiotics, biologics and other chemical drugs except antibiotics (OCD) were 1.1%, 1.2%, and 3.0%, respectively. The first leading cause for noncompliant products was insufficient quantity of major ingredients (283 cases), and the second leading cause was the existence of excess amount of active ingredients (60 cases). Tylosin, spiramycin, ampicillin, tetracyclines and penicillins were most frequently found to be noncompliant among antibiotics. Among the OCD, the noncompliance was found commonly in vitamin A.

Conclusion: The overall trend presented gradually decreasing violation rates, suggesting that the quality of veterinary medicines has improved. Consistent application of the NPMS assessment and the establishment of the Korea Veterinary Good Manufacturing Practice (KVGMP) will help to maintain the good quality of medicine.

Keywords: Veterinary medicine, Quality control, Post-market surveillance assay

Background

Veterinary medicines are concerned with the prevention, control, diagnosis and treatment of diseases that affect the health of companion, domestic, exotic, wildlife, and production animals. They are also used to improve feed efficiency, promote growth of livestock, and prevent the transmission of animal diseases to people. The veterinary medicine industry in Korea has grown following the expansion of livestock industry, and reached a market size of 876 millions USD by 2016. As of 2016, the total number of domestic manufacturers and importers of livestock are 740, consisting of 374 manufacturers, 358 importers, and 8 repair shops of medical devices, while the number of approved products reached a total of 9160 (4000 antibiotics, 2160 biologicals and 3000 other veterinary drugs except antibiotics and biologics [OCD]). In Korea, national product quality control measures for veterinary medicine consists of pre-market government testing system (PMGTS) and the National Post-Market Surveillance (NPMS) assessment on veterinary medicine

* Correspondence: leekwj@korea.kr
Veterinary drugs & Biologics Division, Animal and Plant Quarantine Agency (QIA), 177, Hyeoksin 8-ro, Gimcheon-si, Gyeongsangbuk-do 39660, Republic of Korea

before and after the distribution. Quality controls of antibiotics and biologics are performed by PMGTS prior to reach the products in open market, ensuring that stringent efficacy and safety requirements are met in accordance with the "Handling Rules of Veterinary Medicinal Products" [1, 2].

Meanwhile, local manufacturing facilities and veterinary medicinal products quality have improved owing to the implementation of Korea Veterinary Good Manufacturing Practice (KVGMP) on 1988–05-18 in accordance with the "KVGMP requirement for quality control" resulting in the gradual decrease of the government testing rejection rate [3, 4]. Accordingly, testing of antibiotics by PMGTS was abolished from 2000 to 11-07, while some biologics received partial exemptions from PMGTS as of 2005–04-09. The latter exemptions are limited to KVGMP-designated manufacturers. For biologics, PMGTS is performed on newly approved products, which become exempt from government testing after 10 or more consecutive lots are found to be acceptable. Following acquisition of exempt status, these products are still subject to spot-check government testing when necessary. Moreover, in the case of new antibiotics, the first 5 manufactured lots are designated as priority collection items and collected for testing [3, 5].

In the case of veterinary medicines currently in distribution, the active ingredient quantities of more than 1650 medicines are tested each year in accordance with "Tips for inspecting a veterinary pharmaceutical affair" [5]. The Korean Ministry of Agriculture, Food, and Rural Affairs (MAFRA) has established collection and testing plans designating the number of products, types of active ingredients, and locations from which sampling should take place (Fig. 1). The Korea Animal and Plant Quarantine Agency (QIA) and each individual city/province collects antibiotics, biologics and OCD currently in distribution from manufacturers, importers, and wholesalers of veterinary medicine, veterinary pharmacies, and veterinary hospitals in accordance with these testing plans. During this process, products are collected, with priority given to products with questionable quality, products with sale prices below the cost of production which disrupt the distribution order, identical products sold at widely disparate prices, and products with high market share. Post-marketing quality control measures are implemented on these products through QIA testing and levying of administrative measures such as suspension of marketing authorization and withdrawal of marketing authorization [1, 5]. The present study was performed to analyse the results of these veterinary medicine collections and tests over the past 10 years, between 2006 and 2016, for the purpose of establishing baseline data for future veterinary medicine quality control measures.

Methods

Test sample collection

The tested samples consisted of veterinary medicines stored or distributed by manufacturers, importers, and wholesalers of veterinary medicine, veterinary pharmacies, and veterinary hospitals, and were collected by QIA and local municipalities throughout Korea (9 provinces and 8 cities). In total, 18,213 products were collected and tested from 2006 to 2016. All the drug samples were analysed three times immediately after collecting them, and the results were documented.

Chemicals and reagents

Reference standards were purchased from Sigma-Aldrich (St. Louis, MO, USA) for all the veterinary drugs. All solvents used in chromatographic analysis were of HPLC

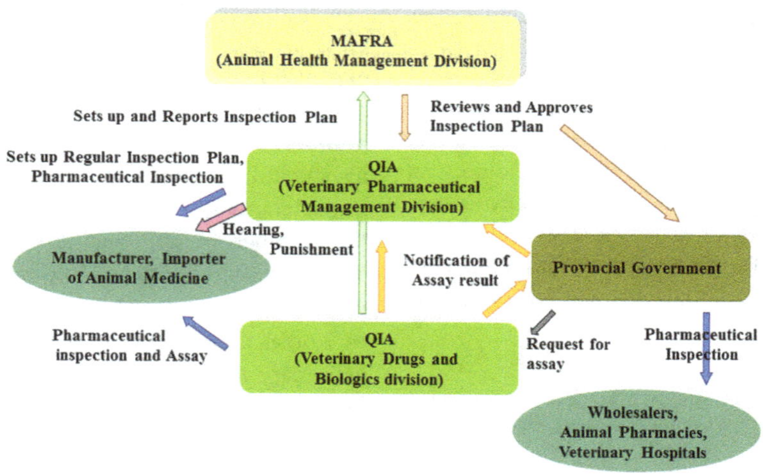

Fig. 1 Schematic figure showing Pharmaceutical inspection of veterinary medicines by post-market surveillance assessment. MAFRA: Ministry of Agriculture, Food and Rural Affairs; QIA: Animal and Plant Quarantine Agency

grade and were purchased from Honeywell Burdick & Jackson (Ulsan 680–160, South Korea). De-ionized water was purified using a Milli-Q System (Millipore, Bedford, MA 01730, USA). Solvents and reagents used in titrimetric assays were reagent grade and were obtained from Duksan Pure Chemical Co., Ltd. (Ansan-si 425–020, South Korea) and Honeywell Burdick & Jackson (Ulsan 680–160, South Korea).

Test methods

Collected veterinary medicine samples were tested by the QIA using various certified methods such as the Korean standards of veterinary pharmaceuticals [6], the Korean pharmacopoeia [7], the Standards of national certification assay of the veterinary biological products [8] and other foreign test methods which are summarized in "Compendial analysis method for veterinary medicines, Animal and Plant Quarantine Agency (QIA), South Korea" (Table 1). [9–13] High Performance Liquid Chromatography (HPLC) and microbial assays were used for antibiotics while HPLC, pH, and titration methods were used for other chemical agents. Finally, vaccines, classified as biologics, were tested using microbial and viral assays.

Results

National post-market surveillance assessment results by year

Testing results for the veterinary medicine samples collected throughout Korea between 2006 and 2016 are shown in Table 2. A total of 18,213 samples, comprising 9504 antibiotics, 8137 OCD, and 572 biologics, were tested, among which a total of 358 samples were found to be noncompliant (average noncompliance rate of 2.0%). The number of noncompliant samples found in different drug groups are antibiotics 103 (1.1%), OCD 248 (3.0%), and biologics 7 (1.2%). The average noncompliance rate by year steadily decreased over the 10 years

Table 1 Outlines of analysis veterinary medicines

Veterinary medicines	Active ingredient	Analytical method (instrumentation)
Antibiotics	Penicillins	HPLC
	Cephalosporins	HPLC
	Tetracyclines	HPLC
	Sulfonamides	HPLC
	Quinolones	HPLC
	Macrolides	HPLC
	Aminoglykosides	HPLC
	Others (avilamycin, colistin, trimethoprim)	HPLC
	Amikacin	Bioassay
OCD	Anthelmintics	HPLC
	Antiprotozoals	HPLC
	Hormones	HPLC
	Paracetamol	HPLC
	Other Antipyretics	Titration
	Vitamins	HPLC
	Nutrition facts	Titration
	Others (tartaric acid, sorbitol)	Titration, pH
	Disinfectants (malic acid, O-Dichlorobenzene, Cresol, Sodium dichloroisocyanurate, Citric acid, Alkylpolyamine ethylglycine, Chlorhexidine digluconate)	HPLC
	Disinfectants (Potassium monopersulphate triple salt, Quaternary ammonium chloride, Alkyldiaminoethylglycine, Hydrogen peroxide, Available chloride, Sodium hypochlorite, Glutaraldehyde, Aldehyde, chlorine dioxide, sodium carbonate, iodine, sodium hydroxide)	Titration
	Probiotics	Bioassay, pH
Biologics	Vaccines	Bioassay, Elisa assay

OCD other chemical drugs except antibiotics

Table 2 Results of national post-market surveillance assay in veterinary medicines from 2006 to 2016

Year	Antibiotics		OCD[a]		Biologics		Total	
	Tested[b]	Noncompliant (%)[c]	Tested[b]	Noncompliant (%)[c]	Tested[b]	Noncompliant (%)[c]	Tested[b]	Noncompliant (%)[c]
2006	606	23 (3.8)	863	24 (2.8)	63	0 (0.0)	1532	47 (3.1)
2007	771	23 (3.0)	687	26 (3.8)	50	0 (0.0)	1508	49 (3.2)
2008	782	5 (0.6)	756	19 (2.5)	45	1 (2.2)	1583	25 (1.6)
2009	916	15 (1.6)	816	43 (5.3)	103	1 (1.0)	1835	59 (3.2)
2010	934	10 (1.1)	663	35 (5.3)	61	1 (1.6)	1658	46 (2.8)
2011	881	17 (1.9)	759	30 (4.0)	55	0 (0.0)	1695	47 (2.8)
2012	918	2 (0.2)	721	22 (3.1)	47	0 (0.0)	1686	24 (1.4)
2013	932	2 (0.2)	664	13 (2.0)	54	1 (1.9)	1650	16 (1.0)
2014	889	4 (0.4)	707	22 (3.1)	70	3 (4.3)	1666	29 (1.7)
2015	1039	1 (0.1)	680	14 (2.1)	24	0 (0.0)	1743	15 (0.9)
2016	836	1 (0.1)	821	0 (0.0)	0	0 (0.0)	1657	1 (0.1)
Total	9504	103 (1.1)	8137	248 (3.0)	572	7 (1.2)	18,213	358 (2.0)

[a]Other chemical drugs except antibiotics (OCD)
[b]The number of tested in the national post-market surveillance assay
[c]The rate of non compliant products, (%) in the national post-market surveillance assay

period, dropping below 1.0% in 2015 and reaching 0.1% in 2016 (Fig. 2).

Reasons for noncompliance in collected and tested veterinary medicines

Table 3 outlines the causes for noncompliance in veterinary medicines collected and tested between 2006 and 2016. From a total of 358 cases, 283 (79.1%) and 60 (16.8%) cases were deemed noncompliant owing to "insufficiency of major ingredient quantity" and "excess of major ingredient quantity", respectively. Moreover, 3 (0.8%), 4 (1.1%), 3 (0.8%), and 5 (1.4%) cases were marked as "inadequate pH," "abnormal characteristics," "violation of marking standards," and "others", respectively.

Noncompliance rate by active ingredient in collected and tested veterinary medicines

Table 4 shows the noncompliance rates for individual compounds in veterinary medicines collected and tested between 2006 and 2016. For antibiotics, the highest number of noncompliant cases (n = 86) were found concerning macrolide drugs, such as tylosin, spiramycin, and erythromycin, followed by 55 cases concerning beta-lactams, such as ampicillin, amoxicillin, and penicillin, and 22 cases concerning tetracyclines. For OCD, the ingredients found to be noncompliant included vitamin A (n = 59), probiotics (n = 9), and topically applied products such as pet shampoos (n = 15), disinfectants (n = 8), and glucocorticoids (n = 10). For biologics, bovine rota-coronavirus live mixed vaccine, canine parvo and coronavirus live mixed vaccines,

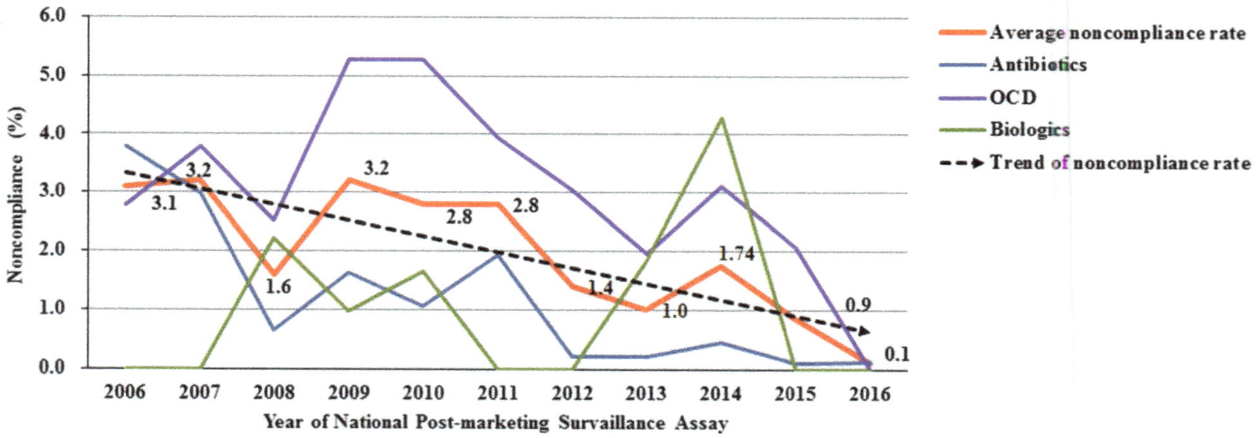

Fig. 2 Violation rate of the post-market surveillance assay in veterinary medicines from 2006 to 2016. OCD: other chemical drugs except antibiotics

Table 3 The causes of noncompliance in veterinary medicines from 2006 to 2016

Case	Antibiotics	OCD[a]	Biologics	Total (%)[b]
Insufficiency of major ingredient content	92	189	2	283 (79.1)
Excess of major ingredient content	11	49	0	60 (16.8)
Inadequate pH	0	3	0	3 (0.8)
Abnormal characteristics	0	2	2	4 (1.1)
Violation of marking standards	1	2	0	3 (0.8)
Others	1	1	3	5 (1.4)
Total	105	246	7	358

[a]Other chemical drugs except antibiotics (OCD)
[b]the rate of noncompliance %

porcine transmissible gastroenteritis rotavirus live mixed vaccine, Newcastle live attenuated vaccine, porcine epidemic diarrhoea vaccine, and classic swine fever virus vaccine were found to be noncompliant which is due to their insufficient efficacy. The biological products which couldn't kill the required number of virus according to the guideline of Animal and Plant Quarantine Agency were listed as non-compliant. Those products also had incorrect pH and may have insufficient concentration of antigens.

Seasonal effect on noncompliance in collected and tested veterinary medicines

An investigation of noncompliant veterinary medicines collected and tested between 2006 and 2016 showed that out of 358 total cases the highest number of noncompliant cases (n = 155) were found during the summer months (June to August). During spring and fall (March to May and September to November, respectively), the number of noncompliant cases were 82 and 80, respectively, while a relatively lower number of noncompliant cases (41) were found during winter (December to February) (Fig. 3).

Discussion

Veterinary medicines are essential for the advancement of the livestock industry, and the importance of quality control is emphasizing more due to the increase in the availability and demand of different types of veterinary medicines. Concentration of active ingredient is the most important characteristic of a drug product, as the amount of active ingredient allows to determine the intensities of treatment and toxicity of that particular drug. Moreover, the noncompliance rates of veterinary medicines are also pertaining in the elevation of contamination and drugs residues in the food products of animal origin [14, 15]. The NPMS assessment was initiated in 1964 for the quality control of OCD which are in distribution. Antibiotics and biologics were previously assessed by both PMGTS and NPMS. The control of antibiotics was abolished from PMGTS on 2000–11-07 and the exception biologics which pass ten times consecutively by PMGTS have been incorporated into the NPMS assessment system on 2005–04-09 [3]. So, NPMS is very important for the quality control of veterinary medicines as there is no other assessment system except NPMS.

Testing methods have greatly improved from traditional bioassay examination owing to continued research and development. Improved HPLC and titration methods are now being used for analysis based on the compendia as shown in Table 1. A small surveillance study in Taiwan in the year of 2013 accounted 6 noncompliant cases out of 343 cases (1.7%), which is comparable with our study [16]. The overall violation rate in Korea in the year 2014 was same as the violation rate in Taiwan in 2013. As shown in Fig. 2, noncompliance rates by year showed an annual trend of gradual decrease from 3.2% to 0.1% which indicates that the implication of NPMS in veterinary medicine is helping to improve the quality of them. In particular, antibiotics have shown very dramatic decrease in noncompliance rates (Table 2), illustrating that veterinary medicine manufacturing facilities and quality control standards have significantly improved over time [3, 4]. That such annual trend reflects the effectiveness of the NPMS assessment and KVGMP programs. Meanwhile, no noncompliant cases for OCD were found in 2016, which was due to the testing of a large proportion of disinfectant samples (700 disinfectants out of 821 OCD) compared to the previous years. The disinfectant reinforcement measure due to the 2016 avian influenza outbreak was the behind cause to test many samples only for disinfectants. Vitamin A, which was often found as a noncompliant product in previous years, did not appear in the list of noncompliant products, as we have tested very few samples of Vitamin A among the OCD in 2016.

Of the 358 noncompliant cases, "insufficiency of active ingredient quantity" was the reason for 283 cases, accounting for approximately 79.1% of all noncompliant cases. The next most frequently observed reason was "excess of active ingredient quantity," with 60 cases observed (approximately 16.8%). In fact, manufacturing facilities cannot always give uniform products. They should have the quality control system and need to check the quality-related parameters batch-wise to comply with the recommended specifications. But, most of the manufacturers do not have quality control system and are unintentionally producing some products which contain less or excess amount of active ingredients. These companies are not also accredited by KVGMP. The second important cause of noncompliance is the using of low quality or potency of active ingredients in veterinary medicine by the manufacturers to reduce the

Table 4 The noncompliant ingredients of products in the post-market surveillance assay from 2006 to 2016

Active ingredients	No. of noncomplience	Noncomplience rate (%)
Vitamin A	59	16.5
Tylosin	48	13.4
Spiramycin	28	7.8
Ampicillin	23	6.4
Amoxicillin	19	5.3
Oxytetracycline	18	5.0
Others	15	4.2
Penicillin	13	3.6
Erythromycin	10	2.8
Gentamicin	9	2.5
Probiotics	8	2.2
Colistin	8	2.2
Dexamethasone	8	2.2
Calcium	5	1.4
Sulfonamides	5	1.4
Chloramphenicol	4	1.1
Doxycycline	4	1.1
Iodine	4	1.1
Ivermectin	4	1.1
Trimethoprim	3	0.8
Cefalexin	3	0.8
Citric acid	3	0.8
Neomycin	3	0.8
Prednisolone	3	0.8
Tiamulin	3	0.8
Amikacin	2	0.6
Apramycin	2	0.6
Benzyl benzoate	2	0.6
Bovine Rota, Corona virus live mixed vaccine	2	0.6
Cefazolin	2	0.6
Cloxacillin	2	0.6
Dicloxacillin	2	0.6
Kanamycin	2	0.6
Melengestrol acetate	2	0.6
Quaternary ammonium salt	2	0.6
Salicylic acid	2	0.6
spectinomycin	2	0.6
Streptomycin	2	0.6
Vitamin B	2	0.6
Amitraz	1	0.3
Newcastle live attenuated vaccine	1	0.3
BPMC	1	0.3
Canine Parvo Corona virus live mixed vaccine	1	0.3
Ceftiofur	1	0.3
Cloprostenol sodium	1	0.3
Enrofloxacin	1	0.3
Florfenicol	1	0.3
Glutaraldehyde	1	0.3
Hydrogen peroxide	1	0.3
Kitasamycin	1	0.3
porcine circo virus vaccine	1	0.3
Phenylbutazone	1	0.3
Porcine transmissible gastroenteritis Rota virus live mixed vaccine	1	0.3
Pyriproxyfen	1	0.3
Tiamphenicol	1	0.3
Trichlorfon	1	0.3
Vitamin E	1	0.3
Porcine Epidemic Diarrhea vaccine	1	0.3
Classic swine fever virus vaccine	1	0.3
Total	358	100

production costs which is investigated by the audit of "Veterinary Management Division" of QIA. So, this report is suggesting to the manufacturers to establish their own quality assurance facilities to produce quality products. Another cause of noncompliance is the storing of the products in improper storage condition particularly in summer season by the sellers and veterinary pharmacies (Fig. 3). It was also recorded in the previous years that the noncompliance rate was increased in summer season due to not maintaining the proper storage condition. This indicates that the seasonal factors, including temperature-related issues during storage and distribution, may act as key factors of noncompliance. Thus, it is suggested to the sellers and distributors to maintain the veterinary medicine in proper storage condition as mention in guidelines.

As shown in Table 4, the noncompliance rate was high among antibiotics with higher molecular weight. The antibiotics were also found to be noncompliant whose active ingredient contain for each dose are high such as tylosin and spiramycin. Among the nutritional supplements, noncompliance was the highest for fat soluble vitamins, such as vitamin A, which has low titre owing to being easily oxidized, as well as a

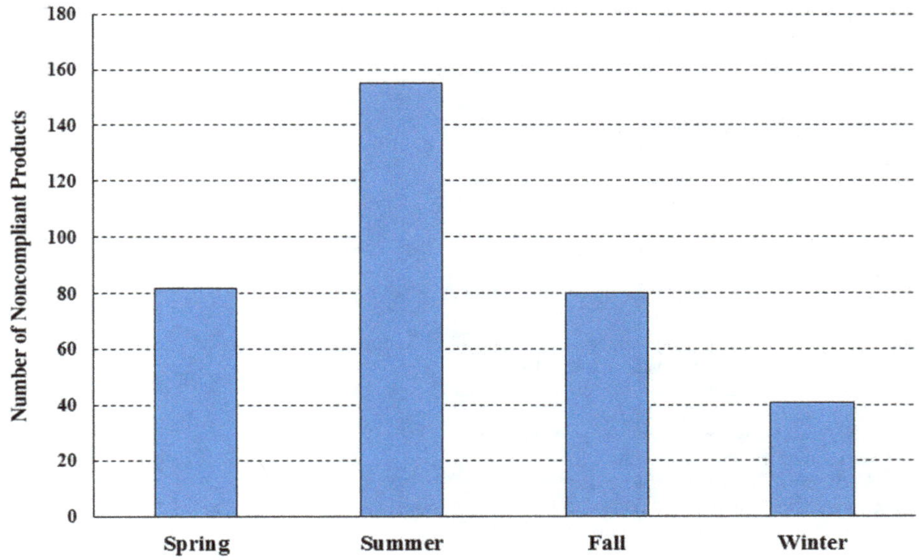

Fig. 3 Seasonal effect on noncompliance in collected and tested veterinary medicines

few probiotics, whose cell count drops quickly when preservation conditions are not adequate. Currently, an average of 60–70 cases of biologics both subject to and exempt from national testing are assessed each year, and among these, noncompliance was reported for 2 cases of bovine rota-coronavirus live mixed vaccine, and 1 case each of Newcastle live attenuated vaccine, canine parvo and coronavirus live mixed vaccines, porcine transmissible gastroenteritis rotavirus live mixed vaccine, porcine epidemic diarrhoea vaccine, and classic swine fever virus vaccine.

Conclusion

Significant improvements in the manufacturing environment and quality control standards have been achieved through the implementation of KVGMP. However, voluntary efforts by manufacturers are still needed to continue the application of KVGMP for the improvement of the quality of veterinary medicines. In particular, OCD showed a high noncompliance rate of about 3%. The Ministry of Agriculture, Food and Rural Affairs (MAFRA) of Korea is expecting to analyse the sales figures from the Korea Animal Health Products Association, and the NPMS assay results from QIA accordingly, to increase the statistical feasibility of the NPMS assessment results. The MAFRA is also expecting to increase the number of test samples for OCD, as they present relatively high noncompliance rates. It is also expected by MAFRA to reinforce testing during the vulnerable summer season. Proactive self-quality control by manufacturers for improved veterinary medicine quality must be promoted; while simultaneously, the efforts to establish an effective quality control system must continue as well.

Abbreviations

HPLC: High performance liquid chromatography.; KVGMP: Korea veterinary good manufacturing practice; MAFRA: Ministry of agriculture, food, and rural affairs; NPMS: National post-market surveillance; OCD: Other chemical drugs except antibiotics; PMGTS: Pre-market government testing system; QIA: Animal and plant quarantine agency

Acknowledgements

Not applicable.

Funding

This work was supported by a grant (No.:101–6200–6240-301-210) from the Animal and Plant Quarantine Agency, Republic of Korea.

Author's contributions

JWK designed the study, analysed the data and submitted the manuscript. KJL was involved in the design of the study and review of the manuscript. HCP, YHJ, MAH, KHJ, MYJ, SJY and SWP contributed to the various assay and analyzed preliminary data. DGK was involved in the critical review and approval of the revised manuscript.

Competing interests

The authors declare that they have no competing interest.

Consent for publication

Not applicable.

References

1. MAFRA. Handling rules of veterinary medicinal products. Notification No. 165. http://www.law.go.kr/%EB%B2%95%EB%A0%B9/%EB%8F%99%EB%AC%BC%EC%9A%A9%EC%9D%98%EC%95%BD%ED%92%88%EB%93%B1%EC%B7%A8%EA%B8%89%EA%B7%9C%EC%B9%99/(00165,20151005) (accessed 29 Jan 2017).
2. Kramer DB, Tan YT, Sato C, Kesselheim AS. Postmarket Surveillance of Medical Devices: A Comparison of Strategies in the US, EU, Japan, and China. PLoS Med. 2013;10(9):e1001519.
3. Lee KJ. GMP Guideline lecture of Veterinary drugs. MAFRA. 2013;37(3):120–4.

4. Jang HJ, Park SW, Yun SM, et al. Post-market surveillance assay of veterinary medicines in Korea. J Vet Publ Hlth. 2009;33(3):147–51.
5. MAFRA. Tip for inspecting a veterinary pharmaceutical affair. Directive No. 78. http://www.law.go.kr/admRulLsInfoP.do?admRulSeq=2000000025687 (accessed 28 Jan 2017).
6. QIA. Korean pharmacopoeia of veterinary medicinal products. Notification No. 2016–16. http://www.law.go.kr/admRulLsInfoP.do?admRulSeq=2100000040880 (accessed 27 Jan 2017).
7. MFDS. Korean pharmacopoeia. Notification No.2016–57. http://www.law.go.kr/admRulLsInfoP.do?admRulSeq=2100000051416 (accessed 30 Jan 2017).
8. QIA. Standards of national certification assay of the veterinary biological products. Notification No. 2016–99. http://www.law.go.kr/admRulLsInfoP.do?admRulSeq=2100000064749 (accessed 26 Jan 2017).
9. The United States Pharmacopoeia convention, 2012. The United States Pharmacopoeia. 36th revision.
10. British Pharmacopoeia Commission, 2012. British Pharmacopoeia.
11. European Pharmacopoeia Commission. European Pharmacopoeia. 7th ed; 2012.
12. Society of Japanese Pharmacopoeia. The Japanese Pharmacopoeia. 16th edition. http://jpdb.nihs.go.jp/jp16e/. Accessed 26 Jan 2017.
13. Compendia of analysis method for veterinary medicines. Animal and Plant Quarantine Agency (QIA), South Korea. http://www.qia.go.kr/viewwebQiaCom.do?id=39863&type=2_14dwyp. Accessed 26 Jan 2017.
14. Kim MK, Cho BH, Lim CM, et al. Chemical residues and contaminants in foods of animal origin in Korea during the past decade. J Agric Food Chem. 2013;61(10):2293–8. doi:10.1021/jf3046297.
15. Kang JW, Park HC, Gedi V, et al. Veterinary drug residues in domestic and imported foods of animal origin in the Republic of Korea. Food Addit Contam Part B. 2015;8(2):106–12. doi:10.1080/19393210.2014.1001795.
16. Annual Report, 2014. ISSN No.: 2409-3335. Food and Drug Administration, Ministry of Health and Welfare, Taiwan, December 2014.

11

Comparison of the effects of ketamine and fentanyl-midazolam-medetomidine for sedation of rhesus macaques (*Macaca mulatta*)

Henri G. M. J. Bertrand[1,2*], Yvette C. Ellen[1,3], Stevie O'Keefe[1] and Paul A. Flecknell[1,4]

Abstract

Background: This study assessed the effects of sedation using a combination of fentanyl, midazolam and medetomidine in comparison to ketamine. Rhesus Macaques (*Macaca mulatta*), ($n = 16$, 5 males and 3 females randomly allocated to each treatment group) received either ketamine (KET) (10 mg.kg^{-1}) or fentanyl-midazolam-medetomidine (FMM) (10 μg/kg^{-1}; 0.5 mg.kg^{-1}; 20 μg.kg^{-1}) both IM. Oxygen (100 %) was provided by mask and heart rate, blood pressure, respiratory rate, $EtCO_2$ and depth of sedation were assessed every 5 min for 20 min. After the last time point, FMM monkeys were reversed with atipamezole-naloxone (0.2 mg.kg^{-1}; 10 μg.kg^{-1}). Recovery was scored using clinical scoring scheme. Differences in physiological parameters and quality of sedation were compared using Area Under the Curve (AUC) method and either Mann-Witney or t-student tests.

Results: Heart rate (beats/min) (Ket = 119 ± 18; FMM = 89 ± 17; $p = 0.0066$), systolic blood pressure (mmHg) (Ket = 109 ± 10; FMM = 97 ± 10; $p = 0.0313$), and respiratory rate (breaths/min) (Ket = 39 ± 9; FMM = 29 ± 10; $p = 0.0416$) were significantly lower in the FMM group. End-tidal CO_2 (mmHg) did not differ between the groups (KET = 33 ± 8; FMM = 42 ± 11; $p = 0.0462$). Although some depression of physiological parameters was seen with FMM, the variables all remained within the normal ranges in both groups. Onset of a sufficient degree of sedation for safe handling was more rapid with ketamine (KET = 2.9 ± 1.4 min; FMM = 7.9 ± 1.2 min; $p = 0.0009$), but FMM recovery was faster (KET = 21.4 ± 13.4 min; FMM = 9.1 ± 3.6 min; $p = 0.0379$) and of better quality (KET = 1.3 ± 0.9; FMM = 7.4 ± 1.9; $p = 0.0009$) most probably because of the effectiveness of the reversal agents used.

Conclusion: FMM provides an easily reversible immobilization with a rapid and good recovery quality and may prove a useful alternative to ketamine.

Keywords: Sedation, Ketamine, Fentanyl, Midazolam, Medetomidine, Recovery macaque

Background

Ketamine, a dissociative anaesthetic, is widely used for the chemical immobilization of non–human primates (NHPs). When administered alone it induces a cataleptic state allowing safe handling as the biting reflex is inhibited [1, 2]. Protective airway reflexes are conserved and voluntary movement can still occur. Ketamine has some analgesic activity, allowing minor procedures such as skin suturing to be undertaken but it is not suitable as a sole agent for more invasive procedures. Ketamine is an NDMA receptor antagonist, and so should prevent "wind-up" associated with noxious stimuli [3], but this effect has never been assessed in NHPs. Several side effects have been described in primates and other species, including pain on injection, muscular and nerve damage at the site of injection [2, 4–6], and rarely, seizures [7–10]. Recovery delirium also occurs but this can be reduced by addition of other agents. Despite these problems, ketamine is widely used in primates, primarily because of its good safety profile and relative lack of

* Correspondence: henri.bertrand@newcastle.ac.uk
[1]Comparative Biology Centre, Newcastle University, Framlington Place, Newcastle Upon Tyne NE2 4HH, UK
[2]Faculty of Veterinary Medicine, University of Liège, Boulevard de Colonster, Liège 4000, Belgium
Full list of author information is available at the end of the article

depression of the cardiovascular and respiratory systems. For some procedures, a greater degree of analgesia and muscle relaxation would be advantageous. Although this can be achieved by the addition of medetomidine, as in other species, recovery is still relatively prolonged even after reversal of the medetomidine with atipamezole [11]. Replacement of ketamine with agents that have less prolonged depressant effects, or are reversible with specific antagonists could therefore be advantageous. In human medicine, the combination of fentanyl and midazolam has been widely used for conscious sedation for minor procedures, and at higher dose rates for surgery [12–15]. Combinations of opioids and benzodiazepines seem to be less effective in Rhesus macaques [16], however in other species, addition of medetomidine to these combinations produces fully reversible anaesthesia [17–19] and an initial report suggests this combination can be used successfully in non-human primates [20].

This study compared the effects of a combination of fentanyl-midazolam-medetomidine (FMM), followed by reversal with naloxone and atipamezole, with ketamine (KET) in rhesus macaques.

Results

Sedation procedure

One female from the KET group started to recover 10 min after administration of the anaesthetic and was placed in a recovery cage. No physiological parameters were recorded after this time point, but the recovery time and the assessment of the recovery quality were assessed. All of the remaining primates were successfully immobilized after the administration of either KET or FMM.

Onset of sedation and recovery times

The onset of a sufficient degree of sedation for safe handling was significantly shorter in the KET group (2.9 ± 1.4 min) than in the FMM group (7.9 ± 1.2 min)*(p* = 0.0009). Recovery was significantly faster in the FMM group (9.1 ± 3.6 min) compared to the KET group (21.4 ± 13.4 min) ($p = 0.0379$) (Fig. 1).

Physiological parameters and depth of sedation

The physiological data are summarised in Table 1. Area under the curves (AUCs) comparisons showed significant differences between the two treatment groups. The heart rate (HR) ($p = 0.0066$), Respiration rate (RR) ($p = 0.0416$), systolic blood pressure (BPsyst) ($p = 0.0313$) and the end-tidal CO_2 ($EtCO_2$) ($p = 0.0462$) AUCs were significantly lower in the FMM group. However, no significant difference was found in SpO_2 between the two groups ($p > 0.1$). The overall degree of sedation over the 20 min procedure was deeper in the FMM group with a

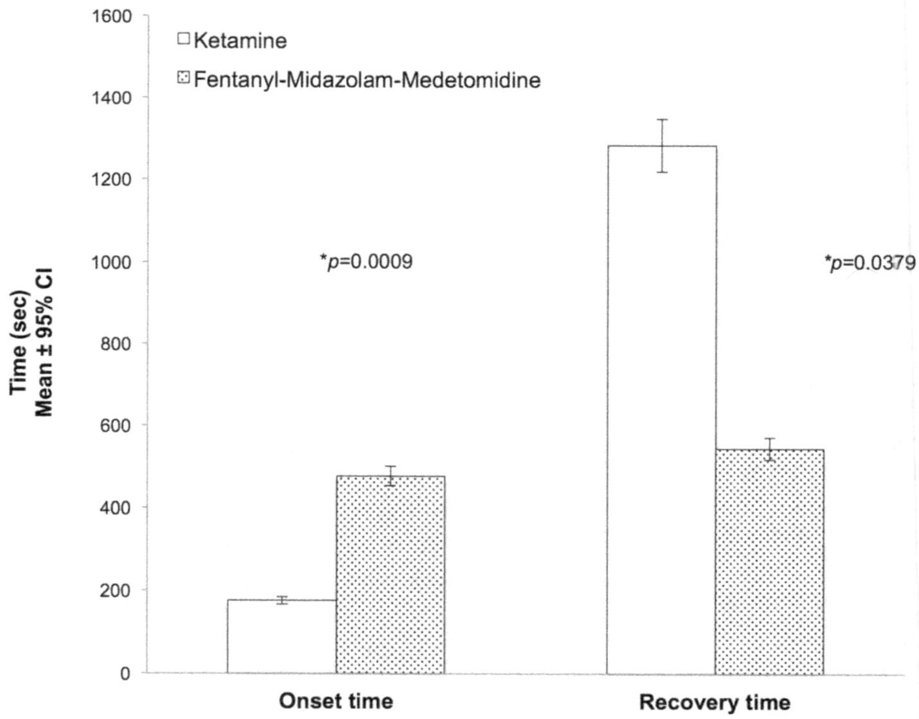

Fig. 1 Onset of sedation and Recovery times in Rhesus macaques receiving ketamine ($n = 8$) or fentanyl-midazolam-medetomidine ($n = 8$) Induction times: Ketamine (KET) 2.9 ± 1.4 min; Fentanyl-midazolam-medetomidine (FMM) 7.9 ± 1.2 min. Recovery times: Ketamine (KET) 21.4 ± 13.4 min; Fentanyl-midazolam-medetomidine (FMM) 9.1 ± 3.6 min. An asterisk next to a *p*-value(*p) indicates a significantly differences

Table 1 Physiological parameters recorded over 20 min for each treatment group

	Treatment groups										*p-value*
	Ketamine					Fentanyl-Midazolam-Fentanyl					
Time	0 *n* = 8	5 *n* = 8	10 *n* = 8	15 *n* = 7	20 *n* = 7	0 *n* = 8	5 *n* = 8	10 *n* = 8	15 *n* = 8	20 *n* = 8	
HR*(beat/min)*	134 ± [illegible]7	121 ± 18	117 ± 17	110 ± 14	112 ± 18	97 ± 17	90 ± 17	87 ± 18	86 ± 18	85 ± 17	0.0066*
SpO_2*(%)*	98.2 ± [illegible].0	99.8 ± 0.7	100 ± 0	99.9 ± 0.4	100 ± 0	96.1 ± 7.8	99.6 ± 0.7	99.8 ± 0.5	99.8 ± 0.7	99.6 ± 0.7	0.7254
RR*(breaths/min)*	36 ± 8	41 ± 8	36 ± 6	40 ± 11	43 ± 11	30 ± 10	28 ± 12	28 ± 11	29 ± 11	29 ± 10	0.0416*
$EtCO_2$*(mmHg)*	36 ± 8	32 ± 9	32 ± 9	34 ± 9	32 ± 8	39 ± 12	44 ± 11	43 ± 11	44 ± 10	42 ± 10	0.0462*
BPsyst*(mmHg)*	111 ± [illegible]0	111 ± 9	107 ± 9	107 ± 11	108 ± 13	101 ± 9	102 ± 10	97 ± 10	93 ± 9	90 ± 8	0.0313*
SD	12 ± 3	12 ± 2	11 ± 3	11 ± 3	11 ± 4	17 ± 1	18 ± 1	18 ± 1	18 ± 1	18 ± 1	0.0009*

Data are shown as mean ± [illegible] SD. *n* represents the number of animals that provide data at the each time point. In the ketamine group one of the primates started to recover after 10 min of sedation and so recording session was stopped. Areas Under the Curve (AUCs) were calculated for each parameter. The Shapiro-wilk test showed a normal distribution for Heart Rate (HR), the Respiration Rate (RR), the Systolic Blood Pressure (BPsyst) and the end-tidal CO_2 ($EtCO_2$). These AUCs parameters were compared with Student t test. The oxygen saturation (SpO_2) and the sedation depth (SD) were compared with the Mann–Whitney U test. An asterisk next to the *p-value* indicates a significant statistical difference at α threshold of 5 %

significantly higher score ($p = 0.0009$) than the KET group.

Recovery quality

Recovery quality was significantly better in the FMM group after administration of reversal agents, than in the ketamine group, as assessed by both the visual analogue scale (VAS) and the recovery clinical scoring scheme (RCS) (Fig. 2). The Bland-Altman plots demonstrated a non-significant bias of 0.1437 and a reasonably good level of agreement between the two tests (Fig. 3). However it also showed a non-homogeneous distribution of the plots that was probably due to the scale difference between the VAS and the RCS. For the Kappa statistic analysis, the average of the two observers for each subject was used. The comparison of recovery group results

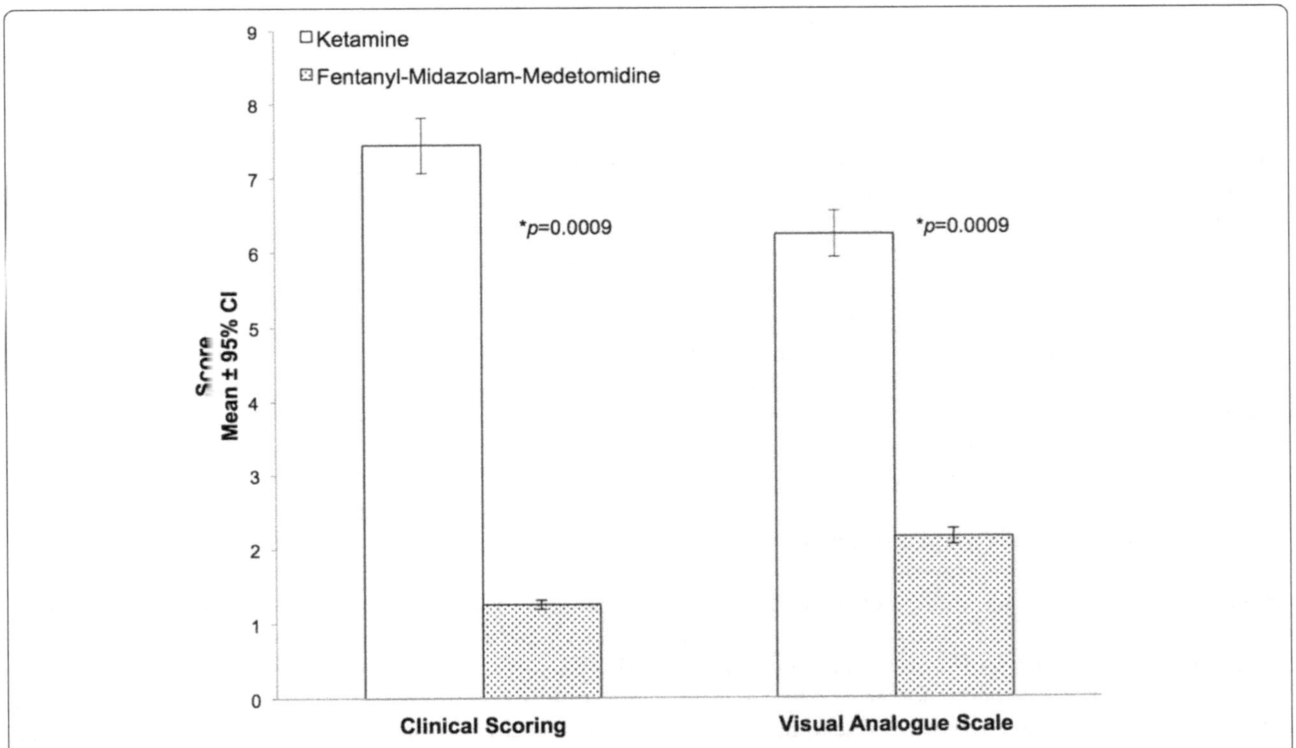

Fig. 2 Recovery quality results in Rhesus macaques receiving ketamine (*n* = 8) or fentanyl-midazolam-medetomidine (*n* = 8). The histograms represent the mean ± 95 % of confidence interval. The results are expressed as mean ± 1 SD. RCS: Ketamine 7 ± 2; Fentanyl-midazolam-medetomidine 1 ± 1. VAS: Ketamine 6.2 ± 0.8; Fentanyl-midazolam-medetomidine 2.2 ± 0.5. An asterisk next to a *p*-value(*p*) indicates a significantly differences

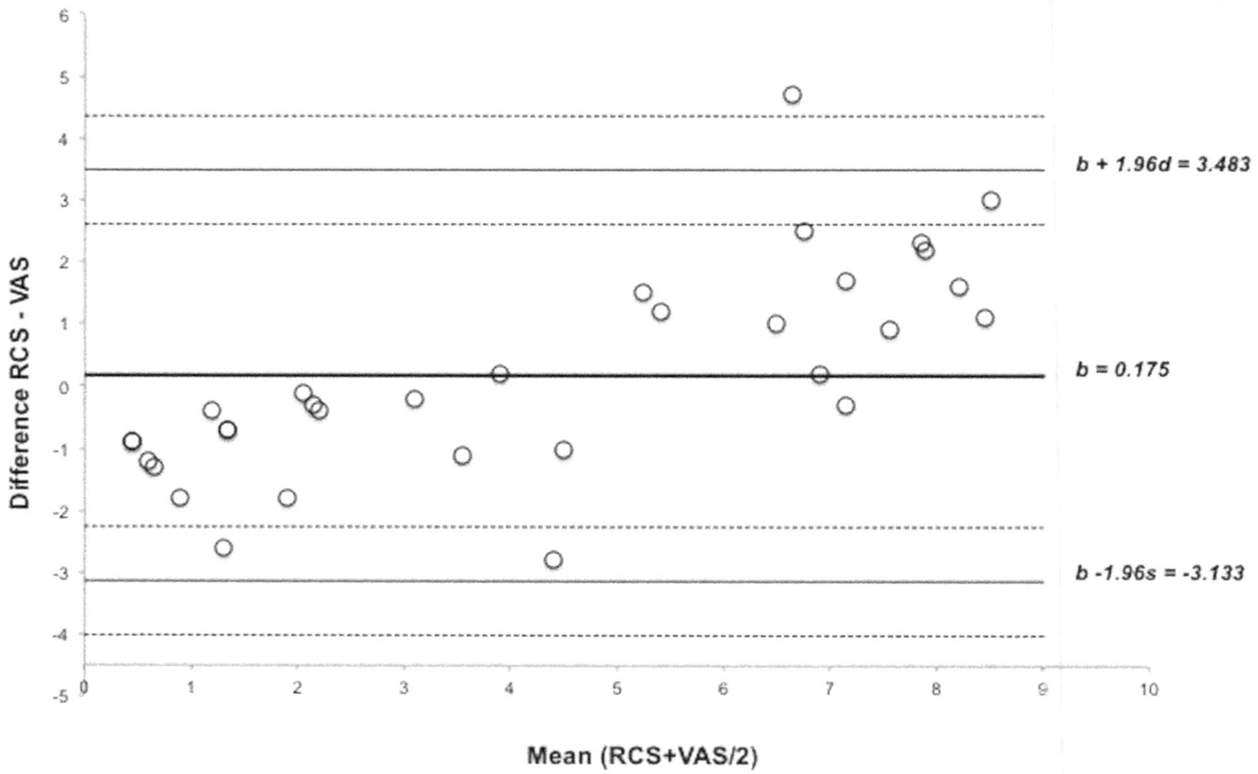

Fig. 3 Bland-Altman plots comparing the quality of recovery in Rhesus macaques receiving ketamine ($n = 8$) or fentanyl-midazolam-medetomidine ($n = 8$). The differences between the scores for each method are plotted against the mean of the two methods. (*b*) = bias; (*b* + *1.96 s*; *b* − *1.96 s*) = Agreement limits. The shaded lines represent the 95 % confidence intervals of the agreement limits

gave a kappa statistic k = 0.662 with a significance of $p =$ 0.01. According to usual interpretation of this result [21], there was a substantial agreement between the RCS and VAS.

Discussion

In this study the administration of the FMM combination to rhesus macaques provided a deeper and more reliable sedation and a better recovery score than ketamine sedation. The impacts of the two regimens on physiological parameters were consistent with the known properties and mechanism of action of the agents used.

High ketamine liposolubility results in rapid bioavailability in the central nervous system, resulting in rapid onset of action [22]. This rapid onset of sedation was observed in the present study and is similar to that reported in previous studies [23–25]. Attainment of sedation sufficient for safe handling was significantly shorter following administration of ketamine than following FMM, likely due to the different rates of absorption and distribution of the components of the combination. The onset of a sufficient degree of sedation to allow safe handling after administration of FMM observed in this study was longer than that reported by Votava *et al.*, using a comparable sedation protocol [20]. This difference may be due to differences in the doses of the agents used in the two studies and the use of hyaluronidase to speed absorption in Votava study. Recovery time in the FMM group was significantly shorter than the KET group, very likely due to the use of specific antagonists to reverse two of the components used for sedation [26, 27]. We chose not to administer flumazenil to reverse midazolam, since our experience has shown that midazolam has minimal sedative effects at the dose used in this species. In this study, because no post-procedural pain was anticipated, naloxone was used to reverse the effects of fentanyl. As an alternative, butorphanol, nalbuphine and buprenorphine have all been shown to be effective antagonists [28–30]. This latter approach has the advantage of providing continued analgesia following reversal of the fentanyl, because of administration of agents with either k agonist/μ antagonist activity, or partial μ agonist actions. A duration of sedation prior to reversal of the FMM regimen of 20 min was chosen as it represented the mean time that NHPs can be safely handled under ketamine sedation [24, 25].

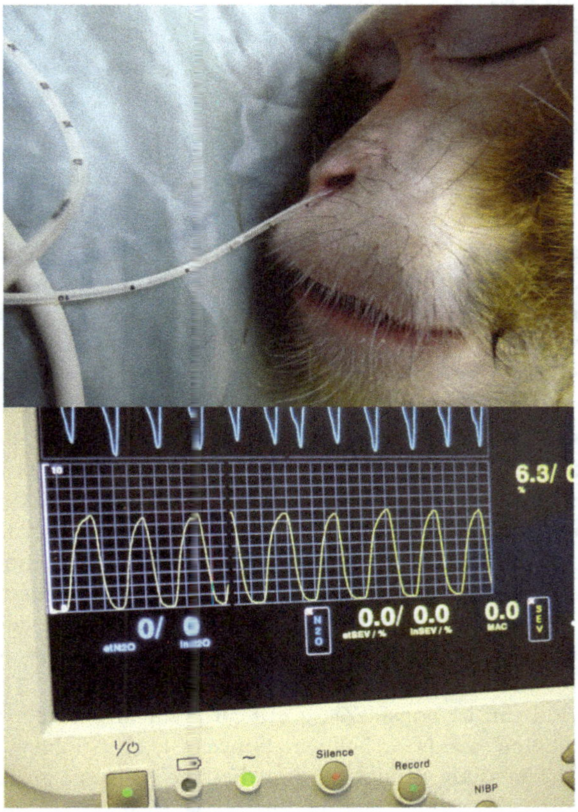

Fig. 4 Respiration monitoring. A soft lubricated tube was inserted in the ventral meatus of one of the nostril. The tube was linked to a side-stream capnograph providing the visualization of a waveform and end-tidal CO_2 value

Anaesthetic agents decrease central nervous system activity and the assessment of somatic withdrawal reflexes is generally accepted as a means of assessing anaesthetic depth [3]. Due to its mechanism of action, ketamine produces a unique cataleptic state, but one which can be considered as light sedation based on the degree of suppression of reflex responses (eg withdrawal reflexes) [3, 4]. Used alone, ketamine increases muscular tone in many species [31–33] but this effect is not as marked in non human primates as in other species [24]. Seizures [7–10] and tissue necrosis [5, 6, 34] can also occur with ketamine injection. In this study, none of these complications occurred, however one of the female primates only remained in lateral recumbency for less than ten minutes post-injection and this has been observed in other studies [24, 25]. Several hypotheses such as the variation of the injection site with incomplete intramuscular administration, individual variability or a possible acquired tolerance to ketamine [25] can explain this observation. In this study, the FMM protocol provided a deeper sedation, comparable to surgical anaesthesia. Following completion of this study, we have used the combination to enable intubation as jaw tone is markedly reduced and laryngeal reflexes absent. We have also repaired deep and superficial wounds, which resulted from fights between cage-mates.

Pulse oximetry was used successfully to assess oxygen saturation, but this technique can be compromised by poor peripheral tissue perfusion [2], such as can occur when $alpha_2$ agonists are administered. This was not a problem in the current study. Systolic blood pressure was measured by a non-invasive oscillometric method. The cuff used to measure the blood pressure followed the general recommendation that the cuff width should equal 40 % of the limb circumference [35]. However, this method has been shown to underestimate systolic and diastolic blood pressures by between 5 and 20 mmHg depending on the cuff location [36–38]. Adequacy of ventilation was assessed using capnography, since this allowed assessment of respiratory rate and pattern and the $EtCO_2$. The $EtCO_2$ is usually measured at the distal extremity of the endo-tracheal tube [39, 40], but in the present study, the $EtCO_2$ was measured in the ventral meatus of the nose with a sample line linked to a side stream capnography device. This approach provided a good waveform and is a technique that could be used routinely for anaesthetic monitoring in this and other primate species

However validation of the approach should be performed as published data comparing the technique are available only in people [41–44].

The significant differences in cardiovascular and respiratory parameters between the sedation protocols in this study are consistent with the mechanism of action of the agents used. Ketamine has a minimal impact on the respiratory system with minimal modification of the ventilation parameters [3]. The breathing rate observed and $EtCO_2$ were similar to those described in a previous study in rhesus macaques but the $EtCO_2$ values recorded were lower [23, 45]. Ketamine affects the cardiovascular system by stimulating the sympathetic pathway and increasing circulating catecholamine concentrations [3]. Heart rate and systolic blood pressure effects were also

Table 2 Sedation Depth Scoring System. A higher score indicates a deeper sedation

Score	Movement	Palpebral reflex	Jaw tone	Withdrawal reflex
1	Whole body	Blinking + others movement	increased	Normal
2	Limb/foot/Hand	Blinking	Normal	Weakly
3	Facial	Weak blinking	Decreased	Delayed
4	Twitching fingers	Delayed blinking	Minimal	Only digits movements
5	No	No	No	No

Table 3 Recovery Clinical Scoring Scheme. System based on 15 points with the principle that a higher score indicates a poorer recovery

•Eyes					
Score	2	1	0	+1	+1
	Close	Semi-close	Open	Nystagmus	Rubbing its eyes
•Mouth					
Score	3	2	1	0	
	Vomitting	Lips smacking/ Nausea sign	Hypersalivation	Nothing	
•Body position					
Score	3	2	1	0	
	Lateral/ ventral recumbency	Unsuccessful attempt to sit	Successful attempt to sit/ Sit but wobbly	Sit and stable	
•Ataxia					
Score	3	2	1	0	
	Strong	Mild	Slight	Absence	
•Environment awareness					
Score	2	1	0		
	No	Partially	Yes		
Total: /15					

consistent with the literature [20, 23, 45, 46]. Due to the known mechanisms and interactions of the individual components of the regimen, it was expected the FMM protocol would have more negative influences on cardiovascular and respiratory functions. Midazolam, has sedative and anxiolytic effects but minimal effects on cardiorespiratory physiology [3, 4], however medetomidine and fentanyl both depress these system and their effects are potentiated when they are combined [3]. Although FMM produced a significant decrease of heart rate, systolic blood pressure and respiratory function, these values stayed within acceptable ranges for deeply sedated primates [1, 3]. There appears to be no previously published information on the impact of fentanyl-midazolam-medetomidine on these parameters in macaques, but the bradycardia noted in this study was similar to that reported by Votava *et al.* [20]. This combination has varying effects in other species. In rats, rabbits, Mongolian gerbils and chinchillas, bradycardia is a consistent finding, whereas effects on blood pressure varied. In contrast to other species in which moderate hypotension was reported, rats developed moderate hypertension [17].

The quality of the recovery was assessed by two methods, a clinical scoring scheme (RCS) and a visual analogue scale (VAS). The VAS is a subjective single-item test that in this study was used only to assess the quality of recovery. VAS assessments are widely used to

Table 4 Recovery quality category

Category	VAS	RCS
Good	0–3.33	0–5
Moderate	3.34–6.67	6–10
Bad	6.68–10	11–15

VAS visual analogue scale, the range are expressed in cm. *RCS* recovery clinical scoring, the ranges are expressed in arbitrary units

assess pain [47], anxiety [48] and other items [49, 50]. Such systems have the advantage of being quick and easy to perform and also to have good reliability [51]. The clinical scoring scheme used in this study was the first attempt to construct and use a multiple-item test to assess recovery in non-human primates. The scale used was based on the Pediatric Anesthesia Emergence Delirium Scale (PAED) [52, 53]. The items chosen to build the RCS were based on their abilities to show modification in cases of excitation or poor recovery and on the facility to observe these modifications. The two methods of assessment demonstrated a strong correlation and a strong agreement with a non-significant bias. The video extracts, used for the scoring the quality of recovery, focused on the period around first attempt to sit. This period can be considered a critical point in recovery as excitation, ataxia or hallucination can lead to injury [3, 54]. The study results showed that the recovery quality was significantly better in the FMM treatment group. There are several possible explanations for this result. The use of specific antagonists in the FMM group may have reversed not only the sedative effects of the three components but also their side effects [26, 27]. The poor quality recovery in the ketamine group may have been the results of ketamine's dissociative effects [3]. Previous studies in dogs and cats, using ketamine, did not report a difference in the quality of recovery compared to other anaesthetic protocols [55, 56]. However the administration of ketamine to children and horses prior the end of anaesthesia resulted in a decrease in the quality of recovery in comparison with the use of α_2-agonists, benzodiazepine or acepromazine [57, 58].

Conclusion

In conclusion, this study demonstrated the efficacy of the combination of fentanyl, medetomidine and midazolam to immobilise rhesus macaques. This regimen offers a potentially useful alternative to ketamine, since specific antagonists can rapidly reverse it, and this results in a better quality of recovery.

Methods

Animals

The animals were purpose bred for research in the UK, and were supplied from the Centre for Macaques to Newcastle University. Animals were housed in a Home

Office (United Kingdom authority) accredited facility and in compliance with the Animal Scientific Procedure Act 1986 and the European Directive 2010/63/EU. Rhesus macaques aged from 3 to 10 years and weighing from 4 to 17.7 kg (n = 16, 10 males and 6 females) scheduled, in November 2014, for annual health checks and tuberculosis testing were used in this study. The animals were housed at Comparative Biology Centre (Newcastle University, United Kingdom), in indoor pens with a solid floor and windows allowing a view on the other pens and the corridors. A minimum floor area 4.40 m^2 was provided for each animal or pair of animals. A smaller pen with a squeeze-back system was located between each housing pen. Enrichment devices and substrate for foraging were provided. Animals were maintained on a light:dark cycle of 12 h:12 h. at a temperature of 22 °C and with 15 air changes per hour and a relative humidity of 24 %. Primates were fed with adapted old world primate diet (Special Diets Service, Witham, United Kingdom) and received tap water *ad libitum* at the time of the study. Forage mix was provided daily to all animals (LBS Biotechnology, United Kingdom). Except for two males, all the primates were paired-housed. The single housing was due to exceptional circumstances unrelated to the research protocols. The primates had not been sedated or anaesthetised during the two weeks prior the start of the study.

Sedation protocols

Animals (5 males and 3 females per group) were assigned randomly to receive either ketamine (KET) or Fentanyl-Midazolam-Medetomidine (FMM). Animals were fasted at least 4 h prior to the administration of the sedative agents. Both sedation protocols were administered by intramuscular injection in the femoral quadriceps, the femoral biceps or the gluteal maximus. Ketamine (Ketaset 100 mg/ml Solution for Injection, Zoetis, London, United Kingdom) was administered at the dose of 10 $mg.kg^{-1}$ [23, 24]. For the FMM protocol, the dose each drug was determined based on a pilot study (data not reported here). Fentanyl (Fentanyl 50 micrograms/ml, Martindale Pharmaceutical, Romford, United Kingdom), midazolam (Midazolam 5 mg/ml, Hameln pharmaceutical ltd, Gloucester, United Kingdom) and medetomidine (Domitor 1 mg/ml, Vetoquinol UK ltd, Buckingham, United Kingdom) were administered at 10 $\mu g.kg^{-1}$, 0.5 $mg.kg^{-1}$ and 20 $\mu g.kg^{-1}$, respectively. Due to the high injection volume 2 injection sites were used. Midazolam and medetomidine were mixed in the same syringe and injected separately from the fentanyl. When primates lost their righting reflex and could be safely handled, they were carried to a room outside of the NHP unit. At the end of the procedure, primates in the KET group were placed in a recovery cage and monitored until the return of the righting reflex. In the FMM group, naloxone at 10 $\mu g.kg^{-1}$ (Naloxone 400 micrograms/ml Solution for injection/infusion, Hameln pharmaceutical ltd, Gloucester, United Kingdom) and atipamezole (Antisedan 5 mg/ml, Vetoquinol UK ltd, Buckingham, United Kingdom) at 0.22 $mg.kg^{-1}$ were mixed in the same syringe and administered by intramuscular injection 20 min after the onset of sedation. Then primates were transferred to a recovery cage and monitored until the return of the righting reflex.

Sedation support and monitoring

Physiological parameters and depth of the sedation were measured every 5 min for 20 min procedure consisting of venous blood sampling, dental examination, an intradermal tuberculosis test and a complete physical examination. Animals were placed in lateral recumbency, covered with a forced-air warming blanket set at 38 °C (Bair hugger model 505, Augustine Medical, USA) and received 100 % oxygen supplementation using a face mask (2 to 4 litres per min). A Vitalogik 4500 monitoring system (Charter-Kontron Ltd, Milton Keynes, United Kingdom) was used to measure vital signs. Heart rate (HR) and oxygen saturation (SpO_2) were assessed using an absorbance pulse oxymeter probe placed on a finger. Blood pressure was assessed using an oscillometric method with a blood pressure cuff (Critikon Dura-Cuf, GE Healthcare, Hatfield, United Kingdom) appropriate for the size of the animal. The cuff was placed on the opposite arm to that used for pulse oximetry to record the blood pressure from the brachial artery. Two measures were taken at each time point and the mean calculated. The respiration rate (RR) and the end-tidal CO_2 ($EtCO_2$), were measured by the side stream gas analyser integrated in the electronic monitoring system. The gas sampling rate was 50 ml/min. A soft neonatal feeding tube with 1.7 mm of diameter and 38 cm of length (100 % latex-free Premature Infant Feeding tube, Bard Ltd, Crawley, United Kingdom) attached to the gas sampling line was lubricated with lidocaine gel (Anbesol teething gel, Alliance pharmaceutical, Chippenham, United Kingdom) and gently advanced to a depth of 3 cm into the ventral meatus of one of the nostril (Fig. 4). This operation was repeated at each time point. The depth of the sedation was assessed by a clinical scoring scheme adapted from previous publications (Table 2).

Onset of sedation and recovery times

All of the sedation procedures were videotaped and analysed at a later date. This enabled blinding of the assessor to the treatment given. The time from administration of the sedative to the time at which it was considered that an animal that could be safely handled was recorded. The recovery time was the time between the end of the 20 min procedure and the return of the righting reflex. The end of the procedure was comparable with the injection of the antidote mix in the FMM group

Recovery quality assessment

Samples of the video-recording from 2 min before to 2 min after the first attempt to sit were selected and the quality of recovery assessed by two treatment-blinded observers using two methods. A recovery clinical scoring scheme (RCS) consisting of a multiple-item list (Table 3) and a visual analogue scale (VAS), with a 10 cm line anchored with "best possible recovery" and "worst possible recovery" were used for this assessment. In both scoring schemes, a high score indicated a poor recovery. The observers were veterinary technicians with extensive experience of working with NHPs. Depending on the numeric result, each recovery was classified using the categories in Table 4.

Statistical analysis

For the HR, BPSyst, RR, EtCO2, SpO2 and sedation depth, Area Under the Curves (AUCs) were estimated using the trapezoidal method [59, 60]. The AUCs normality distribution was assessed using the Shapiro-Wilk test. Student's t test was performed where data were normally distributed; otherwise the Mann–Whitney U test was used.

A Mann–Whitney U test was used to compare sedation times and recovery times between the two groups and the RCS and the VAS sedation recovery scores. Bland-Altman plots and Kappa statistic methods were used to assess the agreement between the VAS and RCS results.

Statistical analyses were performed with SPSS statistic software (vers. 22, IBM, USA) and Excel (vers. 14.3.0, Microsoft, USA). A p-value < 0.05 was considered statically significant

Abbreviations

AUC, area under the curve; BPsyst, systolic blood pressure; $EtCO_2$, endt-tidal CO_2; FMM, Fentanyl-Midazolam-Medetomidine; HR, heart rate; IM, intramuscular; KET, ketamine; NHPs, non-human primates; PAED, pediatric anesthesia emergence delirium scale; RCS, Recovery Clinical scoring scheme; RR, respiration rate; VAS, visual analogue scale

Acknowledgement

Authors tank the primate care staff of the comparative Biology Centre and research assistants of the Institute of Neuroscience for their support in the accomplishment of this work. HGMJB would like to thanks Dr Matthew C. Leach for his advices and assistance in data statistical analysis.

Funding

No funding was obtained to support this study

Authors' contribution

HB, YE, SO and PF developed the experimental design of the study, performed the sedations, prepared and interpreted data, created tables and figures, drafted and finalized the manuscript. The final version of the manuscript was read and approved by all authors of this study.

Competing interest

None of the authors of this paper has a financial or personal relationship with other people or organizations that could inappropriately influence or bias the content of the paper. The authors declare that they have no competing interests.

Consent for publication

Not applicable.

Author details

[1]Comparative Biology Centre, Newcastle University, Framlington Place, Newcastle Upon Tyne NE2 4HH, UK. [2]Faculty of Veterinary Medicine, University of Liège, Boulevard de Colonster, Liège 4000, Belgium. [3]School of Veterinary Medicine and Science, University of Nottingham, Sutton Bonington Campus, Loughborough LE12 5RD, UK. [4]Institute of Neuroscience, Newcastle University, Newcastle Upon Tyne NE1 7RU, UK.

References

1. Abee CR, Mansfield K, Tardif SD, Morris T. Nonhuman Primates in Biomedical Research: Biology and Management. London, United Kingdom: Elsevier Science; 2012.
2. Flecknell P. Laboratory Animal Anaesthesia. 4th ed. Oxford: Elsevier Science; 2015.
3. Grimm KA, Lamont LA, Tranquilli WJ, Greene SA, Robertson SA. Veterinary Anesthesia and Analgesia. Oxford: Wiley Blackwell; 2015.
4. Plumb DC. Plumb's Veterinary Drug Handbook: Desk Edition. 6th ed. Ames, IA: Blackwell; 2008.
5. Sun FJ, Wright DE, Pinson DM. Comparison of ketamine versus combination of ketamine and medetomidine in injectable anesthetic protocols: chemical immobilization in macaques and tissue reaction in rats. Contemp Top Lab Anim Sci. 2003;42:32–7.
6. Carrier CA, Donnelly KB. Post-injection sciatic neuropathy in a cynomolgus macaque (Macaca fascicularis). J Med Primatol. 2013;43:52–4.
7. Adami C, Spadavecchia C, Casoni D. Seizure activity occurring in two dogs after S-ketamine-induction. Schweiz Arch Tierheilkd. 2013;155:569–72.
8. Celesia GG, Chen R-C. Effects of Ketamine on EEG activity in cats and monkeys. Electroencephalogr Clin Neurophysiol. 1974;37:345–53.
9. Christe KL, Lee UJ, Lemoy M-J, Havton LA. Generalized Seizure Activity in an Adult Rhesus Macaque (Macaca mulatta) during Ketamine Anesthesia and Urodynamic Studies. Comp Med. 2013;63:445–7.
10. Gourie-Devi M, Cherian L, Shankar SK. Seizures in cats induced by ketamine hydrochloride anaesthesia–a preliminary report. Indian J Med Res. 1983;77:525–8.
11. Baker NJ, Schofield JC, Caswell MD, McLellan AD. Effects of Early Atipamezole Reversal of Medetomidine–Ketamine Anesthesia in Mice. J Am Assoc Lab Anim Sci. 2011;50:916–20.
12. Cevik E, Bilgic S, Kilic E, Cinar O, Hasman H, Acar AY, Eroglu M. Comparison of ketamine–low-dose midozolam with midazolam-fentanyl for orthopedic emergencies: a double-blind randomized trial. Am J Emerg Med. 2013;31:108–13.
13. Mamula P, Markowitz JE, Neiswender K, Zimmerman A, Wood S, Garofolo M, Nieberle M, Trautwein A, Lombardi S, Sargent-Harkins L, Lachewitz G, Farace L, Morgan V, Puma A, Cook-Sather SD, Liacouras CA. Safety of intravenous midazolam and fentanyl for pediatric GI endoscopy: prospective study of 1578 endoscopies. Gastrointest Endosc. 2007;65:203–10.
14. McQueen A, Wright RO, Kido MM, Kaye E, Krauss B. Procedural Sedation and Analgesia Outcomes in Children After Discharge From the Emergency Department: Ketamine Versus Fentanyl/Midazolam. Ann Emerg Med. 2009; 54:191–197.e4.
15. Milić M, Goranović T, Knežević P. Complications of sevoflurane–fentanyl versus midazolam–fentanyl anesthesia in pediatric cleft lip and palate surgery: a randomized comparison study. Int J Oral Maxillofac Surg. 2010;39:5–9.
16. Gerak LR, Brandt MR, France CP. Studies on benzodiazepines and opioids administered alone andin combination in rhesus monkeys: ventilation and drug discrimination. Psychopharmacology (Berl). 1998;137:164–74.
17. Albrecht M, Henke J, Tacke S, Markert M, Guth B. Effects of isoflurane, ketamine-xylazine and a combination of medetomidine, midazolam and fentanyl on physiological variables continuously measured by telemetry in Wistar rats. BMC Vet Res. 2014;10:1–14.
18. Albrecht M. Influence of repeated anaesthesia on physiological parameters in male Wistar rats: a telemetricstudy about isoflurane, ketamine-xylazine

and a combination of medetomidine, midazolam and fentanyl. BMC Vet Res. 2014;10:1–15.
19. Rahmanian-Schwarz A, Held M, Knoeller T, Amr A, Schaller H-E, Jaminet P. The Effect of Repetitive Intraperitoneal Anesthesia by Application of Fentanyl-Medetomidine and Midazolam in Laboratory Rats. J Invest Surg. 2012;25:123–6.
20. Votava M, Hess L, Schreiberová J, Málek J, Štein K. Short term pharmacological immobilization in macaque monkeys. Vet Anaesth Analg. 2011;38:490–3.
21. Viera AJ, Garrett JM. Understanding Interobserver Agreement: The Kappa Statistic. Fam Med. 2005;37:360–3.
22. Kohn DF, Wixson SK, White WJ, Benson GJ. Anesthesia and Analgesia in Laboratory Animals. New York: Elsevier Science; 1997.
23. Lee VK, Flynt KS, Haag LM, Taylor DK. Comparison of the Effects of Ketamine, Ketamine–Medetomidine, and Ketamine– Midazolam on Physiologic Parameters and Anesthesia-Induced Stress in Rhesus (Macaca mulatta) and Cynomolgus (Macaca fascicularis) Macaques. J Am Assoc Lab Anim Sci. 2010;49:57–63.
24. Naccarato EF, Hunter WS. Anaesthetic effects of various ratios of ketamine and xylazine in rhesus monkeys (Macaca mulatta). Lab Anim. 1979;13:317–9.
25. Settle TL, Rico PJ, Lugo-Roman LA. The effect of daily repeated sedation using ketamine or ketamine combined with medetomidine on physiology and anesthetic characteristics in Rhesus Macaques. J Med Primatol. 2010;39: 50–7.
26. Dahan A, Aarts L, Smith TW. Incidence, Reversal, and Prevention of Opioid-induced Respiratory Depression. Anesthesiology. 2010;112:226–38.
27. Sinclair MD. A review of the physiological effects of $α_2$-agonists related to the clinical use of medetomidine in small animal practice. Can Vet J. 2003; 44:885–97.
28. Flecknell PA, Liles JH, Wootton R. Reversal of fentanyl/fluanisone neuroleptanalgesia in the rabbit using mixed agonist/antagonist opioids. Lab Anim. 1989;23:147–55.
29. Hu C, Flecknell PA, Liles JH. Fentanyl and medetomidine anaesthesia in the rat and its reversal using atipamazole and either nalbuphine or butorphanol. Laboratory Animals. 1992;26:15–22.
30. Latasch L, Probst S, Dudziak R. Reversal by Nalbuphine of Respiratory Depression Caused by Fentanyl. Anesth Analg. 1984;63:814–6.
31. Haskins SC, Farver TB, Patz JD. Ketamine in dogs. Am J Vet Res. 1985;46: 1855–60.
32. Moreland AF, Glaser C. Evaluation of ketamine, ketamine-xylazine and ketamine-diazepam anesthesia in the ferret. Lab Anim Sci. 1985;35:287–90.
33. Nowrouzian I, Schels HF, Ghodsian I, Karimi H. Evaluation of the anaesthetic properties of ketamine and a ketamine/xylazine/atropine combination in sheep. Vet Rec. 1981;108:354–6.
34. Wellington D, Mikaelian I, Singer L. Comparison of Ketamine–Xylazine and Ketamine–Dexmedetomidine Anesthesia and Intraperitoneal Tolerance in Rats. J Am Assoc Lab Anim Sci. 2013;52:481–7.
35. Clark JA, Lieh-Lai MW, Sarnaik A, Mattoo TK. Discrepancies Between Direct and Indirect Blood Pressure Measurements Using Various Recommendations for Arm Cuff Selection. Pediatrics. 2002;11:920–3.
36. Chester AE, Dorr AE, Lund KR, Wood LD. Noninvasive measurement of blood pressure in conscious cynomolgus monkeys. Fundam Appl Toxicol. 1992;19:64–8.
37. Wiester MJ, Iltis R. Diastolic and systolic blood pressure measurements in monkeys determined by a noninvasive tail-cuff technique. J Lab Clin Med. 1976;87:354–61.
38. Yeung KR, Lind JM, Heffernan SJ, Sunderland N, Hennessy A, Makris A. Comparison of indirect and direct blood pressure measurements in baboons during ketamine anaesthesia. J Med Primatol. 2014;43:217–24.
39. Belenkiy S, Ivey KM, Batchinsky AI, Langer T, Necsoiu C, Baker W, Salinas J, Cancio LC. Noninvasive Carbon Dioxide Monitoring in a Porcine Model of Acute Lung Injury Due to Smoke Inhalation and Burns. Shock. 2013;39: 495–500.
40. Fierstra J, Winter JD, Machina M, Lukovic J, Duffin J, Kassner A, Fisher JA. Non-invasive accurate measurement of arterial PCO2 in a pediatric animal model. J Clin Monit Comput. 2013;27:147–55.
41. Manifold CA, Davids N, Villers LC, Wampler DA. Capnography for the nonintubated patient in the emergency setting. J Emerg Med. 2013;45:626–32.
42. Fukuda K, Tatsuya J, Kaneko Y. Is Measurement of end-tidal CO_2 through a nasal cannula reliable? Anesth Prog. 1997;1–4.
43. Agus MS, Alexander JL, Mantell PA. Continuous non-invasive end-tidal CO_2 monitoring in pediatric inpatients with diabetic ketoacidosis. Pediatric Diabetes. 2006;7:1–5.
44. Yanagidate F, Dohi S. Modified nasal cannula for simultaneous oxygen delivery and end-tidal CO2 monitoring during spontaneous breathing. Eur J Anaesthesiol. 2006;23:257–60.
45. Winterborn AN, Bates WA, Feng C, Wyatt JD. The efficacy of orally dosed ketamine and ketamine/medetomidine compared with intramuscular ketamine in rhesus macaques (Macaca mulatta) and the effects of dosing route on haematological stress markers. J Med Primatol. 2008;37:116–27.
46. Young SS, Schilling AM, Skeans S, Ritacco G. Short duration anaesthesia with medetomidine and ketamine in cynomolgus monkeys. Lab Anim. 1999;33:162–8.
47. Myrvik MP, Drendel AL, Brandow AM, Yan K, Hoffmann RG, Panepinto JA. A Comparison of Pain Assessment Measures in Pediatric Sickle Cell Disease: Visual Analog Scale Versus Numeric Rating Scale. J Pediatr Hematol Oncol. 2015;37:190–4.
48. Abend R, Dan O, Maoz K, Raz S, Bar-Haim Y. Reliability, validity and sensitivity of a computerized visual analog scale measuring state anxiety. J Behav Ther Exp Psychiatry. 2014;45:447–53.
49. Rausch M, Zehetleitner M. Comparison between a visual analogue scale and a four point scale as measures of conscious experience of motion. Conscious Cogn. 2014;28:126–40.
50. Wehby G, Naderi H, Robbins J, Ansley T, Damiano P. Comparing the Visual Analogue Scale and the Pediatric Quality of Life Inventory for Measuring Health-Related Quality of Life in Children with Oral Clefts. IJERPH. 2014;11: 4280–91.
51. Maxwell C. Sensitivity and Accuracy of the Visual Analogue Scale: A Psycho-Physical Classroom Experiment. Br J Clin Pharmac. 1978;6:15–24.
52. Janssen NJJF, Tan EYL, Staal M, Janssen EPCJ, Leroy PLJM, Lousberg R, van Os J, Schieveld JNM. On the utility of diagnostic instruments for pediatric delirium in critical illness: an evaluation of the Pediatric Anesthesia Emergence Delirium Scale, the Delirium Rating Scale 88, and the Delirium Rating Scale-Revised R-98. Intensive Care Med. 2011;37:1331–7.
53. Sikich N, Lerman J. Development and Psychometric Evaluation of the Pediatric Anesthesia Emergence Delirium Scale. Anesthesiology. 2004;100:1138–45.
54. Costi D, Ahmed S, Stephens K, Strickland P, Ellwood J, Larsson JN, et al. Effects of sevoflurane versus other general anaesthesia on emergence agitation in children (Review). The Cochrane Library. 2014;1–212.
55. Freitas GC, da Cunha MG MCM, Gomes K, da Cunha JP MCM, Togni M, Pippi NL, Carregaro AB. Acid–base and biochemical stabilization and quality of recovery in male cats with urethral obstruction and anesthetized with propofol or a combination of ketamine and diazepam. Can J Vet Res. 2012; 76:201–8.
56. Kennedy MJ, Smith LJ. A comparison of cardiopulmonary function, recovery quality, and total dosages required for induction and total intravenous anesthesia with propofol versusa propofol-ketamine combination in healthy Beagle dogs. Vet Anaesth Analg. 2014;42:350–9.
57. Chen J, Li W, Hu X, Wang D. Emergence agitation after cataract surgery in children: a comparison of midazolam, propofol and ketamine. Pediatr Anesth. 2010;20:873–9.
58. Valverde A, Black B, Cribb NC, Hathway A, Daw A. Assessment of unassisted recovery from repeated general isoflurane anesthesia in horses following post-anesthetic administration of xylazine or acepromazine or a combination of xylazine and ketamine. Vet Anaesth Analg. 2012;40:3–12.
59. Bate ST, Clark RA. The Design and Statistical Analysis of Animal Experiments. Cambridge, United Kingdom: Cambridge University Press; 2014.
60. Liengme B: A Guide to Microsoft Excel 2007 for Scientists and Engineers. Burlington, MA: Elsevier Science; 2008.

12

Glucocorticosteroids and ciclosporin do not significantly impact canine cutaneous microbiota

Giovanni Widmer[1*], Lluís Ferrer[2], Claude Favrot[3], Judy Paps[4], Kevin Huynh[1] and Thierry Olivry[4]

Abstract

Background: As prednisone and ciclosporin can have immunosuppressive effects and have been considered potential predisposing factors for skin infections, we investigated the impact of these drugs on the diversity of the cutaneous microbiota, the abundance of *Malassezia* and infection with *Papillomaviruses.*

Results: Six atopic, asymptomatic Maltese-beagle dogs were treated with ciclosporin for one month and then with prednisone for another month, with a one-month wash-out between treatments. The dogs were sampled on the abdomen and pinna before and after each treatment using a swab. Samples for *Papillomavirus* detection were obtained with cytobrush sticks. The bacterial microbiota was characterized using 16S amplicon high-throughput sequencing. *Malassezia* populations were quantified with nested real-time PCR targeting the ribosomal internal transcribed spacer 1. The diversity and composition of cutaneous microbiota was not impacted in a detectable manner by any of the treatments. As observed for the bacterial microbiota, *Malassezia* populations were not affected by treatment. Three dogs were positive for *Papillomavirus* at more than one timepoint, but an association with treatment was not apparent.

Conclusions: Ciclosporin and prednisone at doses used for the treatment of atopic dermatitis do not impact the canine cutaneous microbiota in a detectable manner.

Keywords: Prednisone, Ciclosporin, 16S amplicon sequencing, Microbiota, *Malassezia*, *Papillomavirus*, Principal coordinates analysis

Background

Cutaneous infections are very prevalent in atopic dogs; in most cases, they are caused by microorganisms that are considered normal inhabitants of the canine skin, such as *Staphylococcus pseudintermedius* or *Malassezia pachydermatis* [1]. The mechanisms that trigger the proliferation of a commensal cutaneous organism and leads to a bona fide infection are poorly understood. As skin infections are thought to worsen the clinical manifestations of atopic dermatitis, understanding the mechanisms underlying their development is of high interest.

Both glucocorticoids and ciclosporin are extensively used to treat atopic dermatitis in dogs. These drugs are recommended as first line therapies in the recently updated guidelines for the management of this disease [2]. As both drugs, depending on their dose, can have immunosuppressive effects, some authors have suggested that their prolonged use could favor the development of skin infections. For instance, treatment with glucocorticoids is considered to predispose to the development of superficial pyoderma in dogs, and relapsing urinary tract infections are recognized as a common side effect of glucocorticoid treatment in this species [1, 3, 4].

There is less evidence for ciclosporin predisposing to skin infections, but an increased rate of urinary tract infections in atopic dogs treated with this drug has been reported [5]. Finally, the development of viral papillomas in dogs has been mentioned in different studies as one on the side effects of ciclosporin therapy, probably due to an alteration of in the immune mechanism controlling viral replication [6, 7].

* Correspondence: giovanni.widmer@tufts.edu
[1]Department of Infectious Diseases and Global Health, Cummings School of Veterinary Medicine at Tufts University, 200 Westboro Road, North Grafton, MA, USA
Full list of author information is available at the end of the article

One way to assess if ciclosporin and glucocorticoids predispose to the development of skin infections is to analyze the impact of such treatments on the skin microbiota using high-throughput sequencing. These techniques enable the evaluation of the relative abundance of cutaneous bacteria and diversity of the skin microbiota [8, 9]. In this approach, changes in the microbiome could be used as proxy to assess the risk for cutaneous infections. In support of this assertion, skin infections were recently shown to be preceded by a diminished bacterial microbiota diversity in human and canine atopic patients [10, 11].

To examine the impact of ciclosporin and prednisone on the canine skin microbiota, we designed a longitudinal study with dosages used to treat canine allergic skin diseases. We found that these treatments have no discernable impact on the diversity of canine bacterial microbiota nor on *Malassezia* or *Papillomavirus* populations of the skin.

Methods

Dogs and treatments

Six co-housed Maltese-beagle crossbred atopic dogs numbered 1 to 6 were used for this study. The dogs are purpose-bred for allergy research. There were three intact males and three females aged between 3 and 8 years (average: 5.7 years . These dogs had been sensitized in preceding years to *Dermatophagoides farinae* house dust mites [12]. For this study, allergen challenges and lesion induction were not performed, and the dogs did not exhibit skin lesions at any time. At first, six dogs were treated orally with 5 mg/kg of ciclosporin once daily for one month. After a 1-month wash out, the dogs were treated with 0.75 mg/kg of prednisone per os once daily for one month. The interventions were approved by the Institutional Animal Care and Use Committee at NC State University. Drugs used in this study were those commercially available. They were purchased from this university's Veterinary Hospital Pharmacy. No anesthesia was used and the dogs were not euthanized upon conclusion of the in vivo study.

Sample collection

Samples were collected aseptically at six timepoints over a period of 7 months. These timepoints are numbered T0 (pre-treatment) - T5, where T0 samples were collected 19 days before initiation of ciclosporin treatment, T1 on the day ciclosporin was first administered, T2 at conclusion of ciclosporin treatment, T3 44 days after the end of ciclosporin treatment and upon initiation of prednisone treatment, T4 at the end of the prednisone treatment and T5 after a 30-day washout period. Samples were collected in all cases from two sites: ventral pinna and inguinal skin. For the bacterial microbiota and for the *Malassezia* analyses, a sterile swab was used (Isohelix, Harrietsham, Kent, UK). Swabs were rubbed for 15 s on each side of the swab within an area of approximately 4 cm^2. For the evaluation of *Papillomavirus*, the samples were obtained using sterile cytobrush sticks (CytoSmear, Purfybr, Munster, Indiana) [13]. Samples were stored at 4 °C for no more than 72 h before extraction and final storage at − 80 °C.

16S rRNA amplicon sequencing for bacterial microbiota characterization

DNA was extracted from swabs using the Power Soil DNA isolation kit (MoBio, Carlsbad, CA). Bacterial populations were characterized using 16S ribosomal RNA (rRNA) amplicon high-throughput sequencing. A portion of the bacterial 16S rRNA ribosomal rRNA gene from the V1 V2 variable region was amplified using primers 27F and 338R [14], generating an amplicon of > 300 nucleotides (nt). A first PCR of 20 cycles using primer 27F (AGAGTTTGATYMTGGCTCAG) and 338R (TGCTGCCTCCCGTAGGAGT) was followed by a second PCR of 20 cycles to incorporate Illumina adapters and a unique 6-nt barcode. All PCR experiments included a positive and negative control reaction. Barcoded PCR products were electrophoresed on 2.5% agarose gel to check for the presence of amplification product of the correct size. The concentration of amplicon DNA was quantified by measuring absorbance at 260 and 280 nm. Amplicons were pooled at approximately equal concentration and the pooled library sequenced at the Tufts University Genomics core facility (tucf.org) using an Illumina MiSeq sequencer and a custom sequencing primer [15]. Amplicons were sequenced single-end, 300 nt. An average of 92,567 (standard deviation (SD) = 72,127) sequence reads were obtained per barcode. FASTQ files were deposited in the European Nucleotide Archive under accession number PRJEB15158. To assess the level of experimental noise in the sequence data, we duplicated three samples (Additional file 1). Duplicates were amplified separately from the same DNA sample and each amplicon tagged with a unique 6-nt barcode.

Bioinformatics and statistical analysis

Bioinformatics analysis was performed using mothur essentially as described [16–18]. Briefly, random subsamples of 5000 sequences were aligned using Clustal Omega [19] and curated to remove sequencing errors. Chimeras were removed using Uchime [20] as implemented in mothur. Sequences were denoised using program pre.cluster [18] using a difference threshold of 2 nt. Differences between bacterial populations (β diversity) were quantified using the weighted Unifrac phylogenetic distance [21]. Unifrac is a metric of pairwise phylogenetic dissimilarity frequently used in microbial ecology. It is a measure of the fraction of branches in a phylogenetic tree which are unique to either of the two populations being compared. Matrices of pairwise distance between 89 samples were computed in *mothur* and visualized on Principal Coordinate Analysis (PCoA) plots using GenAlEx [22]. Sequences were classified using the Naïve Bayesian classifier [23] with template and taxonomy reference files downloaded from the Ribosomal Database Project [24]. The minimum bootstrap value for taxonomic assigment was set at 70%.

To measure α diversity, we used the Shannon and Berger-Parker indices. The latter index is equal to the proportion of the most abundant Operational Taxonomic Unit (OTU), where an OTU is a collection of similar sequences and can be viewed as a proxy of species. In contrast to Shannon diversity, increasing Berger-Parker diversity indicates decreasing diversity.

The significance of clustering of samples based on Unifrac distance was tested using ANOSIM [16]. Variation Partitioning Analysis [25] as implemented in CANOCO [26] was used to assess the relative contribution of two independent variables, dog and time, to the microbiome profile.

Malassezia nested PCR

A nested PCR protocol was developed and used to amplify a 142-nt fragment of the *Malassezia* Internal Transcribed Spacer (ITS) 1. The following primers targeting the ribosomal repeat sequence of *M. pachydermatis* were used; outside primer forward: AGGTTTCCGTAGGTGACCT, outside primer reverse: TTCGCTGCGTTCTTCATCGA [27]. The inside, nested, forward primer (unpublished) was AACCCGTGTGCACTT, and the reverse nested primer CGTTGTCGAAAGTTG. To quantify *Malassezia* DNA, amplification curves were generated with a RT PCR assay on a Roche LightCycler instrument. PCR experiments were controlled with positive and negative controls and specificity of the amplification confirmed by sequencing a representative amplicon. As a positive control, a sample from a dog with severe *Malassezia* overgrowth (20–25 organisms/high power field) was used. The number of PCR cycles needed to reach the instrument's detection threshold, known as the Crossing Point (C_t), was used as a measure of relative *Malassezia* DNA concentration. A standard curve was calculated to convert C_t values to *Malassezia* DNA copy number. Seven 10-fold serial dilutions of a *Malassezia* DNA reference sample with an average of 41.7 cells per high-power field were prepared and PCR amplified using the nested primer sets described above. A first order linear regression with the equation

$$Ct = -4.06^* \log(\text{copy number}) + 43.94$$

and $r^2 = 0.998$ was obtained and used to convert PCR C_t values to ITS1 copy number.

Papillomavirus PCR

Samples collected with a cytobrush were kept at 4 °C for no longer than 24 h and stored at − 18 °C until extraction. To pellet cells and debris, tubes (still containing the cytobrush tip) were centrifuged at 15000 *g* for 10 min. The cytobrush tip was removed and the saline supernatant aspirated leaving 25 μl in the tube. DNA was extracted using the DNeasy extraction kit (Qiagen, Hilden, Germany) following the manufacturer's instructions. DNA was eluted in 100 μl sterile water. RT PCR was used to identify and quantify *Papillomavirus* DNA in the samples. The PCR amplified a region of the L1 gene (canPVf/FAP64; CTTCCTGAWCCTAAYMAKTTTGC/CCWATATCWVHCATNTCNCCATC). This probe detects all viruses belonging to the genus *Papillomavirus*. The papillomavirus PCR was performed at the Veterinary School of the University of Zurich, Switzerland, as described elsewhere [13].

Results

Analysis of bacterial microbiota

Impact of treatments

We used PCoA of pairwise weighted Unifrac distance matrices to display differences in 16S rRNA sequence profile in different dog skin swabs. Figure 1 shows three versions of the same PCoA of 89 samples. The plots are colored according to date of collection (A), dog (B) and body site (C). There is no visible indication that ciclosporin or prednisone treatment, initiated at timepoint T1 and T3, respectively, affected the skin bacterial microbiota (panel A). Statistical analysis of weighted Unifrac distances between samples collected at the six timepoints confirmed this interpretation (Table 1). T1 and T2 samples, and T3 and T4 samples were not significantly different ($p = 0.262$ and $p = 0.345$, respectively). Only two comparisons, T0 versus T2 and T0 versus T5 were significantly different. Since these timepoints do not bracket the treatments, we suspected a temporal effect unrelated to treatment and concluded that the tested interventions had not discernable effect on microbiota.

To investigate another possible effect of the tested drugs, we estimated the α-diversity of the bacterial populations in swabbed samples using the Shannon [28] and Berger-Parker diversity index [29]. Altogether, the skin bacterial diversity was not signifcantly impacted by ciclosporin and prednisone treatment (Fig. 2).

Shannon diversity indices ranged in value between 3.4 and 5.1 regardless of treatment. We used Kruskal-Wallis one-way ANOVA on ranks to test whether microbiota diversity collected on the various dates differed. The test

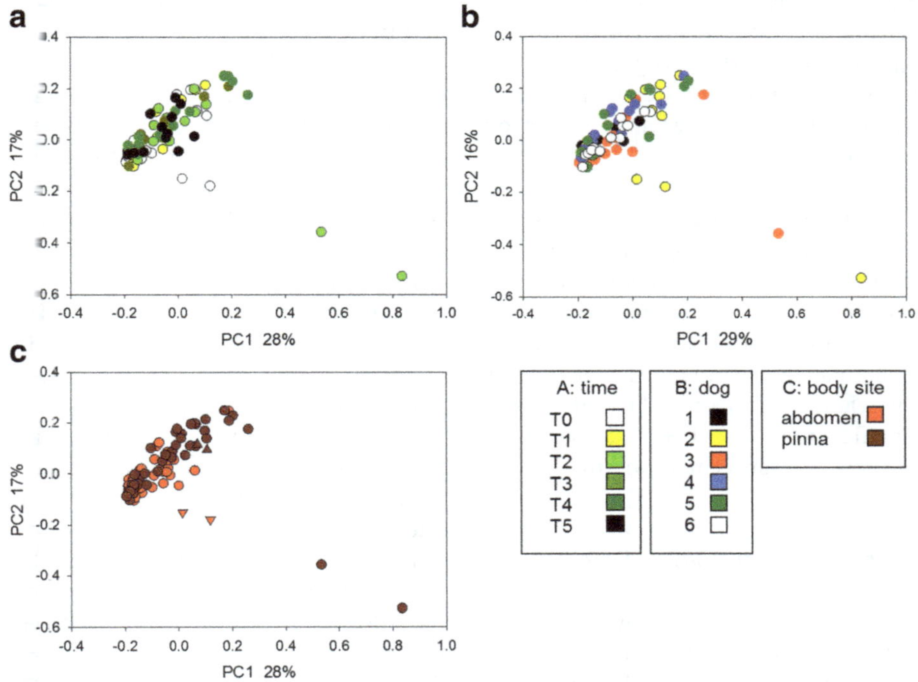

Fig. 1 Principal Coordinates Analysis of 89 swab samples. Colors represent time of collection (**a**), dog (**b**) and body site (**c**) as shown in the key. The complete list of samples is shown in supplementary material. Duplicated samples extracted from the same sample and barcoded separately are indicated with matching triangles in plot C (see also Additional file 1)

Table 1 ANOSIM R values and statistical significance of pairwise weighted Unifrac distance between microbiota collected at six timepoints

Comparison[a]	R	p
T0-T1	0.26	0.023
T0-T2	0.54	0.001[b]
T0-T3	0.08	0.217
T0-T4	0.25	0.039
T0-T5	0.25	0.001[b]
T1-T2	0.06	0.262[c]
T1-T3	−0.04	0.624
T1-T4	−0.04	0.579
T1-T5	0	0.375
T2-T3	0.15	0.138
T2-T4	−0.06	0.726
T2-T5	0.01	0.417
T3-T4	0.01	0.345[c]
T3-T5	0.12	0.094
T4-T5	−0.05	0.694

[a] timepoint abbreviations as described in Materials and Methods
[b] statistically significant R after correction for multiple comparisons
[c] comparisons of samples collected immediately before and after ciclosporin and prednisone treatment

returned a significant *P*-value ($P = 0.02$). As for ANOSIM described above, comparisons between sampling dates were not significantly different when comparing samples collected immediately before and immediately after each treatment. Similarly, the analogous analysis based on Berger-Parker α-diversity showed no significant difference between pre- and post-treatment samples. In

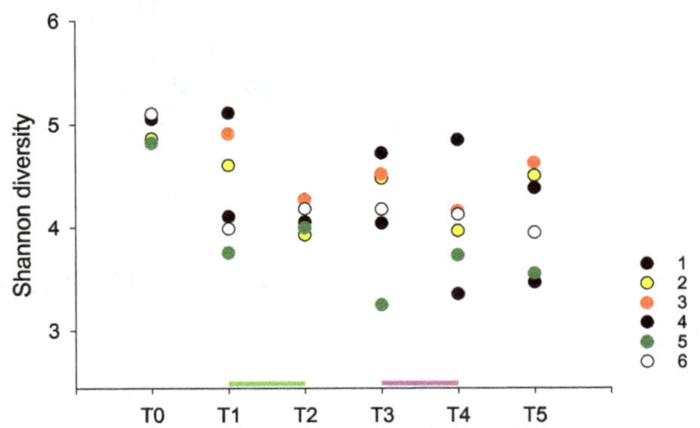

Fig. 2 Microbiome diversity over time. Mean Shannon diversity for each animal is represented for each collection date. The means were calculated for samples collected from each dog at each timepoint ($n = 2–6$). Times of collection are represented on the x axis as defined in Materials and Methods. Dogs are colored as shown in the key. Green and pink bars indicate ciclosporin and prednisone treatment, respectively

contrast to the analysis of Shannon diversity, no overall difference between sampling dates was found using one-way ANOVA ($F_{5,30} = 2.205$, $p = 0.08$). Together, Unifrac distances and diversity values indicate that neither ciclosporin nor prednisone had a detectable impact on the skin bacterial microbiota.

The phylum-level classification of 85 swab samples is shown in Fig. 3. Consistent with PCoAs, neither ciclosporin nor prednisone induced any apparent change in microbiota taxonomy. A lower-level taxonomic classification shows the same lack of treatment effect (Additional files 2 and 3). Figure 3 shows a temporal trend of increasing relative abundance of Firmicutes over time. A linear regression of relative Firmicutes abundance over time was highly significant ($F_{1,23} = 20.8$, $P < 0.001$), but this trend appears to be unrelated to the tested interventions.

Diversity of skin microbiota between dogs and anatomical location

We analyzed 16S sequences to explore whether skin microbiota differed by dogs. Since all animals where subjected to the same treatment, this analysis is not central to the topic investigated here, but is relevant to understanding the evolution of skin microbiota and the extent to which co-housed animals may harbor different microbiota. Clustering by dog was found to be statistically significant (ANOSIM, $n = 6$, $R = 0.25$, $P < 0.0001$). Variation Partitioning Analysis was used to further evaluate the relative contribution of two independent variables, dog and time, on the microbiome profile. The results of this analysis show that variable "dog" explains 27.5% of the explained variation, which is 10 times more than the variation explained by variable "time" (2.6%). This outcome is consistent with the PCoA and ANOSIM results described above and in Additional file 4 in showing that time of sample collection had a relatively small impact on the skin microbiome.

When the samples from six dogs were separated by anatomical site, clustering of skin microbiota by dog became apparent by PCoA (Additional file 4) and was statistically significant when all dogs were compared (abdomen, $n = 6$, ANOSIM $R = 0.40$, $P < 0.0001$; pinna $n = 6$ ANOSIM $R = 0.24$, $P < 0.001$). After Bonferroni correction, 8/15 pairwise comparisons of abdomen microbiota were significantly different. For the pinna, only two out of 15 pairwise comparisons between dogs were significantly different (Additional file 5). α and β diversity was analyzed in relation to body site and to compare intra-dog vs inter-dog diversity. Based on Shannon diversity, samples collected from the abdomen and from the pinna were equally diverse ($n = 93$, t test $P = 0.079$). In contrast, samples collected from the same dog, whether from the pinna or the abdomen, were less different from each other than samples from different dogs (Kruskal-Wallis ANOVA on ranks, $P < 0.001$). This analysis indicates that in spite of the animals being housed together, the skin microbiota populating different

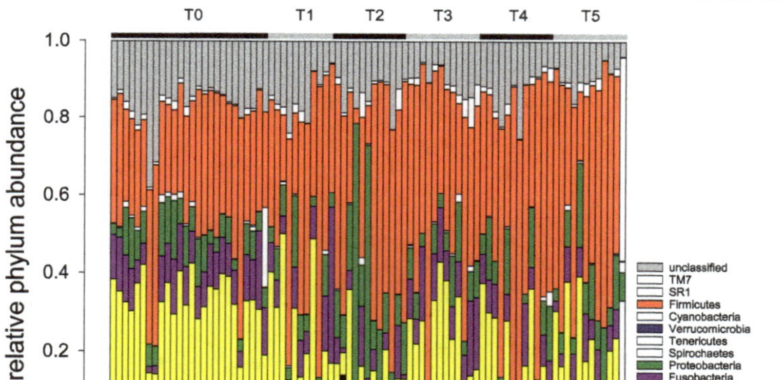

Fig. 3 Phylum-level classification of bacterial microbiota from 85 skin swabs shows no apparent impact of treatment. Each bar represents a different sample. The most abundant phyla are colored as shown in the key. Timepoints are indicated uppermost. T1 and T2 indicate beginning and end of ciclosporin treatment, respectively; T3 and T4 indicate beginning and end of prednisone treatment, respectively. Within each timepoint (T), samples are ordered by dog (1 - > 6). The samples are from left to right: **T0**, 1_ing1, 1_ing2, 1_pinna1, 1_pinna2, 2_ing1, 2_ing2, 2_pinna1, 2_pinna2, 3_ing1, 3_ing2, 3_ing3, 3_pinna1, 3_pinna2, 3_pinna3, 4_ing1, 4_ing2, 4_pinna1, 4_pinna2, 5_ing1, 5_ing2, 5_pinna1, 5_pinna2, 6_ing1, 6_ing2, 6_pinna1, 6_pinna2. **T1**, 1_ing1, 1_pinna1, 2_ing1, 2_pinna1, 3_ing1, 3_pinna1, 4_ing1, 5_ing1, 5_pinna1, 6_ing1, 6_pinna1. **T2**, 1_ing1, 1_pinna1, 2_ing1, 2_pinna1, 3_ing1, 3_pinna1, 4_ing1, 4_pinna1, 5_ing1, 5_pinna1, 6_ing1, 6_pinna1. **T3**, 4_ing1, 4_pinna1, 5_ing1, 5_pinna1, 6_ing1, 6_pinna1, 1_ing1, 1_pinna1, 2_ing1, 2_pinna1, 3_ing1, 3_pinna1. **T4**, 1_ing1, 1_pinna1, 2_ing1, 2_pinna1, 3_ing1, 3_pinna1, 4_ing1, 4_pinna1, 5_ing1, 5_pinna1, 6_ing1, 6_pinna1. **T5**, 1_ing1, 1_pinna1, 2_ing1, 2_pinna1, 3_ing1, 3_pinna1, 4_ing1, 4_pinna1, 5_ing1, 5_pinna1, 6_ing1, 6_pinna1, where the number before the underscore indicates dog number and the final number within each code indicates left (1) and right (2) side. On timepoint T0 dog 3 was sampled three times, as indicated by (3)

animals tends to diverge, and that each dog is populated by a distinct bacterial microbiota.

Quantification of *Malassezia* and association with bacterial diversity

A nested real-time PCR assay was used to quantify *Malassezia* DNA in the same swab samples as used for 16S rRNA sequencing. *Malassezia* carriage varied among dogs. At time T0, before initiation of treatment, some dogs had high *Malassezia* loads (i.e., dog 5) (Additional file 6). In contrast, other dogs showed very low loads (dogs 3, 6). Despite this trend, high inter-sample variability was observed among samples from a same dog. The density of *Malassezia* was higher on the pinnae than on the abdomen (Mann-Whitney Rank sum test, U = 2016, n = 72, P = 0.021). *Malassezia* populations significantly varied in the course of the experiment (ANOVA on Ranks, n = 24/group, H = 20.1, 5 d.f., P < 0.001). However, such variation did not appear to be a result of treatment (Additional file 6). Neither of the two pairwise comparisons between C_t values from samples taken immediately before and after the treatment were significantly different (Tukey's test).

We analyzed *Malassezia* PCR C_t values and 16S rRNA diversity for an association between *Malassezia* infestation and bacterial diversity. For this analysis, we used both Shannon and Berger-Parker diversity indices. Bacterial diversity and *Malassezia* relative abundance were not significantly correlated (Additional file 7). Although none of the regressions were statistically significant, we observed a slight yet non-significant increase in bacterial diversity with increasing *Malassezia* C_t (decreasing *Malassezia* relative abundance) for the abdominal samples and an opposite trend for those collected on the pinnae.

Detection of *Papillomavirus* DNA

The results of PCR to detect *Papillomavirus* DNA in the skin samples are summarized in Table 2; these results are in agreement with those from previous studies that had demonstrated that *Papillomavirus* DNA is detectable on the skin of healthy dogs. Dogs 2 and 4 were positive once and dog 3 was positive on two consecutive sampling points. As observed for the bacterial microbiota and *Malassezia* infestation, the results did not correlate with the treatments administered.

Table 2 Results of Papillomavirus PCR

Dog number and sampling site	Timepoint					
	T0	T1	T2	T3	T4	T5
1 Pinna	–	–	–	–	–	–
1 Abdomen	–	–	–	–	–	–
2 Pinna	–	–	–	–	+	–
2 Abdomen	–	–	–	–	–	–
3 Pinna	–	+	+	–	–	–
3 Abdomen	–	–	–	–	–	–
4 Pinna	–	–	–	–	–	–
4 Abdomen	–	–	–	+	–	–
5 Pinna	–	–	–	–	–	–
5 Abdomen	–	–	–	–	–	–
6 Pinna	–	–	–	–	–	–
6 Abdomen	–	–	–	–	–	–

Discussion

The cutaneous microbiota of six atopic dogs was analyzed at six timepoints over a 7-months period. This study is unique because of its comprehensive examination of microbiota, including bacteria, *Malassezia and Papillomavirus.* To our knowledge, this is the first study that investigated the impact of non-antimicrobial treatments on the canine cutaneous microbiome. The major limitation of this study is the small number of dogs investigated. However, as we found no apparent trend when pre- and post-treatment samples were compared, it is unlikely that a study with more animals would lead to a different conclusion.

Our original hypothesis was that ciclosporin or glucocorticoids would reduce bacterial diversity, facilitating overgrowth of pathogens and the development of overt skin infections. Our results show that the treatment with ciclosporin at 5 mg/kg/q 24 h or with prednisone at 0.75 mg/kg/q 24 h does not impact the profile or the diversity of the cutaneous bacterial microbiome of the dog. Therefore, it is unlikely that treatment itself directly increases the risk of secondary bacterial infections commonly observed in atopic dogs. The specific trigger(s) of *Staphylococcus pseudintermedius* proliferation ending in pyoderma in an atopic dog remain unclear, but the leading hypothesis is that abnormalities in the skin barrier or immunologic changes linked to atopic dermatitis [30] lead to a reduction in bacterial diversity and facilitate bacterial infections, as reported in humans [10] and more recently in dogs [11]. In this study, we did not challenge dogs with the allergen to which they are sensitized, because the main objective was to assess the impact of the treatment - and not allergic inflammation - on the bacterial microbiota, on *Malassezia* and on *Papillomavirus* infection. The assessment of the bacterial microbiome after an allergen challenge in this acute canine atopic dermatitis model has been reported previously [31].

The detection and relative quantification of *Malassezia* DNA was successful using the PCR primers reported by Makimura et al. [27] which are specific for *Malassezia pachydermatis.* A nested PCR protocol was used to increase the sensitivity of this test. None of the two treatments had an impact on the relative abundance of *Malassezia* yeast and thus we concluded that ciclosporin and prednisolone do not affect cutaneous *Malassezia* populations under the conditions tested. The outbreaks of *M. pachydermatis* frequently observed in atopic dogs probably should be better attributed to changes in the cutaneous ecosystem caused by the atopic disease rather than to treatment itself. Previous studies have reported that in human atopic patients different *Malassezia* species are present on the skin, which is typically not the case in healthy individuals [32, 33]. Importantly, in this study, we only investigated the most common and clinically important *Malassezia* species in the dog (*M. pachydermatis*) and therefore cannot draw conclusions on the diversity of the entire *Malassezia* population, as reported in atopic humans [34]. A recent study based on high-throughput sequence data of the ribosomal internal transcribed spacer I analyzed the fungal population of the skin in healthy and atopic dogs [35]. This study found that the relative abundance of *Malassezia* was not impacted by the dog's health status. This observation and our study are however difficult to compare. While Meason-Smith et al. used high-throughput sequencing to infer relative abundance, we quantified *Malassezia* using real-time PCR. In contrast to the earlier study, our experiments were not designed to assess differences in skin microbial populations between atopic and healthy animals.

As for the analysis of bacterial microbiota and *Malassezia*, we found that the treatments did not increase the presence of detectable *Papillomavirus* in the skin. As expected, papillomavirus DNA was detected in some dogs at different points of the study (Table 2), but all dogs were negative for this group of commensals at the end of the study.

Conclusions

Ciclosporin and prednisone, used at typical dosages prescribed for the treatment of atopic dermatitis for one month did not impact the canine cutaneous microbiota in a detectable manner. The data suggest that these treatments are unlikely to increase the risk of secondary microbial infections commonly observed in atopic dogs. Whether a longer treatment would change the skin microbiota remains undetermined but deserving of further study.

Additional files

Additional file 1: Sample replication and experimental noise. Three samples were replicated to estimate the level of technical variation. Replicated samples are shown in black. For clarity some black data points were slightly shifted on the plot to eliminate symbol overlap. The distance between replicates represents the experimental noise caused by PCR and sequencing. The mean weighted Unifrac distance among 4275 non-replicated pairwise comparisons ($93 \times 92/2-3 = 4275$) was 0.383, whereas the mean for the three pairwise distance between replicates was 0.186. Unifrac distance values originating from experimental noise was thus significantly smaller than the average Unifrac distance from different samples (Mann-Whitney Rank Sum Test $U = 456$, $p = 0.005$). Triangle up, dog 1 abdomen; triangle down, dog 2 pinna; diamond, dog 3 abdomen. The percent variation explained by the first two principal axes is indicated.

Additional file 2: Example of lower-level classification of skin microbiota over time for dog 1 and dog 3. Bars are arranged from left to right in chronological order grouped by anatomical site. Stacks are arranged from bottom to top in order of diminishing cumulative taxon abundance across all samples. The 20 most abundant taxa are shown. Bars height is < 1 because less abundant taxa are not shown. Sequences classified at the genus level with 70% probability value were assigned to the next higher taxonomic level i.e., family, order, class or phylum. The dates when the samples were collected are abbreviated as DDMMYY. On 5/21/14 (T1), dog 1 samples were collected in duplicate and dog 3 samples in triplicate. Replicate samples were barcoded individually to visualize experimental variation (see Additional file 1). The dogs showed a different composition of the microbiome, which remained relatively constant over time. As seen in the other analyses, no effect of treatment on microbiota composition was apparent.

Additional file 3: Genus-level classification of abdomen and pinna skin microbiota from six dogs.

Additional file 4: Principal Coordinates Analysis by body site. When two sampling locations are considered separately, clustering by dog is significant (pinna $n = 6$, ANOSIM $R = 0.24$, $P < 0.001$; abdomen, $n = 6$, ANOSIM $R = 0.40$, $P < 0.0001$). The data points are color-coded by dog as shown in Fig. S1. A, pinna; B, abdomen.

Additional file 5: Pairwise ANOSIM R values and statistical significance level for comparisons of weighted Unifrac distance between microbiota from six dogs and two body sites.

Additional file 6: Temporal evolution of *Malassezia* infestation of pinna and inguinal area of six dogs. The timepoints are labelled as indicated in Materials and Methods. Data points are colored according to dog as in Fig. 1. Swabs from the left and right side were analyzed individually as shown by duplicated lines of same color. Ciclosporin and prednisone treatment are represented with a green and a pink bar, respectively. Crossing points exceeding 41 cycles (< 10 copies) were deemed negative and are not represented in graphs. Triangles indicate positive control. Crossing points were converted to number of ITS1 copies using the standard curve.

Additional file 7: Lack of significant association between *Malassezia* abundance and bacterial diversity. Left and right graph show the analysis of inguinal and pinna samples, respectively. Full symbols indicate Shannon diversity, empty symbols Berger-Parker diversity. Linear regression model is indicated by lines.

Abbreviations

ANOVA: Analysis of Variance; nt: nucleotide; OTU: Operational Taxonomic Unit; PCoA: Principal Coordinates Analysis; rRNA: ribosomal RNA; SD: standard deviation

Acknowledgments

The authors gratefully acknowledge Elanco for funding the study, and Albert Tai and the Tufts Genomics staff for sequencing.

Funding

Elanco reviewed and approved the study protocol, and funded the study; it had no part in the execution of the study, data analysis or writing of the manuscript.

Authors' contributions

LF and TO designed the experiment and obtained the funding. JSP contributed to the design and performed the in vivo study. GW supervised the bench work and analyzed the 16S sequence data. KH processed the samples, prepared the 16S amplicon libraries and performed the Malassezia PCR analyses. CF performed the Papillomavirus analysis and analyzed the data. GW and LF wrote the manuscript, which was reviewed and revised by the other authors. All authors read and approved the final revision.

Consent for publication

Not applicable

Competing interests

TO declares having received consulting honoraria and previous research support from Elanco or one of its founding companies (Novartis Animal Health).

Author details

[1]Department of Infectious Diseases and Global Health, Cummings School of Veterinary Medicine at Tufts University, 200 Westboro Road, North Grafton, MA, USA. [2]Department of Clinical Sciences, Cummings School of Veterinary Medicine at Tufts University, 200 Westboro Road, North Grafton, MA, USA. [3]Clinic for Small Animal Internal Medicine, Vetsuisse Faculty, University of Zürich, Winterthurerstrasse 260, -8057 Zürich, CH, Switzerland. [4]Department of Clinical Sciences, College of Veterinary Medicine, North Carolina State University, 1060 William Moore Drive, Raleigh, NC 27607, USA.

References

1. Miller WH, Griffin CE, Campbell KL. Muller & Kirk's small animal dermatology. St Louis: Elsevier; 201[illegible]
2. Olivry T, DeBoer DJ, Favrot C, Jackson H, Mueller RS, Nuttall T, et al. Treatment of canine atopic dermatitis: 2015 updated guidelines from the international committee on allergic diseases of animals. BMC vet. Res. 2015;11:210.
3. Ihrke PJ, Norton AL, Ling GV, Stannard AA. Urinary tract infection associated with long-term corticosteroid administration in dogs with chronic skin diseases. J Am Vet Med Assoc. 1985;186:43–6.
4. Peterson AL, Torres SM, Rendahl A, Koch S. Frequency of urinary tract infection in dogs with inflammatory skin disorders treated with glucocorticoid therapy: a retrospective study. Vet Dermatol. 2012;23:201–e43.
5. Radowicz SN, Power HT. Long-term use of ciclosporin in the treatment of canine atopic dermatitis. Vet Dermatol. 2005;16:81–6.
6. Seibel W, Sundberg JP, Lesko LJ, Sauk JJ, McCleary LB, Hassell TM. Cutaneous papillomatous hyperplasia in ciclosporin-a treated beagles. J Invest Dermatol. 198[illegible];93:224–30.
7. Favrot C, Olivry T, Werner AH, Nespecca G, Utiger A, Grest P, et al. Evaluation of papillomaviruses associated with cyclosporine-induced hyperplastic verrucous lesions in dogs. Am J Vet Res. 2005;66:1764–9.
8. Rodrigues-Hoffman A, Patterson AP, Diesel A, Lawhon SD, Lu HJ, Elkins Stephenson C, et al. The skin microbiome in healthy and allergic dogs. PLoS One. 2014;9:e83197.
9. Weese JS. The canine and feline skin microbioma in health and disease. Vet Dermatol. 2013;24:1[illegible]–e31e.
10. Kong HH, Oh J, Deming C, Conlan S, Grice EA, Beatson MA, et al. Temporal shifts in the skin microbiome associated with disease flares and treatment in children with atopic dermatitis. Genome Res. 2012;22:850–9.
11. Bradley CW, Morris DO, Rankin SC, Cain CL, Misic AM, Houser T, et al. Longitudinal evaluation of the skin microbiome and association with microenvironment and treatment in canine atopic dermatitis. J Invest Dermatol. 2016;136:1[illegible]82–90.
12. Olivry T, Wofford J, Paps JS, Dunston SM. Stratum corneum removal facilitates experimental sensitization to mite allergens in atopic dogs. Vet Dermatol. 2011;22:1[illegible]8–96.
13. Lange C, Zollinger S, Tobler K, Ackerman M, Favrot C. Clinically healthy skin of dogs is a potential reservoir for canine papillomaviruses. J Clin Microbiol. 2011;49:707–9.
14. Koenig JE, Spor A, Scalfone N, Fricker AD, Stombaugh J, Knight R, et al. Succession of microbial consortia in the developing infant gut microbiome. Proc Natl Acad Sci U S A. 2011;108(Suppl 1):4578–85.
15. Luo X, Jellison KL, Huyn K, Widmer G. Impact of bioreactor environment and recovery method on the profile of bacterial populations from water distribution systems. PLoS One. 2015;10:e0133427.
16. Clark KR. Non-parametric multivariate analyses of changes in community structure. Aust J Ecol. 1993;18:117–43.
17. Ras R, Huyhn K, Desoky E, Badawy A, Widmer G. Perturbation of the intestinal microbiota of mice infected with Cryptosporidium Parvum. Int J Parasitol. 2015;45:567–73.
18. Schloss PD, Westcott SL, Ryabin T, Hall JR, Hartmann M, Lesniewski RA, et al. Introducing mothur: open-source, platform-independent, community-supported software for describing and comparing microbial communities. Appl Environ Microbiol. 2009;75:7537–41.
19. Sievers F, Wilm A, Dineen D, Gibson TJ, Karplus K, Li W, et al. Fast, scalable generation of high-quality protein multiple sequence alignments using Clustal omega. Mol Syst Biol. 2011;7:539.
20. Edgar RC, Haas BJ, Clemente JC, Quince C, Knight R. UCHIME improves sensitivity and speed of chimera detection. Bioinformatics. 2011;27:2194–200.
21. Lozupone C, Hamady M, Knight R. UniFrac - An online tool for comparing microbial community diversity in a phylogenetic context. BMC Bioinformatics. 2006;7:371–85.
22. Peakall R, Smouse PE. GenAlEx 6.5: genetic analysis in excel. Population genetic software for teaching and research–an update. Bioinformatics. 2012;28:2537–9.
23. Wang Q, Garrity GM, Tiedje JM, Cole JR. Naive Bayesian classifier for rapid assignment of rRNA sequences into the new bacterial taxonomy. Appl Environ Microbiol. 2007;73:5261–7.
24. Cole JR, Wang Q, Fish JA, Chai B, McGarrell DM, Sun Y, et al. Ribosomal database project: data and tools for high throughput rRNA analysis. Nucl Acids Res. 2014;42:D633–D42.
25. Brocard D, Legendre P, Drapeau P. Partialling out the spacial component of ecological variation. Ecology. 1992;73:1045–55.
26. ter Braak CJF, Šmilauer P. Canoco reference manual and user guide. Biometris: Wageningen and České Budějovice; 2012.
27. Makimura K, Tamura Y, Kudo M, Uchida K, Salto H, Yamaguchi H. Species identification and strain typing of Malassezia species stock strains and clinical isolates based on the DNA sequences of nuclear ribosomal internal transcribed spacer 1 regions. J Med Microbiol. 2000;49:29–35.
28. Shannon C, Weaver W. Biodiversity measurements. *The Mathematical Theory of Communication. Urbana University Press, Illinois* 1948;117–27.
29. Berger WH, Parker FL. Diversity of planktonic foraminifera in deep-sea sediments. Science. 1970;168:1345–7.
30. Santoro D, Marsella R, Pucheu-Haston CM, Eisenschenk MN, Nuttall T, Bizikova P. Review: pathogenesis of canine atopic dermatitis: skin barrier and host–micro-organism interaction. Vet Dermatol. 2015;26(2):84–e25.
31. Pierezan F, Olivry T, Paps JS, Lawhon SD, Wu J, Steiner JM, Suchodolski JS, Rodrigues Hoffmann A. The skin microbiome in allergen-induced canine atopic dermatitis. Vet Dermatol. 2016;27:332–e82.
32. Han SH, Cheon HI, Hur MS, Kim MJ, Jung WH, Lee YW et al. Analysis of the skin mycobiome in adult patients with atopic dermatitis. Exp Dermatol. 2018; Jan 21.
33. Yim SM, Kim JY, Ko JH, Lee YW, Choe YB, Ahn KJ. Molecular analysis of *Malassezia* microflora on the skin of patients with atopic dermatitis. Ann Dermatol. 2010;22:41–7.
34. Sugita T, Suto H, Unno T, Tsuboi R, Ogawa H, Shinoda T. Molecular analysis of *Malassezia* microflora on the skin of atopic dermatitis patients and healthy subjects. Nihon Ishinkin Gakkai Zasshi. 2001;42:217–8.
35. Meason-Smith C, Diesel A, Patterson A, Older CE, Mansell JM, Suchodolski JS et al. What is living on your dog's skin? Characterization of the canine cutaneous mycobiota and fungal dysbiosis in canine allergic dermatitis. FEMS Microbiol Ecol. 2015;Dec91(12).

13

How to transport veterinary drugs in insulated boxes to avoid thermal damage by heating or freezing

Johannes Horak[1,2], Astrid Haberleitner[3] and Günther Schauberger[1*]

Abstract

Background: The transport of veterinary drugs must comply with the general standards for drug storage. Although many vehicles are equipped with active heating and/or cooling devices assuring recommended storage conditions, simple insulated transport boxes are also often used. In this study, measurements for typical transport boxes were performed under laboratory conditions by the use of a climate chamber for a temperature of −20 °C and 45 °C to investigate the impact of box size, insulation material, liquid vs. dry filling products, filling degree and other parameters on the thermal performance of insulated boxes. Model calculations and instructions are presented to predict the retention time of recommended drug storage temperatures.

Results: The measurements and the model calculations showed that the loading of the transport boxes with additional water bottles to increase the heat capacity is appropriate to prolong the retention time of the recommended temperature range of the drugs. Insulated transport boxes are not suitable to store drugs over a period of more than approximately 12 h. For practical use a recipe is presented to measure the thermal properties of a transport box and the related retention time for which the recommended storage temperatures can be assured.

Conclusions: The following principles for drug transportation in vehicles are recommended: (1) Before transfer into boxes, drugs should always be thermally preconditioned (2) Increase the filling degree of the boxes with thermally preconditioned water bottles or re-usable thermal packs will increase the heat capacity. Do not deep-freeze the bottles or packs below 0 °C to avoid drug freezing due to contact. (3) Open the lid of the boxes only to uncase drugs that are immediately needed. (4) The bigger the box and the higher the filling degree, the longer the retention time of the transport box. (5) Wherever possible, place the drug box at a cool site inside the vehicle. (6) The monitoring of the inside temperature of the transport boxes is recommended. By the proper use of such transport boxes the recommended temperatures can be maintained over one working day.

Keywords: Storage recommendations, Drug, Thermal conditions, Transport

Background

The transport of veterinary drugs in vehicles must comply with the general standards for drug storage in veterinary dispensaries. Although many veterinary vehicles are equipped with active heating and/or cooling devices (active systems [1]) assuring recommended drug storage conditions, simple insulated transport boxes (passive systems [1]) are also often used in veterinary vehicles [2] as well as in emergency medical service (EMS) vehicles [3]. Such boxes are especially needed for the time when the engine is in non-operating state and the air conditioning of the vehicles is not working (parking time, during consultancy). However, such "simple" transport boxes must assure the maintenance of the appropriate storage temperatures of the drugs kept in them. The thermal properties of the transport boxes, which are exposed to the thermal conditions inside the vehicles, are major factors controlling the retention time for which the recommended storage temperatures can be assured.

The quality of medicines can be negatively affected when subjected to inadequate storage temperatures; thermal

* Correspondence: Gunther.schauberger@vetmeduni.ac.at
[1]WG Environmental Health, Division for Physiology and Biophysics, Department for Biomedical Sciences, University of Veterinary Medicine Vienna, Veterinärplatz 1, A 1210 Vienna, Austria
Full list of author information is available at the end of the article

degradation and the loss of potency of drugs have been reported following the exceedance of certain temperature thresholds [4–6]. Küppers et al. [7] recommended that temperature-sensitive drugs should be replaced after any temperature stress beyond the limits given by the manufacturers (e.g., 25 °C) and that the drugs should be replaced at least once per year. The inactivation process is described by the Arrhenius equation: the higher the temperature, the higher the degradation of active substances [5, 8–10]. The recommendations distinguish in general between cool (controlled room temperature) and cold storage conditions defined by the ranges 2 °C to 25 °C and 2 °C to 8 °C, respectively [11, 12].

Beside bags [13], although boxes are used to transport and store temperature-sensitive drugs in veterinary vehicles [2, 3, 14], it often remains unclear whether they are appropriate for this purpose. However, to the knowledge of the authors, no systematic investigations on the suitability or practicability of passive storage boxes for drug transport in vehicles have been published so far. Both exceedance of the upper temperature limit and a shortfall of the temperature to below the lower limit (e.g., freezing) must be considered. The discrepancy between the thermal needs and requirements to store drugs and the realities was shown by Haberleitner et al. [2] and Ondrak et al. [14] for veterinary vehicles.

The dynamic behaviour of the inside temperature of the box depends on two main features. (1) The heat flow rate through the walls of the box depends of the temperature difference between inside and outside temperature, the insulation of the box (wall thickness and thermal conductivity), and the area of the box walls. (2) The heat content depends on the mass and the thermal capacity of the filling. The lower the heat flow rate (1) and the higher the heat capacity of the box (2), the slower the change of the inside temperature.

In this study, the thermal performance of typical transport boxes were specifically investigated under laboratory conditions to reveal the impact of box size, insulation material, liquid vs. dry filling products, filling degree and other parameters. For practical use, a recipe is presented to measure the thermal properties of a transport box and the related retention time for which the recommended storage temperatures can be assured. With this simple model it can be assessed whether a certain transport box is appropriate to carry veterinary drugs without exceeding a certain threshold temperature. The objective of this paper is to contribute to the quality assurance of veterinary drug storage especially in vehicles.

Methods

Six insulated boxes considered typical for drug storage use in veterinary vehicles were investigated under laboratory conditions.

Transport boxes

The transport boxes differed in the type of insulation material, volume, surface area, wall thickness, and colour (Table 1). With the exception of one box (A), which employed a different insulation technique (vacuum plates), the insulation material was expanded polystyrene with a heat conductivity of $\lambda = 0.028\ \text{W K}^{-1}\ \text{m}^{-1}$, whereas for a vacuum insulated plate, a value of $\lambda = 0.005\ \text{W K}^{-1}\ \text{m}^{-1}$ was assumed [15]. A vacuum insulated plate consists of an outer layer of expanded polypropylene foam (EPP) with openings for a vacuum insulated panel which is a form of thermal insulation consisting of a gas-tight enclosure surrounding a rigid core, from which the air has been evacuated [15].

Figure 1 shows two typical transport boxes used in the experiments.

Measurements

To determine the thermal properties of the boxes, the time courses of the inner temperature of water-filled 100 mL bottles, which simulate injection vials, at defined positions in the box were measured in a heating (45 °C) or cooling chamber (−20 °C) to provide a constant ambient temperature. The contact area of the box to the wall of the climate chamber was minimised to prevent heat exchange due to conduction, by the use of point bearings.

The temperature was measured at positions P1 to P6 as depicted in Fig. 2. Measurements were performed using a calibrated Fluke Hydra 2620A with 7 channels in 15 s intervals, with channel 7 recording the ambient temperature.

Determination of the thermal properties of the boxes

The time course of the temperature difference $T_B = \Theta_B - \Theta_A$ between the inside temperature Θ_B (water bottle) and the ambient temperature Θ_A of the heating chamber (Θ_A = 45 °C) or cooling chamber (Θ_A = −20 °C) is given by the Newton's law of cooling $T_B = T_{B,0} \exp(-\gamma\ t)$ with the temperature difference $T_{B,0}$ for $t = 0$ [16]. The thermal constant γ is given by $\gamma = A\, U_m / c$ and specifies the thermal properties of the transport box. This factor was used to characterise the box and depends on its geometry, the overall coefficient of heat transmission U_m (U-value) and the entire heat capacity of its content c (transported drugs). The weighted mean of the overall coefficient of heat

Table 1 Properties of the studied transport boxes

Box	Volume V [dm^3]	Outside surface area A [m^2]	Wall thickness d [cm]
A	60	1.06	4
B	32	0.60	2
C	44	0.80	4
D	54	0.90	4
E	75	1.10	4
F	10	1.13	14

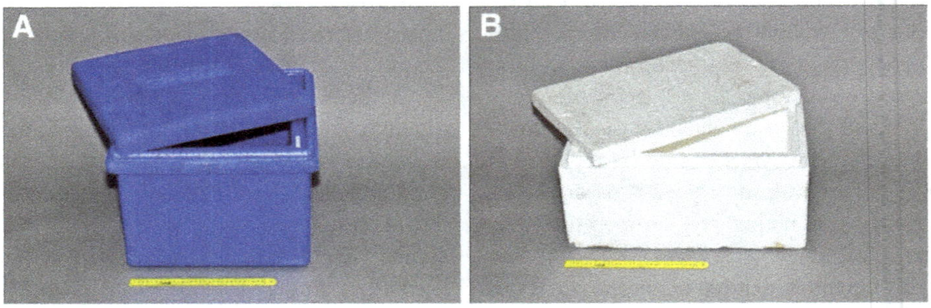

Fig. 1 Typical drug transportation boxes. The insulation of box **a** (*left*) consists of vacuum plates, and box **b** (*right*) is insulated only with polystyrene (EPS). The length of the scale is 33 cm

transmission U_m was calculated with $U_m = \sum_{i=1}^{n} A_i U_i / \sum_{i=1}^{n} A_i$, where U_i is the coefficient of heat transmission of each box wall, and A_i is the corresponding wall surface area. The coefficient of heat transmission of a box wall U_i is given by $U_i = 1/\left(1/\alpha_i + \sum_{j=0}^{n} \frac{d_j}{\lambda_j} + 1/\alpha_o\right)$, where α_i (α_o) are the coefficients of heat transfer between the air inside (outside) the box and the adjacent surface. The thickness of a material layer is given by d_j, and its thermal conductivity by λ_j. Since there is almost no forced convection inside the box and in the heating or cooling chamber, the value of α_i and α_o can be assumed to be $\alpha_i = \alpha_o = 3$ W m^{-2} K^{-1} [17]. The content's heat capacity is $c = \sum m_i c_i$ depending on the mass of the drugs m_i and their heat capacity c_i.

Following the determination of the time course of the temperature difference T_B during a cooling or heating process, the thermal constant γ was determined by a regression analysis. The temperature was measured at the positions depicted in Fig. 2, and the thermal constant γ_i was determined for each of these positions i. The maximum value of the thermal constant was selected for further analysis to reflect a worst-case scenario.

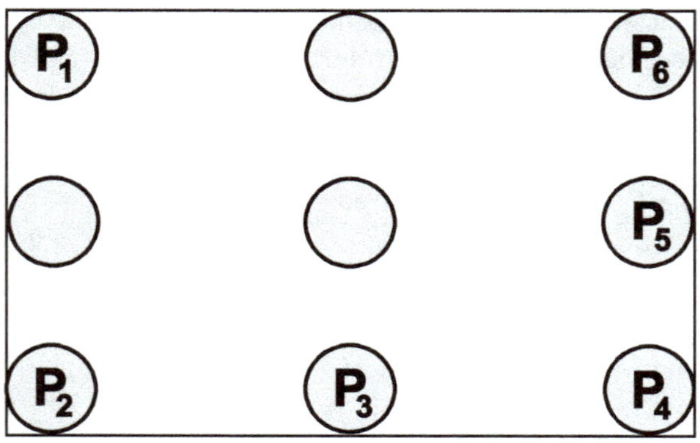

Fig. 2 Measurement points inside a transport box. Points P_1 to P_6 denote the 100 mL water-filled bottles (simulating injection vials) in which the temperature sensors were placed

The value of γ was also calculated using the mechanical and thermal properties given in Table 2. For the calculation of the entire heat capacity of the content (stored drugs) of the boxes, two different types of drugs were distinguished: liquid drugs, which show a high specific heat capacity close to that of water, and dry drugs (e.g., powder, tablets). For dry drugs, the specific heat capacity was estimated to be c_d = 1100 kJ kg^{-1} K^{-1}; for liquid drugs (independently if the drugs are hydrophilic or lipophilic), it was estimated to be c_l = 4000 kJ kg^{-1} K^{-1}. To increase the heat capacity of the entire box, resulting in a lower thermal constant γ, additional water bottles with a volume of 1000 mL were added.

The total heat capacity of a box's content was calculated as $c = m_d\ c_d + m_l\ c_l + m_w\ c_w$ where m_d and m_l denote the mass of dry and liquid drugs (simulated by 100 mL bottles) respectively, and m_w the mass of additional 1000 mL water bottles. The corresponding specific heat capacities are shown in Table 2.

Table 2 Mechanical and thermal properties of the materials of the insulated boxes and the drugs inside [15–17]

Mechanical and thermal properties	Symbol	Value
Density (kg m^{-3})		
Glass	ρ_G	2600
Air	ρ_A	1.2
Water	ρ_W	1003
Specific heat capacity (J K^{-1} kg^{-1})		
Glass	c_G	750
Air	c_A	1000
Water	c_W	4190
Drugs (dry) (drugs, blister pack, card)	c_d	~1100
Drug (liquid) (drugs, bottle)	c_l	~4000
Heat conductivity (W K^{-1} m^{-1})		
Expanded polystyrene (EPS)	λ	0.028
Vacuum plates	λ	0.005
Heat transfer coefficient (W K^{-1} m^{-2})		
Inside and outside	α_i and α_o	3.0

The filling degree F was defined as $F = c/c_{max}$ with the maximum heat capacity of a box $c_{max} = V_i \rho_w c_w$. This assumes that the box's volume V_i is filled entirely with water (water density ρ_w = 1000 kg m^{-3}, and specific heat capacity of water c_w = 4.18 kJ kg^{-1} K^{-1}). The heat capacity of the air inside a box was neglected. For the measurements inside the climate chamber, the 100 mL bottles as well as the additional 1000 mL water bottles were preconditioned.

Model calculations

Two boxes were modelled (Table 3): box X with a volume of 27 dm^3 (inner dimension 3 × 3 × 3 dm^3), and box Y with a volume of 54 dm^3 (inside dimension 6 × 3 × 3 dm^3). The wall thickness is 5 cm, which results in an outside surface area of 0.96 m^2 and 1.44 m^2, respectively. The coefficient of heat transmission was calculated for expanded polystyrene (EPS) with U_m = 0.408 W m^{-2} K^{-1}.

For the first calculation, the two boxes, X and Y, were filled only with three 100 mL bottles (as used for injectables), and in the second calculation, the remaining volume was filled with 1000 mL water bottles, resulting in a total of 24 to 49 bottles for boxes X and Y respectively. The mass of a full 100 mL bottle totals approximately 190 g. This yielded a heat capacity of 2.28 kJ K^{-1} for the two boxes filled only with drugs and 102.6 kJ K^{-1} for box X and 207.1 kJ K^{-1} for box Y when filled with additional 1000 mL water bottles (Table 3).

Results

Measurements

The measurements in the heating (Θ_A = 45 °C) and cooling chamber (Θ_A = −20 °C) were used to determine the thermal constant γ_{meas} which was then compared to corresponding calculated values γ_{calc} (Table 4). The calculations were carried out with the mechanical and thermal properties (Table 2) of the transport boxes. A comparison of measured and calculated γ values by a regression analyses showed a high agreement with a coefficient of determination of r^2 = 0.843, which is significant at the 0.001 level. The filling degree varied between 4.5% and 17.9%. A mean relative deviation of 22% between γ_{meas} and γ_{calc} was found which we attribute to geometric factors (e.g., thermal bridges due to corners, edges and the cover plate). These are not accounted for the chosen model of the coefficient of heat transmission which assumes a plane wall.

Table 3 Parameters for the model calculation for the two transport boxes X and Y

Box properties	Box X	Box Y
Filling volume V (dm^3)	27	54
Surface area A (m^2)	0.96	1.44
Coefficient of heat transmission U_m (W m^{-2} K^{-1}) (U-value)	0.408	
Only Drugs (three 100 mL water bottles)		
Heat capacity c (kJ K^{-1})	2.28	
Thermal constant γ (h^{-1})	0.6184	0.9277
Filling degree F (heat capacity) (%)	2	1
Drugs and additional water bottles		
Heat capacity c (kJ K^{-1})	102.6	207.1
Thermal constant γ (h^{-1})	0.0137	0.0102
Filling degree F (heat capacity) (%)	91	92

Table 4 Comparison of the measured γ_{meas} and the calculated γ_{calc} thermal constant for the six transport boxes and various relative heat capacities, measured in the heating (30 °C) and/or cooling (−10 °C) chamber

Box	Filling degree F [%]	Thermal constant γ [h^{-1}]	
		Measured γ_{meas}	Calculated γ_{calc}
A	7.2	0.0256	0.0340
	7.2	0.0319	0.0370
B	3.9	0.2570	0.3090
	9.8	0.1448	0.1200
	13.6	0.1080	0.0870
	13.6	0.0950	0.0870
C	4.6	0.1700	0.1500
	9.9	0.1000	0.0710
D	4.7	0.1250	0.1440
	10.3	0.0670	0.0660
	12.1	0.0711	0.0660
E	4.5	0.1700	0.1300
	8.2	0.1011	0.0730
	10.7	0.1080	0.0660
F	17.9	0.0702	0.0800

Model calculations

Model calculations were performed to demonstrate the impact of box size and their degree of filling on thermal performance for the two boxes X and Y (Table 3).

These calculations were performed for two different environmental conditions: Summer with an ambient temperature of Θ_A = 30 °C and winter with Θ_A = −10 °C. The retention time, defined as the time period during which the storage requirements are fulfilled, was then calculated for the two boxes under the assumption that the box content was thermally preconditioned. For summer calculations it was assumed to have an initial temperature of 2 °C, equal to the lower threshold of cold and cool storage conditions. For winter the corresponding upper thresholds where chosen yielding initial temperatures of 8 °C and 25 °C respectively. The resulting time courses of the drug's temperatures are plotted in Fig. 3, for a (A) summer scenario and (B) winter scenario.

Retention time calculation and various filling degrees for the two boxes are summarised in Table 5. Values below 12 h were marked in bold to show possible drug storage problems during a working day. These calculations show the high impact of the filling degree on retention time, especially for cold storage conditions (2 °C and 8 °C).

Calculations for boxes X and Y also demonstrate the influence of a box's size. The ratio of surface area (responsible for the heat exchange between box and environment) to volume decreases with box size. For the same degree of filling *F*, the retention time is greater for the larger box, Y, as compared to the smaller box, X (Table 5).

Due to the fact that Table 5 represents model calculations we added high filling degrees to show the importance of this parameter for the retention time, even if these cannot be reached in reality. This demonstrates that the filling degree *F* should be as big as possible to maximise the retention time of a transport box.

Discussion

The proper transport of temperature-sensitive drugs in vehicles is a widespread and notorious problem [18–21]. For veterinary vehicles a one year field study was

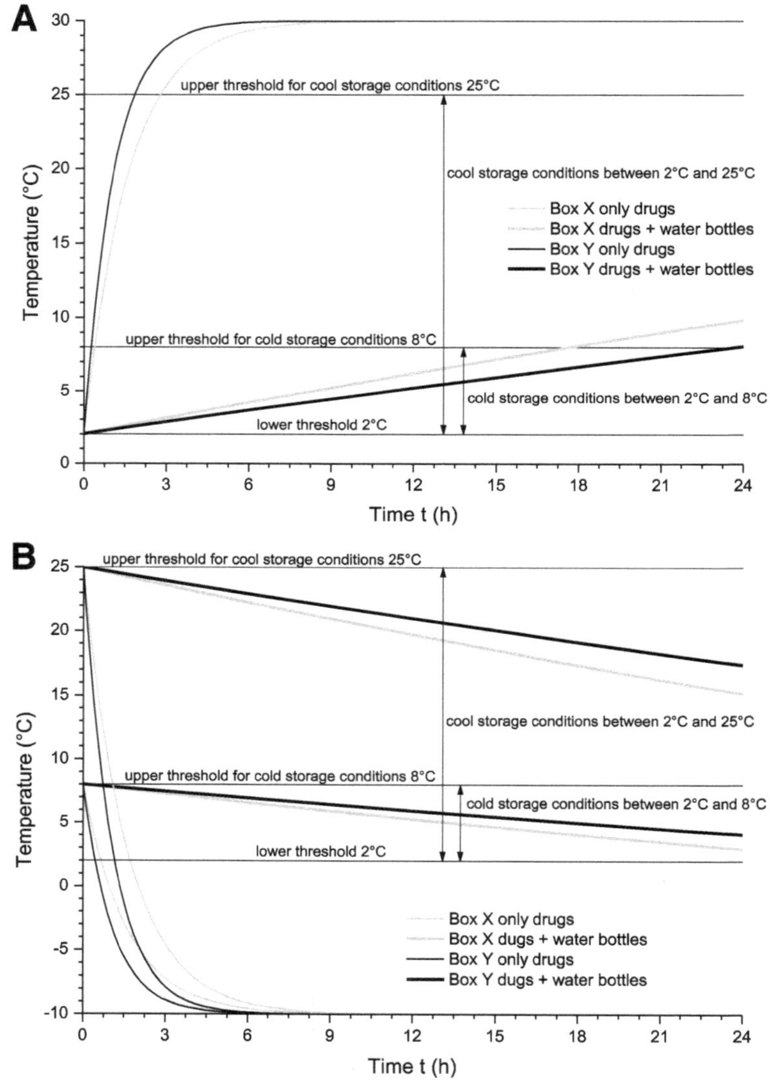

Fig. 3 Model calculation of the time course of the inside temperature Θ_B of the two virtual boxes X and Y depending on the size and the filling degree (heat capacity) of the boxes. The chosen parameters represent a summer (**a**) and a winter scenario (**b**) for drugs that must be stored either in a cool (2 °C ≤ Θ_B ≤ 25 °C) or cold environment (2 °C ≤ Θ_B ≤ 8 °C). For the summer scenario, the environmental temperature was Θ_A = 30 °C and the initial temperature Θ_B = 2 °C at *t* = 0 h. For the winter scenario, the environmental temperature was Θ_A = −10 °C, and the initial temperature (*t* = 0 h), depending on the storage conditions (*cool or cold*), was Θ_B = 25 °C and Θ_B = 8 °C, respectively

Table 5 Retention time (h) of the inside temperature in the recommended temperature range (cool storage conditions 2 °C – 25 °C and cold storage conditions 2 °C – 8 °C) in the insulated boxes X and Y for thermal summer and winter conditions with an ambient temperature of Θ_A = 30 °C and Θ_A = 30 °C, respectively

Box X										
No of additional 1000 mL water bottles	0	1	2	4	6	10	14	15	20	24
Heat capacity of the additional water bottles c_W (kJ K^{-1})	0.0	4.2	8.4	16.7	25.1	41.8	58.5	62.7	83.6	100.3
Entire heat capacity c (kJ K^{-1})	2.3	6.5	10.6	19.0	27.4	44.1	60.8	65.0	85.9	102.6
Filling degree F (%)	2	6	9	17	24	39	54	58	76	91
Thermal constant γ (h^{-1})	0.6184	0.2183	0.1325	0.0742	0.0515	0.0320	0.0232	0.0217	0.0164	0.0137
	Retention time of the inside temperature in the recommended range (h)									
Winter cool 2 °C – 25 °C	**1.7**	**4.9**	**8.1**	14.4	20.8	33.5	46.2	49.3	65.2	77.9
Winter cold 2 °C – 8 °C	**0.7**	**1.9**	**3.1**	**5.5**	**7.9**	12.7	17.5	18.7	24.7	29.5
Summer cool 2 °C – 25 °C	**2.8**	**7.9**	13.0	23.2	33.4	53.9	74.3	79.4	104.9	125.4
Summer cold 2 °C – 8 °C	**0.4**	**1.1**	**1.8**	**3.2**	**4.7**	**7.5**	**10.4**	**11.1**	14.7	17.5
Box Y										
No of additional 1000 mL water bottles	0	1	2	4	6	10	20	30	40	49
Heat capacity of the additional water bottles c_W (kJ K^{-1})	0.0	4.2	8.4	16.7	25.1	41.8	83.6	125.4	167.2	204.8
Entire heat capacity c (kJ K^{-1})	2.3	6.5	10.6	19.0	27.4	44.1	85.9	127.7	169.5	207.1
Filling degree F (%)	1	3	5	9	13	21	41	61	81	99
Thermal constant γ (h^{-1})	0.9277	0.3274	0.1988	0.1113	0.0773	0.0480	0.0246	0.0166	0.0125	0.0102
	Retention time of the inside temperature in the recommended range (h)									
Winter cool 2 °C – 25 °C	**1.2**	**3.3**	**5.4**	**9.6**	13.8	22.3	43.5	64.6	85.8	104.8
Winter cold 2 °C – 8 °C	**0.4**	**1.2**	**2.0**	**3.6**	**5.2**	**8.5**	16.5	24.5	32.5	39.7
Summer cool 2 °C – 25 °C	**1.9**	**5.3**	**8.7**	15.5	22.3	35.9	70.0	104.0	138.0	168.7
Summer cold 2 °C – 8 °C	**0.3**	**0.7**	**1.2**	**2.2**	**3.1**	**5.0**	**9.8**	14.6	19.3	23.6

The drugs and the water bottles were preconditioned for summer and winter conditions at a temperature at the lower (2 °C) and upper (8 °C or 25 °C) limit of the recommended temperature range. Values below a retention time of 12 h were marked in bold

published recently by Haberleitner et al. [2] showing that the drugs are frequently exposed to temperatures not compliant with recommended storage conditions. In many vehicles, drugs are stored in boxes without an active cooling or heating supply. Field measurements showed transport temperatures for emergency medical technician (EMS) vehicles far outside of the recommended temperature range, as summarised by Brown et al. [20]. For summer conditions, maximum inner temperatures up to 60 °C were determined, and for wintertime, minimum temperatures significantly below the freezing point [18, 21]. It became evident that either active heating or cooling systems should be used [18, 22] or other efforts made to maintain the recommended temperatures when passive storage systems are used. However, to the knowledge of the authors, no systematic investigations on the suitability or practicability of passive storage boxes for drug transport in vehicles have been published so far.

Storage temperatures outside the recommended range can affect the quality of drugs [6]. Exceedance of the upper limit of the recommended temperature range may cause a loss of drug quality due to degradation processes. The inactivation process is described by the Arrhenius equation, the higher the temperature the higher the degradation of active substances using the mean kinetic temperature [5, 8–10]. The mandatory shelf life of a temperature-sensitive drug allows for a degradation of active substances of less than 5% during correct storage [7, 9, 23]. For a typical drug, an increase in the mean kinetic temperature of 5 °C will decrease the drug's shelf life by a factor of two [21]. For the US the storage standards of the US Pharmacopeial Convention are summarised by Brown and Campagna [24].

The lower limit of 2 °C for the storage temperature was selected in this study to avoid freezing the drugs, even though the freezing point is an individual constant of each drug and may differ over a wide range [7]. In particular, injection preparations and vaccines are sensitive to freezing and lose quality and efficacy after thawing. Because "frozen" and "not frozen" distinguish between "(potentially) usable" and "not usable" [7, 12], we selected this limit of 2 °C for pragmatic reasons.

To investigate the practicability of insulated boxes for storing drugs in vehicles, we measured the retention time for winter conditions and summer conditions with an experimental ambient temperature of −10 °C and 30 °C, respectively. The measuring protocol of the World Health Organisation [25] for vaccines suggested the ambient temperatures of −5 °C and 43 °C, respectively. The filling degree of the transport boxes, which describes the heat capacity load, was defined in a similar way as proposed by the German [26] and French [27] standards. The measuring points inside the boxes were selected according to the World Health Organisation [25], and the most adverse measuring point was selected for the calculation [28].

The results obtained from the experiments were compared with the values of the thermal constant γ obtained from the model calculation (Table 4). The high coefficient of determination r^2 showed that the selected exponential model corresponds well with the measured time course data for the inner temperature of the box and demonstrates that the thermal constant of practically any transport box can analogously be determined. Thus, the time course and the retention time of any box can be predicted by its geometry, the thermal properties, and the heat capacity of the box as determined by the drugs and the additional water bottles.

Model calculations were performed for two boxes that differ significantly in size and volume to show the influence of these parameters. The time course of the inner temperature of the two boxes differs only slightly (by the constant filling degree of the volume) because the dominant factor is the entire heat capacity of a box. By adding 1000 mL water bottles, the filling degree F can be increased up to 90%, and the retention time can be increased by a factor of approximately 45 and 80 for box X and box Y, respectively. This shows the dominant influence of the filling degree on the retention time [25–27]. Insulated transport boxes cannot be considered appropriate to store drugs over a period of more than 12 h (Table 5). This means that after a "working day", the content of the transport boxes must be stored under appropriate conditions (e.g., transfer into a refrigerator) and thermally preconditioned according to the recommended temperatures before it is transferred back into the box for the next tour. A Haberleitner, G Schauberger, J Horak and I Schmerold [2] were able to show that a proper management of the storage of drugs by using solely styrofoam transport boxes can guarantee the requirements to the thermal storage conditions.

The ambient temperature of the transport boxes is the inside temperature of the vehicles being itself predominantly subjected to the outdoor temperature and the radiation balance if no additional heating and cooling (air-conditioning) is in operation. As long as the incoming solar radiation and the outgoing long-wave radiation is nearly balanced, the indoor temperature of the vehicles is close to the ambient temperature (e.g., during an overcast sky, under a car port, or inside a garage).

If the radiation balance is dominated by the incoming solar radiation, the temperature inside the car stabilises within a range between 20 and 35 K above the outside temperature [29–36]. Marty et al. [37] found a temperature difference even close to 60 K. As a rough estimation, they assessed the inside temperature due to solar radiation could reach 30 °C for winter time, 60 °C for spring and autumn and up to 90 °C during summer time. The harsh environment inside parked vehicles can cause heat stroke as a life-threatening syndrome observed in human and animals [38, 39] which is documented in the US, by 37 lethal heat stokes by children per year (1998–2015) [33, 40].

Grundstein et al. [31] developed simple models to calculate the inside steady state temperature of the cabin as a function of the outside air temperature, the irradiance of the solar radiation, and the cloud cover. The dynamic behaviour of the temperature increase after parking a vehicle in the sun was also measured by several authors [29, 30, 32–34, 36]. A dynamic model for the cabin temperature, which is driven by outside air temperature, solar radiation and wind velocity was presented recently [41]. In most cases, a value close to the maximum temperature is achieved 20 min after stopping the ventilation. The most effective measure to reduce the inside temperature is to increase the ventilation by partly opened windows [32, 34–36]. The protection of the windows by a cover to reduce the incoming solar radiation was investigated by Jascha and Keck [36] (paper fabrics and tin foil) and Devonshire and Sayer [42] using infrared reflecting foils. They found a reduction up to 11 K [36] and a higher score of thermal comfort [42], compared to the unprotected windows. Veterinary vehicles should, therefore, always be parked during daytime (solar radiation) in the shade. The direct exposure of the transport box to solar radiation through car windows should be strictly avoided during summer conditions. The additional heat flow rate could reach up to 1000 W/m^2. This additional heat load would reduce the retention time of a transport box drastically. Therefore the box should be stored also inside the cabin in the shade.

The use of passive boxes for drug transportation should only be a temporary substitute for air conditioning of the cabin to avoid heating as well as freezing. Estimation and knowledge of the thermal properties of the boxes used is a crucial factor for appropriate drug transport in vehicles and an important contribution to quality assurance in veterinary practice.

Conclusion

Observing the physical rules governing the thermal performance of passive boxes, the following principles for drug transportation in vehicles can be recommended:

- Before transfer into boxes, the drugs should always be thermally preconditioned (i) at the upper limit of the recommended temperature range for ambient temperatures below the recommended temperature ("winter") or (ii) at the lower limit for ambient conditions above the recommended temperature ("summer"). The most critical storage condition is the range between 2 °C and 8 °C
- Increase the filling degree of the box as much as possible by thermally preconditioned water bottles or re-usable thermal packs to increase the heat capacity of the transport box. Do not deep-freeze the bottles or packs below 0 °C to avoid drug freezing due to contact. This recommendation applies also to active devices (e.g., refrigerators).
- Open the lid of the boxes only to uncase needed drugs. Avoid air exchange especially due to wind effects and due to the thermal rise of the warmer air from inside the boxes during cold outside conditions.
- The bigger the box and the higher the filling degree, the longer the retention time of the transport box.
- Wherever possible, place the drug box at a cool site. The vehicle should always be parked in the shade or, if possible, inside a well ventilated car port. The transport box should not be exposed to direct solar radiation.
- The monitoring of the inside temperature of the transport boxes is recommended using remote temperature sensors and/or temperature data loggers to avoid and/or detect violation of recommended storage temperatures.

Appendix

Recipe to measure thermal properties of a box and to calculate the retention time

For practical use, a recipe is described to calculate the retention time, for a transport box to avoid an exceedance of a temperature threshold. The recipe includes two steps: (1) measurement of the thermal properties of the box, and (2) calculation of the retention time.

In a first step the thermal constant γ of a selected transport box is measured. The box is filled in the same way as it is proposed for practical use. For the application of the transport box the retention time is calculated for a certain ambient temperature. This retention time gives the reliability that the storage temperature of the transported drugs will not exceed the recommended temperature range.

Step 1: Measurement of the thermal properties of a box

For the measurements and the calculation the following equipment is required (1) the transport box, (2) water bottles, to simulate the expected filling degree of the box, (3) thermometer (unit: degree Celsius), and (4) calculator. Bottles of arbitrary size are to be filled with water. The mass of water should equal the mass of the pharmaceuticals that are usually transported inside the box at hand. The filled bottles should be cooled in a refrigerator to about 4 °C. It is crucial that none of the water is frozen.

After the cooldown to the preconditioned temperature, the initial box (water) temperature $\Theta_{B,i}$ of at least one of the bottles is measured. Afterwards the box that is to be tested is loaded with the cooled water bottles.

The box should now be placed in a room that fulfils the following requirements (1) low temperature fluctuation, (2) no direct solar radiation, and (3) no draught. The box should stay about 1 m away from corners or walls and the ambient room temperature Θ_A has to be measured.

After about 8 h (depending on the filling degree (Table 5)), the final box (water) temperature $\Theta_{B,f}$ has to be measured. If the difference between $\Theta_{B,f}$ and $\Theta_{B,i}$ is at least 5 °C the experiment is finished, otherwise the duration of 8 h has to be expanded and a new value of the final box temperature $\Theta_{B,f}$ has to be measured. The time t is the duration that the box was left in the room in hours. All four parameters $\Theta_{B,i}$, $\Theta_{B,f}$, Θ_A, and t, which have to be measured, are listed in the highlighted Box of Step 1. The measurement procedure in short: (1) Measure the initial temperature inside the box $\Theta_{B,i}$, (2) leave the box for several hours in a room with constant ambient temperature Θ_A, (3) measure the final temperature inside the box $\Theta_{B,f}$, and (4) determine the duration for the measurements inside the room t.

These temperatures and the duration of the experiment are inserted into the following equation:

$$\gamma_C = \left| \ln\left(\frac{\Theta_{B,f}-\Theta_A}{\Theta_{B,i}-\Theta_A}\right) \right| \cdot \frac{1}{t}$$

This yields the constant γ_C which characterises the thermal properties of the investigated box. To be on the safe side, a correction factor κ = 1.45 has to be applied which yields

$$\gamma = \kappa \gamma_C$$

Step 1: Measurement of the thermal properties of a box

Calculation of the retention time t_{th}

Initial temperature	$\Theta_{B,i} = 8°C$
Threshold temperature (which should not exceeded)	$\Theta_{th} = 20\ °C$
Assumed ambient temperature inside the vehicles	$\Theta_A = 32\ °C$
Thermal constant γ (calculated in Step1)	$\gamma = 0.0463\ h^{-1}$

$$t_{th} = \left|\ln\left(\frac{20\ -\ 32}{8\ -\ 32}\right)\right| \cdot \frac{1}{0.0463} = 15\ \text{h}$$

This means that in a vehicle compartment with an ambient temperature of $\Theta_A = 32°C$ the temperature of the drugs inside the box would rise above the threshold temperature Θ_{th}= 20°C after approximately 15 hours.

Attention: the filling degree of the transport box must be similar to the situation during the measurement of the thermal constant γ (step 1)

Step 2: Calculation of the retention time

In step 2, the retention time t_{th} (in hours) is calculated. Based on the drugs which are transported in the box, the threshold temperature Θ_{th} has to be selected. The initial temperature is the temperature inside the transport box, before the box is moved to the vehicle $\Theta_{B,i}$.The assumed cabin temperature during the day is used as ambient temperature Θ_A. The thermal constant γ of the box was calculated in step 1. These values are to be inserted into the following equation

$$t_{th} = \left|\ln\left(\frac{\Theta_{th}-\Theta_A}{\Theta_{B,i}-\Theta_A}\right)\right| \cdot \frac{1}{\gamma}$$

The retention time t_{th} can be used as estimation if the box can be used to transport the drugs inside the vehicle without risk, that the threshold temperature Θ_{th} will be exceeded.

Step 2: Calculation of the retention time

Measurement of the four parameters

Initial temperature	$\Theta_{B,i} = 5°C$
Final temperature	$\Theta_{B,f} = 10°C$
Mean ambient temperature	$\Theta_A = 25°C$
Experiment duration	$t = 9$ h

Measurement of the thermal constant γ

$$\gamma_C = \left|\ln\left(\frac{10\text{-}25}{5\text{-}25}\right)\right| \cdot \frac{1}{9} = 0.0320\ h^{-1}$$

Finally the safety factor $\kappa = 1.45$ is applied and yields $\gamma = 0.0320 \quad 1.45 = 0.0463\ h^{-1}$

Acknowledgements

We want to thank Prof. Ivo Schmerold for providing the funding. We are grateful to Kurt Wimmer, who supported the measurements.

Funding

This study was supported by funds of the Austrian Federal Ministry of Health, Family and Youth (BMGFJ-70420/0303-I/A/15/2007) and the Austrian Federal Chamber of Veterinarians.

Authors' contributions

JH acquired, analysed, and interpreted the data, drafted and revised the manuscript. AH collated and analysed the data and revised the manuscript. GS conceived the design of the study, drafted and revised the article. All authors read and approved the final manuscript.

Authors' information

JH is a PhD student at the Institute of Atmospheric and Cryospheric Sciences, University of Innsbruck. AH is a PhD student at the Institute of Pharmacology and Toxicology, Department for Biomedical Sciences, University of Veterinary Medicine Vienna. She is working at the veterinary services of the Federal Province of Lower Austria. GS is professor and head of the WG Environmental Health at Division for Physiology and Biophysics, Department for Biomedical Sciences at the University of Veterinary Medicine Vienna.

Competing interests

The authors declare that they have no competing interests.

Consent for publication

Not applicable.

Author details

[1]WG Environmental Health, Division for Physiology and Biophysics, Department for Biomedical Sciences, University of Veterinary Medicine Vienna, Veterinärplatz 1, A 1210 Vienna, Austria. [2]Institute of Atmospheric and Cryospheric Sciences, University of Innsbruck, Innrain 52f, A-6020 Innsbruck, Austria. [3]Institute of Pharmacology and Toxicology, Department for Biomedical Sciences, University of Veterinary Medicine Vienna, Veterinärplatz 1, A 1210 Vienna, Austria.

References

1. WHO. Appendix 9, model guidance for the storage and transport of time- and temperature-sensitive pharmaceutical products. In: Forty-fifth report of the WHO expert committee on specifi cations for pharmaceutical preparations. Geneva: World Health Organization; 2011.
2. Haberleitner A, Schauberger G, Horak J, Schmerold I. Thermal drug storage conditions in veterinary vehicles - a one-year field study in Austria. Wien Tierärztl Monatsschr. 2014;101(5–6):110–9.
3. Mejia J: Vehicular Based Drug Box Temperature Control Study. Norfolk, VA: Old Dominion University, Unpublished master's thesis. Old Dominion University, Norfolk, VA. Retrieved from http://www.digital.lib.odu.edu; 2006.
4. Grant TA, Carroll RG, Church WH, Henry A, Prasad NH, Abdel-Rahman AA, et al. Environmental temperature variations cause degradations in epinephrine concentration and biological activity. Am J Emerg Med. 1994;12(3):319–22.
5. De Winter S, Vanbrabant P, Vi NTT, Deng X, Spriet I, Van Schepdael A, et al. Impact of temperature exposure on stability of drugs in a real-world out-of-hospital setting. Ann Emerg Med. 2013;62(4):380–7. e381
6. Gammon DL, Su S, Huckfeldt R, Jordan J, Patterson R, Finley PJ, et al. Alteration in prehospital drug concentration after thermal exposure. Am J Emerg Med. 2008;26(5):566–73.
7. Küpper TEAH, Schraut B, Rieke B, Hemmerling AV, Schöffl V, Steffgen J. Drugs and drug administration in extreme environments. J Travel Med. 2006;13(1):35–47.
8. Haynes JD. Worldwide virtual temperatures for product stability testing. J Pharm Sci. 1971;60(6):927–9.
9. ICH Q1A(R2). Stability testing of new drug substances and products Q1A(R2) step 4. In: Geneva: international conference on harmonisation of Technical requirements for registration of pharmaceuticals for human use; 2003.
10. Nakamura T, Yamaji T, Takayama K. Effects of packaging and heat transfer kinetics on drug-product stability during storage under uncontrolled temperature conditions. J Pharm Sci. 2013;102(5):1495–503.
11. Summerhays GES. Monitoring of temperature in cars with regard to the pharmaceutical precautions of medicine storage. Equine Vet Educ. 2000; 12(6):307–11.

12. Taylor J. Recommendations on the control and monitoring of storage and transportation temperatures of medicinal products. Pharm J. 2001;267(7158): 128–31.
13. Rudland SV, Jacobs AG. Visiting bags: a labile thermal environment. Br Med J. 1994;308(6934):954–6
14. Ondrak J, Jones M, Fajt V. Temperatures of storage areas in large animal veterinary practice vehicles in the summer and comparison with drug manufacturers' storage recommendations. BMC Vet Res. 2015;11(1):248.
15. Fricke J, Heinemann U, Ebert HP. Vacuum insulation panels-from research to market. Vacuum. 2008;82(7):680–90.
16. Gröber H, Erk S, Grigull U. Fundamentals of heat transfer. Berlin, Heidelberg: Springer-Verlag; 1961.
17. ASHRAE. Heat transfer (chapter 4). In: ASHRAE handbook—fundamentals volume chapter 4 SI edn. Atlanta, USA: American Society of Heating, Refrigerating and Air-Conditioning Engineers Inc.; 2009.
18. Brown LH, Bailey LC, Medwick T, Okeke CC, Krumperman K, Tran CD. Medication storage temperatures on U.S. ambulances: a prospective multicenter observational study. Pharm Forum. 2003;29(2):540–4.
19. Brown LH, Wojcik SM, Bailey LC, Tran CD. Can stock rotation effectively mitigate EMS medication exposure to excessive heat and cold? Am J Emerg Med. 2006;24(1):14–8.
20. Brown LH, Krumperman K, Fullagar CJ. Out-of-hospital medication storage temperatures: a review of the literature and directions for the future. Prehosp Emerg Care. 2004;8(2):200–6.
21. Allegra JR, Brennan J, Lanier V, Lavery R, MacKenzie B. Storage temperatures of out-of-hospital medications. Acad Emerg Med. 1999;6(11):1098–103.
22. Helm M, Castner T, Lampl L. Environmental temperature stress on drugs in prehospital emergency medical service. Acta Anaesthesiol Scand. 2003;47(4):425–9.
23. ICH Q1E. Evaluation for stability data Q1E. In: Geneva international conference on harmonisation of Technical requirements for registration of pharmaceuticals for human use; 2003.
24. Brown LH, Campagna JD. Medication storage in the EMS environment: understanding the science and meeting the standards. Emerg Med Serv. 2005;34(3):71. 73–77, 90
25. World Health Organisation. Guidelines on the international packaging and shipping of vaccines in., vol. WHO / IVB / 05.23. Geneva: WHO; 2005.
26. DIN 55545–1. Packagings - Packagings with insulating properties - part 1: initial evaluation testing. Berlin: Beuth Verlag; 2006.
27. AFNOR NF S99-700. Emballages isothermes et emballages réfrigérants pour produits de santé. Méthode de qualification des performances thermiques. Paris: Association Française de Normalisation; 2007.
28. WHO. WHO good distribution practices for pharmaceutical products. WHO Technical report series, no. 957, 2010, annex 5. Geneva: WHO; 2010.
29. Gibbs LI, Lawrence DW, Kohn MA. Heat exposure in an enclosed automobile. J Louisiana State Med Soc. 1995;147(12):545–6.
30. Gregory NG, Constantine E. Hyperthermia in dogs left in cars. Vet Rec. 1996; 139(14):349–50.
31. Grundstein A, Meentemeyer V, Dowd J. Maximum vehicle cabin temperatures under different meteorological conditions. Int J Biometeorol. 2009;53(3):255–61.
32. King K, Negus K, Vance JC. Heat stress in motor vehicles: a problem in infancy. Pediatrics. 1981;68(4):579–82.
33. McLaren C, Null J, Quinn J. Heat stress from enclosed vehicles: moderate ambient temperatures cause significant temperature rise in enclosed vehicles. Pediatrics. 2005;116(1):e109–12.
34. Roberts KB, Roberts EC. The automobile and heat stress. Pediatrics. 1976; 58(1):101–4.
35. Surpure JS. Heat-related illness and the automobile. Ann Emerg Med. 1982; 11(5):263–5.
36. Jascha I, Keck G. Klima im Personenkraftwagen-ein Beitrag zum Tierschutz. Wien Tierärztl Monatschr. 1984;71(8/9):227–37.
37. Marty W, Sigrist T, Wyler D. Temperature variations in automobiles in various weather conditions: an experimental contribution to the determination of time of death. Am J Forensic Med Pathol. 2001;22(3):215–9.
38. Grundstein AJ, Duzinski SV, Dolinak D, Null J, Iyer SS. Evaluating infant core temperature response in a hot car using a heat balance model. Forensic Sci Med Pathol. 2015;11(1):13–9.
39. Grundstein A, Duzinski S, Null J, Impact of dangerous microclimate conditions within an enclosed vehicle on pediatric thermoregulation. Theor Appl Climatology. 2014. doi:10.1007/s00704-015-1636-2.
40. Hyperthermia Deaths of Children in Vehicles. [www.ggweather.com/heat], retrieved: May 19, 2017.
41. Horak J, Schmerold I, Wimmer K, Schauberger G. Cabin air temperature of parked vehicles in summer conditions: life-threatening environment for children and pets calculated by a dynamic model. Theor Appl Climatology. 2016. doi:10.1007/s00704-016-1861-3.
42. Devonshire JM, Sayer JR. Radiant heat and thermal comfort in vehicles. Hum Factors. 2005;47(4):827–39.

14

Evaluation on antithrombotic effect of aspirin eugenol ester from the view of platelet aggregation, hemorheology, TXB_2/6-keto-$PGF_{1\alpha}$ and blood biochemistry in rat model

Ning Ma, Xi-Wang Liu, Ya-Jun Yang, Dong-Shuai Shen, Xiao-Le Zhao, Isam Mohamed, Xiao-Jun Kong and Jian-Yong Li*

Abstract

Background: Based on the prodrug principle, aspirin and eugenol, as starting precursors, were esterified to synthesize aspirin eugenol ester (AEE). The aim of the present study was to evaluate the antithrombotic effect of AEE in an animal disease model. In order to compare the therapeutic effects of AEE and its precursors, aspirin, eugenol and a combination of aspirin and eugenol were designed at the same molar quantities as the AEE medium dose in the control group.

Methods: After oral administration of AEE (dosed at 18, 36 and 72 mg/kg) for seven days, rats were treated with k-carrageenan to induce tail thrombosis. Following the same method, aspirin (20 mg/kg), eugenol (18 mg/kg) and 0.5 % CMC-Na (30 mg/kg) were administered as control drug. Different drug effects on platelet aggregation, hemorheology, TXB_2/6-keto-$PGF_{1\alpha}$ ratio and blood biochemistry were studied.

Results: AEE significantly inhibited ADP and AA-induced platelet aggregation in vivo. AEE also significantly reduced blood and plasma viscosity. Moreover, AEE down-regulated TXB_2 and up-regulated 6-keto-$PGF_{1\alpha}$, normalizing the TXB_2/6-keto-$PGF_{1\alpha}$ ratio and blood biochemical profile. In comparison with aspirin and eugenol, AEE produced more positive therapeutic effects than its precursors under the same molar quantity.

Conclusion: It may be concluded that AEE was a good candidate for new antithrombotic and antiplatelet medicine. Additionally, this study may help to understand how AEE works on antithrombosis in different ways.

Keywords: Aspirin eugenol ester (AEE), Thrombosis, k-carrageenan, Rat, Platelet aggregation, Blood viscosity

Background

In the last century, remarkable increases of life spans in dogs and cats have promoted the development of geriatric veterinary medicine [1, 2]. The findings have proved that age-related thrombin was a possible risk factor in dogs and cats [3, 4]. Thus, there is a need for anti-thrombotic drugs for animals. The physiological process of thrombosis is complex and influenced by many factors such as platelet aggregation, ratio of thromboxane B_2 (TXB_2) to 6-keto prostaglandin $F_{1\alpha}$ (6-keto-$PGF_{1\alpha}$), biochemical and hemorheological parameters [5–8]. Therefore, the impacts of drugs on platelet aggregation, hemorheology, TXB_2/6-keto-$PGF_{1\alpha}$ ratio and blood biochemistry can be employed for examining the effect of compound in thrombosis prevention [9].

Aspirin is extensively used in human and veterinary medicine to reduce inflammation, pain and fever. In cats, aspirin is not well tolerated because of the deficient in

* Correspondence: lijy1971@163.com
Key Lab of New Animal Drug Project of Gansu Province, Key Lab of Veterinary Pharmaceutical Development, Ministry of Agriculture, Lanzhou Institute of Husbandry and Pharmaceutical Science of CAAS, No.335, Jiangouyan, Qilihe district, Lanzhou 730050, China

glucuronate and has a prolonged elimination half-time. The pharmacodynamics of aspirin are similar in human and dogs. Related researches have proved that prophylactic use of aspirin can reduce the risk of heart attack, stroke and some cancers [10, 11]. A number of reports have showed that eugenol has antiseptic, analgesic, antibacterial, anti-platelet aggregation and anticancer properties [12–14]. Notably, aspirin and eugenol produce similar pharmacological effects especially on inflammation and platelet aggregation.

Gastrointestinal damage caused by aspirin and vulnerability of eugenol limit their application. These side effects and structural instability are related to chemically carboxyl group of aspirin and hydroxyl group of eugenol. In order to increase therapeutic effect and stabilization, aspirin and eugenol as starting precursors were esterified to synthesize aspirin eugenol ester (AEE). AEE, a pale yellow, odorless crystal, overcomes the disadvantages of its precursors. Anti-ulcerogenic activity of eugenol has been confirmed in a previous study, in which eugenol (100 mg/kg, p.o.) significantly and dose-dependently reduced gastric ulcers induced by platelet activating factor and ethanol in Wistar rats [15]. So a combination of eugenol and aspirin could play complementary roles to reduce gastrointestinal damage and enhance the therapeutic effects. A 15-day sub-chronic toxicity study identified that no histopathological changes was observed in any organ from the rats following low-dose AEE (50 mg/kg), whereas mucosa height of stomach, duodenum and ileum were increased in rats following high-dose AEE exposure (2000 mg/kg) [16].

Carrageenan-induced rat tail thrombosis model has been widely used to evaluate whether substances have antithrombotic effects during the drug discovery stage [17–20]. The length of thrombosis in rat tail directly reflects the effects of drug on thrombosis formation [21, 22].

The preventive effects of AEE on thrombosis formation have been confirmed in k-carrageenan-induced rat tail thrombosis model in which AEE significantly inhibited thrombus formation and reduced the tail thrombosis length [23]. However, investigations of the preventive effects of AEE against thrombosis are not sufficient. In order to understand and illustrate the possible underlying mechanism of AEE, a follow-up study was carried out using the same animal disease model and drug dosage. The aim of the present study was to evaluate the effects of AEE on platelet aggregation, hemorheology, blood biochemistry and TXB_2/6-keto-$PGF_{1\alpha}$ ratio. To compare the effects of AEE and its precursors, equimolar doses of aspirin, eugenol and combination of aspirin and eugenol were also administered in the experiment.

Methods

Chemicals and reagents

AEE (transparent crystal, 99.5 % purity with RP-HPLC) was prepared in Key Lab of New Animal Drug Project of Gansu Province, Key Lab of Veterinary Pharmaceutical Development of Agricultural Ministry, Lanzhou Institute of Husbandry and Pharmaceutical Sciences of CAAS. CMC-Na was supplied by Tianjin Chemical Reagent Company (Tianjin, China). Aspirin and Tween-80 were obtained from Aladdin Industrial Corporation (Shanghai China). Eugenol was supplied by Sinopharm Chemical Reagent Co., Ltd. (Shanghai China). Adenosine diphosphate (ADP), arachidonic acid (AA) and k-carrageenan were purchased from Sigma (St. Louis, USA). Blood biochemical analysis reagents were obtained from Meikang Co., Ltd (Zhejiang, China). All chemical reagents were of analytical reagent grade. A Thermo Fisher Scientific Multiskan Go 1510 was used for spectrophotometry (USA).

Animals and treatment

Ninety male Wistar rats (approximately 160 g) were purchased from the animal breeding facilities of Lanzhou Army General Hospital (Lanzhou, China). Animals were housed in plastic cages (size: 50 × 35 × 20 cm, 10 rats per cage) with stainless steel wire cover and chopped bedding in a ventilated room. The light/dark regime was 12/12 h and living temperature was maintained at 22 ± 2 °C with relative humidity of 55 ± 10 %. The animals had free access to a standard diet and tap water (Standard compressed rat feed from Keao Xieli Co., Ltd., Beijing, China). Rats were allowed a 2-week acclimation period prior to the start of experiment.

Drug preparation

AEE and aspirin suspensions were prepared in 0.5 % of CMC-Na. Eugenol and Tween-80 (mass ratio of 1:2) were mixed with distilled water. Kappa-carrageenan (k-carrageenan) was dissolved in physiological saline.

Study design

Ninety rats were divided into 9 groups in the study. According to individual body weight (BW), rats were intragastrically (i.g.) administered with 18, 36 and 72 mg/kg AEE, 20 mg/kg aspirin or 18 mg/kg eugenol. For the comparability of the experimental results, medium-dose AEE, aspirin and eugenol were administered at the dose of 0.11 mmol. In order to compare AEE with its precursors, an equimolar combination of aspirin and eugenol was designed in the experiment. Rats in CMC-Na group were given 0.5 % CMC-Na at the dose of 30 mg/kg BW, and the volume of CMC-Na was nearly equal in comparison with other drug suspensions. A detailed description of the study design is shown in Table 1. All drugs and CMC-Na were administered intragastrically for seven days, after which the rats were intraperitoneally injected with 20 mg/kg k-carrageenan to induce thrombosis.

Table 1 Design of the experiment

Groups	Drug	Dosage (mg/kg)	Molar quantity (mmol)
Control	–	–	–
Model	–	–	–
CMC-Na	CMC-Na	30	–
Aspirin	aspirin	20	0.11
Eugenol	eugenol	18	0.11
AEE L	AEE	18	0.06
AEE M	AEE	36	0.11
AEE H	AEE	72	0.22
Combination	aspirin + eugenol	20 + 18	0.11

Ninety rats were divided into 9 groups ($n = 10$). CMC-Na was used as the vehicle. The volumes of CMC-Na and drug suspension were nearly equal. The molar quantity of medium-dose AEE, aspirin and eugenol are same at 0.11 mmol. An equimolar combination of aspirin and eugenol was used in the study. Rats in the model, CMC-Na, aspirin, eugenol, AEE and combination groups were intraperitoneally injected with 20 mg/kg k-carrageenan to induce thrombosis

Carrageenan-induced rat tail thrombosis model

Carrageenan-induced rat tail thrombosis was induced as described in the previous study [23].

Measurement of rat tail thrombosis length

After the last treatment with different drugs, each rat was intraperitoneally injected with k-carrageenan. Swelling and redness in rat tail were monitored. Thrombus lengths were measured and photographed at 24 and 48 h.

Blood sampling

After the last measurement of thrombosis length at 48 h, rats were anesthetized with 10 % chloral hydrate and blood samples were taken from the heart. According to the requirement of the experiment, blood samples were collected in different volume with different anticoagulants. Serum for biochemical analysis and plasma for ELISA were stored at −80 °C until the day of analysis. All platelet aggregation and hemorheological tests were performed within 3 h of blood collection.

Hemorheological tests

Blood samples of approximately 2 mL were collected and anticoagulated with EDTA-K_2, after which 0.8 mL whole blood samples were prepared for whole blood viscosity examination. The remaining blood samples were centrifuged at 1000 g for 10 min to obtain plasma, after which 0.5 mL of plasma was used for plasma viscosity examination. A kone plate viscometer LBY-N6A analytical instrument (Precil Company, Beijing, China) was used for the measurement of whole blood viscosity and plasma viscosity at 37.0 ± 0.5 °C. For whole blood viscosity, measurements were made at three shear rates: 5, 100 and 200 s^{-1}. Plasma viscosity was measured at a shear rate of 100 s^{-1}.

Assay of platelet aggregation

In vivo assessment of the anti-platelet aggregation effect of AEE was performed using light transmission aggregometry in platelet-rich plasma (PRP). About 2 mL blood samples were collected and diluted by 3.8 % sodium citrate on the proportion of 9:1 in vacuum tubes, which were prepared for platelet aggregation analysis. Platelet aggregation was assessed in PRP, which was obtained by centrifugation of citrated whole blood at room temperature for 10 min at 1000 rpm. Then, PRP was placed into two cuvettes (0.25 mL PRP in each cuvette) and stirred with a rotor at 37 °C for 5 min, after which 5 μM ADP and 5 mM AA was added, respectively. The platelet-poor plasma (PPP) was obtained by centrifugation of PRP at room temperature for 10 min at 3000 rpm, which was used to set zero. Aggregation was measured with a Chrono-log Platelet Aggregometer Model 700 (Chrono-log Corp., USA). After the addition of an aggregating agent, light transmission at maximal aggregation was recorded. The results are expressed as percentage of maximal aggregation.

Blood biochemical analysis

Blood samples of approximate 1 mL were collected into vacuum tubes without anticoagulant, and centrifuged at 4000 rpm for 10 min to obtain serum. Serum was analyzed using an XL-640 automatic biochemistry analyzer (Erba, German). Levels of total bilirubin (T-BIL), total protein (TP), albumin (ALB), alanine transaminase (ALT), aspartate aminotransferase (AST), alkaline phosphatase (ALP), gamma glutamyl transpeptidase (GGT), lactate dehydrogenase (LDH), blood urea nitrogen (BUN), creatinine (CR), glucose (GLU), glutamic pyruvic transaminase (GPT), creatine kinase (CK), calcium (Ca), phosphorus (P), triglycerides (TG) and total cholesterol (TCH) were analyzed in the experiment.

Measurement of plasma TXB_2 and 6-keto-$PGF_{1\alpha}$

Samples anticoagulated with EDTA-K_2 were centrifuged at 1000 g for 10 min to obtain 200 μL of plasma for TXB_2 and 6-keto-$PGF_{1\alpha}$ measurements. ELISA kit of TXB_2 was purchased from U.S.A TSZ Biological Trade Co., Ltd. (New Jersey, USA) and 6-keto-$PGF_{1\alpha}$ ELISA kit was from Abcam Co., Ltd (Cambridge, UK). The ELISA operation was followed the protocols included with each kit.

Statistical analysis

Statistical analyses were carried out using SPSS (Statistical Product and Service Solutions,IBM. Co., Armonk, NY, USA). Data obtained from experiment was expressed as mean ± standard deviation (SD). Statistical differences were evaluated by ANOVA with least significant difference (LSD) test. *P*-values less than 0.05 were considered to indicate statistical significance.

Results

Effects on hemorheology

Hemorheological parameters were analyzed by routine laboratory assays. The results are shown in Table 2. In comparison with the control group, whole blood viscosity and plasma viscosity were significantly increased in model group ($P < 0.01$, or $P < 0.05$). There was no statistical difference between CMC-Na and model groups. In order to eliminate the influence of the vehicle, drug-treated groups were compared with CMC-Na group. Aspirin reduced whole blood viscosity at low shear rate ($P < 0.05$), but did not influence whole blood viscosity at medium and high shear rates. Whole blood viscosity at low and medium shear rates in groups supplemented with AEE were significantly lower than that of CMC-Na group ($P < 0.01$). Whole blood viscosity at high shear rate was also significantly reduced by low-dose AEE ($P < 0.05$). Aspirin and eugenol remarkably reduced plasma viscosity (aspirin: $P < 0.01$; eugenol: $P < 0.05$). Low and high doses of AEE showed strong effects on reducing the plasma viscosity values ($P < 0.01$). No change was observed on whole blood viscosity and plasma viscosity between CMC-Na and combination groups.

In order to find out the difference in results between AEE and its precursors, multiple comparisons were carried out. In the experiment, the molar quantities of aspirin, eugenol and medium-dose AEE were same. The results are shown in Fig. 1. AEE showed stronger effects on whole blood viscosity reduction at low shear rate than eugenol and combination groups ($P < 0.01$, Fig. 1a). In comparison with aspirin, eugenol and the combination groups, AEE significantly reduced whole blood viscosity at medium and high shear rates ($P < 0.01$ or $P < 0.05$ Fig. 1b and c). Interestingly, the plasma viscosity values of each AEE group was significantly lower than that of combination group ($P < 0.01$, Fig. 1d). Moreover, the mean values of whole blood viscosity and plasma viscosity in AEE groups were lower than other drug-treated groups. Medium-dose AEE reduced whole blood viscosity more effectively than eugenol ($P < 0.01$ or $P < 0.05$ Fig. 1a, b and c). Moreover, medium-dose AEE showed better effects than aspirin on whole blood viscosity at medium shear rate ($P < 0.01$ Fig. 1b). There were significant differences on plasma viscosity and whole blood viscosity (at low and medium shear rates) between AEE M and combination groups ($P < 0.01$ Fig. 1a, b and d). To varying degrees, under the equimolar quantity of drugs, medium-dose AEE stronger reduced whole blood viscosity and plasma viscosity than aspirin, eugenol and combination of them from the different hemorheological parameters.

Effect of AEE on platelet aggregation in vivo

The results of platelet aggregation are shown in Table 3. Platelet aggregation induced by AA and ADP was significantly increased in model group ($P < 0.01$). No difference was observed between model and CMC-Na groups. AEE, eugenol and aspirin remarkably reduced AA-induced platelet aggregation than CMC-Na in varying degrees ($P < 0.05$ or $P < 0.01$). The mean values in aspirin and eugenol groups were 20.44 and 27.10, which indicated aspirin had stronger effects than eugenol on inhibiting AA-induced platelet aggregation. In regard to ADP-induced platelet aggregation, the values in aspirin, combination, medium and high-dose AEE groups were lower than CMC-Na group ($P < 0.01$).

The effects of different drug on platelet aggregation were evaluated in the study (seen in Fig. 2). Medium- and high-dose AEE showed stronger effects than aspirin on reducing AA-induced platelet aggregation values ($P < 0.01$). Meanwhile, three different doses of AEE displayed better effects than eugenol ($P < 0.01$). ADP-induced platelet aggregation values in low-dose AEE group were higher than aspirin and combination groups ($P < 0.01$). Medium- and

Table 2 Drug effects on hemorheological parameters in k-carrageenan-induced rat tail thrombosis model ($n = 10$)

Groups	WBV (mPa.s)			PV (mPa.s)
	Low shear rate (5 s^{-1})	Medium shear rate (100 s^{-1})	High shear rate (200 s^{-1})	
Control	$18.56 \pm 3.03^{##}$	$4.63 \pm 0.77^{##}$	$3.55 \pm 0.79^{##}$	$1.55 \pm 0.28^{#}$
Model	27.75 ± 3.27	6.74 ± 0.78	5.24 ± 0.63	2.04 ± 0.47
CMC-Na	26.42 ± 2.66	6.87 ± 0.62	5.22 ± 0.52	1.97 ± 0.25
Aspirin	$22.75 \pm 3.57^{*}$	6.21 ± 0.62	5.21 ± 0.35	$1.39 \pm 0.13^{**}$
Eugenol	28.69 ± 2.93	6.87 ± 0.72	5.52 ± 0.79	$1.63 \pm 0.25^{*}$
AEE L	$20.03 \pm 2.75^{**}$	$5.38 \pm 0.78^{**}$	$4.58 \pm 0.67^{*}$	$1.32 \pm 0.12^{**}$
AEE M	$22.60 \pm 2.28^{**}$	$5.48 \pm 0.86^{**}$	4.74 ± 0.52	1.68 ± 0.61
AEE H	$22.25 \pm 3.60^{**}$	$5.14 \pm 0.69^{**}$	4.63 ± 0.62	$1.50 \pm 0.14^{**}$
Combination	27.45 ± 2.90	6.58 ± 1.06	5.28 ± 0.63	2.19 ± 0.30

After the last measurement of rat tail thrombosis length at 48 h, 0.8 mL of whole blood and 0.5 mL of plasma were collected for hemorheological parameter tests. Data are expressed as mean ± SD. $^{#}P < 0.05$, $^{##}P < 0.01$ compared with model group. $^{*}P < 0.05$, $^{**}P < 0.01$ compared with CMC-Na group. *WBV* whole blood viscosity, *PV* plasma viscosity. AEE L: AEE 18 mg/kg; AEE M: 36 mg/kg; AEE H: AEE 72 mg/kg; Combination: combination of aspirin and eugenol (molar ratio 1:1)

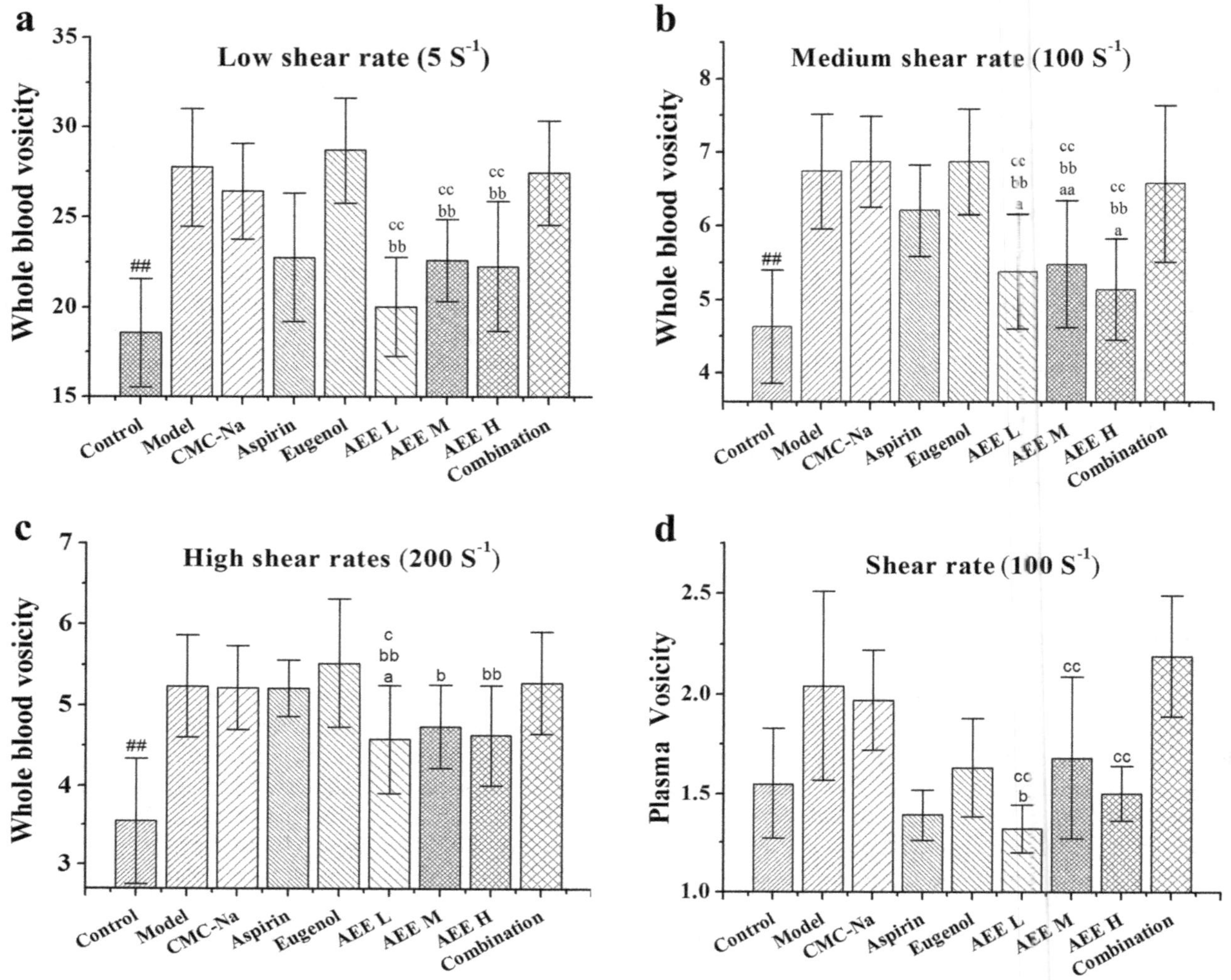

Fig. 1 Comparative effects of aspirin, eugenol and AEE on hemorheological parameters ($n = 10$). (**a-c**): whole blood viscosity at the shear rates of 5 s^{-1}, 100 s^{-1} and 200 s^{-1}. (**d**): plasma viscosity at the shear rate of 100 s^{-1}. $^{\#}P < 0.05$, $^{\#\#}P < 0.01$ compared with model group. $^{a}P < 0.05$, $^{aa}P < 0.01$ compared with aspirin group. $^{b}P < 0.05$, $^{bb}P < 0.01$ compared with eugenol group. $^{c}P < 0.05$, $^{cc}P < 0.01$ compared with combination group. Under the same molar quantity, medium dose of AEE showed better effects than its precursors on whole blood viscosity and plasma viscosity reduction in varying degrees. AEE L: AEE 18 mg/kg; AEE M: 36 mg/kg; AEE H: AEE 72 mg/kg. Combination: combination of aspirin and eugenol (molar ratio 1:1)

high-dose AEE significantly inhibited ADP-induced platelet aggregation more effectively than eugenol ($P < 0.01$). The values of ADP-induced platelet aggregation in high-dose AEE group were lower than that in combination group ($P < 0.05$). Based on these results, under the same molar quantity, medium-dose AEE showed better effects than aspirin and eugenol on AA-induced platelet aggregation and possessed more effective effects of inhibiting ADP-induced platelet aggregation than eugenol.

Blood biochemical results

The results of blood biochemistry are given in Table 4. In comparison with control group, TP, ALB, ALP, ALT, Ca and TG in model group were significantly reduced ($P < 0.01$), AST and TCH were remarkably elevated ($P < 0.05$ and $P < 0.01$). The results of ALB, ALT and LDH between model and CMC-Na groups showed some differences ($P < 0.05$, or $P < 0.01$). When compared with CMC-Na group, aspirin significantly reduced the levels of T-BIL, AST, LDH, TG and TCH, and elevated the levels of TP, ALB, BUN and Ca ($P < 0.05$, or $P < 0.01$). In addition, there was no significant difference between CMC-Na and eugenol groups.

In comparison with CMC-Na group, the levels of ALB and Ca were significantly increased in AEE groups ($P < 0.05$, or $P < 0.01$), whereas TCH was significantly reduced ($P < 0.05$, or $P < 0.01$). Low- and medium-dose AEE significantly increased the level of TP and reduced the level of T-BIL ($P < 0.01$). The TG and BUN levels in high-dose AEE group were significantly reduced ($P < 0.05$). In

Table 3 Effect of AEE on platelet aggregation in k-carrageenan-induced rat tail thrombosis model ($n = 10$)

Groups	AA-induced PAg	ADP-induced PAg
Control	8.70 ± 1.34##	31.90 ± 2.77##
Model	29.00 ± 1.49	50.10 ± 3.34
CMC-Na	30.10 ± 2.13	51.90 ± 2.28
Aspirin	20.44 ± 2.74**	40.89 ± 4.26**
Eugenol	27.10 ± 3.14*	50.10 ± 2.23
AEE L	18.70 ± 3.49**	49.30 ± 2.79
AEE M	11.80 ± 3.70**	43.30 ± 3.13**
AEE H	15.70 ± 3.43**	42.20 ± 3.26**
Combination	11.50 ± 2.50**	45.50 ± 3.17**

5 μM ADP and 5 mM AA were added separately to platelet-rich plasma (PRP), which was used to assess platelet aggregation. Results are expressed as the percentage of maximal aggregation. Data are expressed as mean ± SD. #$P < 0.05$, ##$P < 0.01$ compared with the model group. *$P < 0.05$, **$P < 0.01$ compared with the CMC-Na group. PAg: platelet aggregation. AEE L: AEE 18 mg/kg; AEE M: 36 mg/kg; AEE H: AEE 72 mg/kg; Combination: combination of aspirin and eugenol (molar ratio 1:1)

comparison with the CMC-Na group, the levels of ALB, AST, LDH and BUN in combination group were significantly elevated ($P < 0.01$). The differences in blood biochemical indexes among the groups treated with three doses of AEE were dose-independent.

Effects of AEE on TXB_2 and 6-keto-$PGF_{1α}$

The results of TXB_2 and 6-keto-PGF_{1a} are shown in Table 5. TXB_2 and TXB_2/6-keto-$PGF_{1α}$ ratio were elevated in model group in comparison with those in control group, but 6-keto-$PGF_{1α}$ was declined ($P < 0.01$). There was no difference in TXB_2 between CMC-Na and model groups. However, a significant decrease of 6-keto-$PGF_{1α}$ and an increase of TXB_2/6-keto-$PGF_{1α}$ ratio were observed ($P < 0.01$). Eugenol and aspirin significantly increased 6-keto-$PGF_{1α}$ and lowered TXB_2/6-keto-$PGF_{1α}$ ratio than CMC-Na ($P < 0.01$). In comparison with CMC-Na group, low-, medium- and high-dose AEE had significantly increased 6-keto-$PGF_{1α}$ and reduced TXB_2 with a drop of TXB_2/6-keto-$PGF_{1α}$ ratio ($P < 0.01$). No dose response relationship was observed in AEE groups on TXB_2 and 6-keto-$PGF_{1α}$.

Figure 3 shows the effects different drugs on TXB_2 and 6-keto-$PGF_{1α}$. In comparison with aspirin and eugenol, AEE reduced TXB_2 and 6-keto-$PGF_{1α}$ to varying degrees with the exception of 6-keto-$PGF_{1α}$ in medium-dose AEE group. TXB_2 in high-dose AEE group were higher than combination group ($P < 0.05$). Three different doses of AEE remarkably lowered 6-keto-$PGF_{1α}$ in comparison with combination group ($P < 0.05$ or $P < 0.01$). Under the same molar quantity, medium-dose AEE significantly reduced TXB_2 than aspirin and eugenol ($P < 0.05$ or $P < 0.01$). Results of 6-keto-$PGF_{1α}$ in medium-dose AEE group were higher than eugenol and combination groups. Meanwhile, the TXB_2/6-keto-$PGF_{1α}$ ratio in medium-dose AEE group was significantly lower than that in eugenol ($P < 0.01$). Therefore, equimolar AEE possessed better effects on reducing TXB_2, increasing 6-keto-$PGF_{1α}$ and regulation of TXB_2/6-keto-$PGF_{1α}$ ratio than its precursors.

Discussion

Several chemical drugs are used to prevent or treat thrombosis such as clopidogrel, ticlopidine, dabigatran and apixaban. However, available antithrombosis agents still have some limitations such as gastrointestinal damage and hemorrhage. Therefore, there is an obvious need for more efficacious and alternative treatment options for thrombosis. A previous study showed that AEE could reduce platelet aggregation in vitro, fibrinogen concentration and regulate coagulation parameters, indicating that AEE was a promising drug candidate for

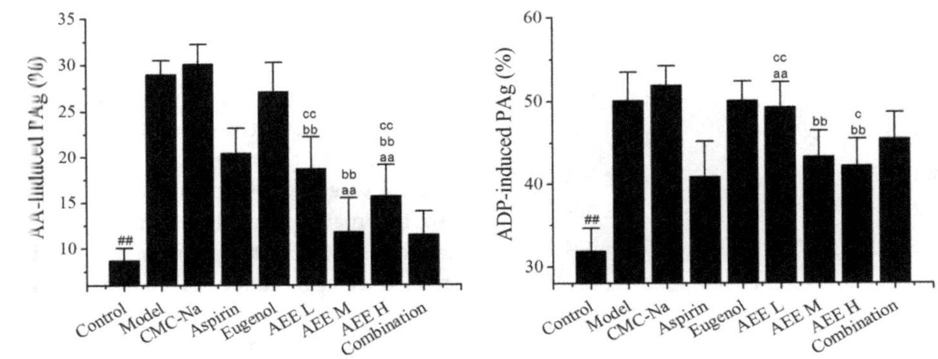

Fig. 2 Comparative effects of aspirin, eugenol and AEE on platelet aggregation in k-carrageenan-induced rat tail thrombosis model ($n = 10$). #$P < 0.05$, ##$P < 0.01$ compared with model group. a$P < 0.05$, aa$P < 0.01$ compared with aspirin group. b$P < 0.05$, bb$P < 0.01$ compared with eugenol group. c$P < 0.05$, cc$P < 0.01$ compared with combination group. No difference was observed between model and CMC-Na groups, which indicated that CMC-Na made no influence on PAg index. AEE showed strong effects than aspirin and eugenol at the same molar quantity. PAg:platelet aggregation. AEE L: AEE 18 mg/kg; AEE M: 36 mg/kg; AEE H: AEE 72 mg/kg; Combination: combination of aspirin and eugenol (molar ratio 1:1)

Table 4 Biochemical parameters in rats intragastrically administered different drugs ($n = 10$)

Variables	Unit	Control	Model	CMC-Na	Aspirin	Eugenol	AEE L	AEE M	AEE H	Combination
T-BIL	umol/L	0.90 ± 0.13	0.97 ± 0.19	1.00 ± 0.17	0.74 ± 0.12**	1.11 ± 0.17	0.72 ± 0.15**	0.65 ± 0.10**	0.86 ± 0.12	1.17 ± 0.17*
TP	g/L	58 ± 2.9##	53 ± 4.3	50 ± 3.4	60 ± 2.2**	50 ± 4.7	59 ± 2.4**	60 ± 3.3**	58 ± 4.1**	61 ± 3.9**
ALB	g/L	23 ± 1.0##	20 ± 1.4	18 ± 1.1##	20 ± 0.8*	19 ± 1.4	21 ± 2.3**	21 ± 0.7**	20 ± 1.1*	22 ± 1.2**
ALT	U/L	69 ± 10##	57 ± 9	67 ± 12#	61 ± 5	68 ± 13	65 ± 6	65 ± 6	58 ± 14	67 ± 13
AST	U/L	79 ± 11#	93 ± 10	85 ± 12	65 ± 8**	96 ± 14	76 ± 10	75 ± 16	74 ± 12	120 ± 14**
ALP	U/L	240 ± 19##	145 ± 22	156 ± 22	178 ± 27	137 ± 23	180 ± 25	181 ± 21	177 ± 11	172 ± 54
GGT	U/L	3.16 ± 0.49	3.34 ± 0.44	3.20 ± 0.25	3.44 ± 0.45	3.15 ± 0.67	3.55 ± 0.57	3.72 ± 0.64	3.61 ± 0.51	3.62 ± 0.60
LDH	U/L	141 ± 28	129 ± 29	161 ± 18#	123 ± 31*	190 ± 27	128 ± 20	126 ± 22	140 ± 38	227 ± 36**
BUN	mmol/L	8.0 ± 0.6	8.9 ± 1.7	9.9 ± 1.7	11.5 ± 1.4*	10.3 ± 1.9	9.4 ± 0.7	9.7 ± 1.5	8.3 ± 0.9 *	12.5 ± 1.3**
CR	umol/L	27.3 ± 4.6	29.3 ± 4.9	29.0 ± 4.8	37.4 ± 3.6*	31.6 ± 4.1	24.9 ± 3.8	32.1 ± 4.6	25.2 ± 3.2	36.4 ± 4.7**
Glu	mmol/L	8.01 ± 0.68	8.11 ± 0.68	7.98 ± 0.53	7.78 ± 0.38	7.52 ± 0.30	7.50 ± 0.81	7.40 ± 0.25	7.57 ± 0.62	7.90 ± 0.81
Ca	mmol/L	2.42 ± 0.06##	2.08 ± 0.10	2.12 ± 0.15	2.30 ± 0.05**	2.12 ± 0.12	2.47 ± 0.12**	2.35 ± 0.05**	2.24 ± 0.14*	2.19 ± 0.06
P	mmol/L	3.31 ± 0.19	3.47 ± 0.25	3.50 ± 0.60	3.36 ± 0.40	3.64 ± 0.43	3.23 ± 0.45	3.36 ± 0.20	3.54 ± 0.15	3.53 ± 0.22
TG	mmol/L	1.19 ± 0.21##	0.66 ± 0.09	0.78 ± 0.06	0.56 ± 0.09*	0.69 ± 0.16	0.71 ± 0.19	0.59 ± 0.15	0.58 ± 0.27*	0.77 ± 0.21
TCH	mmol/L	1.37 ± 0.07##	1.98 ± 0.08	1.81 ± 0.23	1.53 ± 0.17**	1.93 ± 0.18	1.62 ± 0.12*	1.56 ± 0.18*	1.55 ± 0.26**	1.96 ± 0.29

After the last measurement of thrombosis length at 48 h, blood was drawn from the heart. Serum samples were prepared by centrifugation and analyzed using an automatic biochemistry analyzer. #$P < 0.05$, ##$P < 0.01$ compared with the model group. *$P < 0.05$, **$P < 0.01$ compared with the CMC-Na group. AEE L: AEE 18 mg/kg; AEE M: 36 mg/kg; AEE H: AEE 72 mg/kg; Combination: combination of aspirin and eugenol (molar ratio 1:1)

preventing cardiovascular diseases [23]. It was important to characterize its possible mechanism from different views.

Blood hemorheology is an integrated branch of physics and medicine. Increased blood viscosity is a risk factor for thrombosis, atherosclerosis and other cardiovascular events [24]. The increased blood and plasma viscosity in model group can be related to the acute inflammation caused by k-carrageenan injection [23, 25]. AEE decreased whole blood and plasma viscosity, which contributed to ameliorating blood circulation. It also proved that AEE could reduce fibrinogen concentration and normalize blood components [23]. Changes of blood components, especially the reduction of hematocrit, may be responsible for the decrease of viscosity. Additionally, blood viscosity is also determined by shear rate, red blood cell deformability and aggregation. The effects of AEE and its dosage influence on hemorheological parameters should be assessed in the future studies. Some differences were observed between aspirin and combination groups in hemorheological parameters. The mean values of plasma component such as TP, ALB, TG and TCH in aspirin group were lower than those in combination group, which may be the reason for the decrease in plasma viscosity. It was speculated that the differences in RBC deformability and aggregation in aspirin and combination groups were responsible for the different results in whole blood viscosity.

Table 5 Effects of each treatment on TXB_2, 6-keto-$PGF_{1\alpha}$ and the TXB_2/6-keto-$PGF_{1\alpha}$ ratio in k-carrageenan-induced rat tail thrombosis model ($n = 10$)

Groups	TXB_2	6-keto-$PGF_{1\alpha}$	TXB_2/6-keto-$PGF_{1\alpha}$
Control	498 ± 32##	889 ± 28##	0.56 ± 0.04##
Model	696 ± 39	586 ± 24	1.19 ± 0.08
CMC-Na	703 ± 37	550 ± 22##	1.28 ± 0.08##
Aspirin	658 ± 44*	741 ± 23**	0.89 ± 0.06**
Eugenol	678 ± 58	699 ± 30**	0.97 ± 0.09**
AEE L	605 ± 22**	667 ± 17**	0.91 ± 0.04**
AEE M	612 ± 45**	737 ± 13**	0.83 ± 0.07**
AEE H	644 ± 23**	599 ± 26**	1.08 ± 0.07**
Combination	598 ± 51**	701 ± 31**	0.86 ± 0.10**

Blood samples anticoagulated with EDTA-K_2 were centrifuged at 1000 g for 10 min to obtain plasma, which was analyzed using ELISA kits. Data are expressed as mean ± SD. ##$P < 0.01$ compared with the model group. *$P < 0.05$, **$P < 0.01$ compared with the CMC-Na group. AEE L: AEE 18 mg/kg; AEE M: 36 mg/kg; AEE H: AEE 72 mg/kg; Combination: combination of aspirin and eugenol (molar ratio 1:1)

Salicylic acid is the major metabolite of AEE confirmed by in vivo and in vitro experiments [26]. As a classic drug, aspirin is used therapeutically in the prevention of cardiovascular disease by blocking TXA_2 synthesis. Salicylic acid, also the main metabolite of aspirin, is the primary substance responsible for pharmacological function of aspirin on platelet aggregation. AEE and aspirin share the same metabolite as salicylic acid; therefore, AEE and aspirin likely inhibit platelet aggregation via similar mechanism. The effects of eugenol on human platelet aggregation had been investigated and proved that eugenol was a strong platelet aggregation inhibitor [12, 13]. Vascular endothelial cell damage caused by k-carrageenan may be the reason for the increased platelet aggregation in

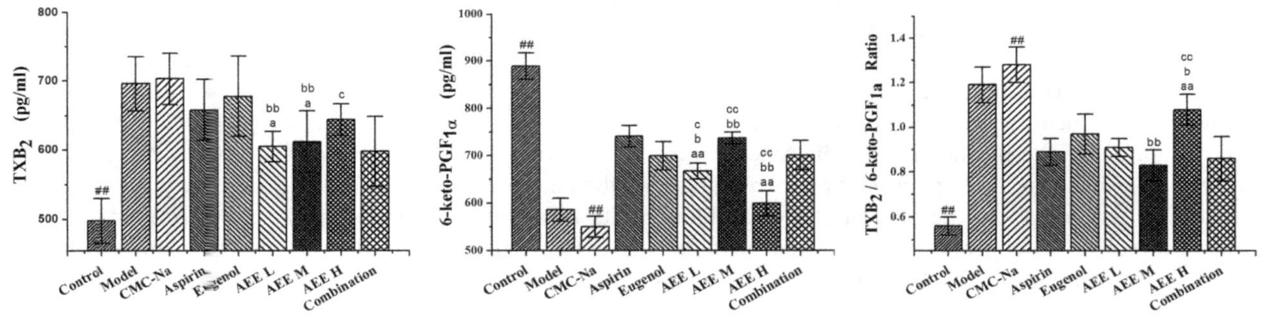

Fig. 3 Comparative effects of aspirin, eugenol and AEE on TXB_2, 6-keto-$PGF_{1\alpha}$ and TXB_2/6-keto-$PGF_{1\alpha}$ ratio in different groups ($n = 10$). $^{\#}P < 0.05$, $^{\#\#}P < 0.01$ compared with model group. $^{a}P < 0.05$, $^{aa}P < 0.01$ compared with aspirin group. $^{b}P < 0.05$, $^{bb}P < 0.01$ compared with eugenol group. $^{c}P < 0.05$, $^{cc}P < 0.01$ compared with combination group. AEE L: AEE 18 mg/kg; AEE M: 36 mg/kg; AEE H: AEE 72 mg/kg; Combination: combination of aspirin and eugenol (molar ratio 1:1)

model group [18]. The vehicle, CMC-Na, had no effect on platelet aggregation. In the case of equal molar quantity, AEE inhibited the platelet aggregation and showed stronger effects than eugenol on AA and ADP-induced platelet aggregation, and better effects than aspirin on AA-induced platelet aggregation. Based on the results, the effect of AEE on platelet aggregation is likely produced by both salicylic acid and eugenol. AEE is decomposed into salicylic acid and eugenol by the enzyme after absorption, after which salicylic acid and eugenol as the major metabolites showed their original activities and acted synergistically to increase the inhibitory effect on platelet aggregation. Previous studies have confirmed that platelet aggregation is an important influence in blood viscosity [27]. Thus, the reduced platelet aggregation caused by AEE was another factor contributing to the decreases of blood and plasma viscosity.

In order to explore the further mechanisms of inhibiting platelet aggregation, the levels of TXB_2 and 6-keto-$PGF_{1\alpha}$ in plasma were measured. TXB_2 and 6-keto-$PGF_{1\alpha}$ are the stable hydrolysis products of thromboxane A2 (TXA_2) and prostacyclin I2 (PGI_2), respectively. TXA_2 is a potent inducer of platelet aggregation and vasoconstriction [6]. PGI_2 is a powerful vasodilator that inhibits platelet aggregation [28]. Arachidonate is a precursor of both PGI_2 and TXA_2. Cyclooxygenase (COX) plays an important role in arachidonate metabolic pathways to generate PGI_2 and TXA_2 [29]. Some evidences have demonstrated that both aspirin and eugenol inhibit COX activity [30–32]. Aspirin, as an inhibitor of COX, could reduce both the level of TXB_2 and 6-keto-$PGF_{1\alpha}$. However, the level of 6-keto-$PGF_{1\alpha}$ in aspirin group was higher than that of CMC-Na group. The previous study showed that aspirin significantly decreased the length of rat tail thrombosis [23]. Thrombosis formation may produce the reductive effects on 6-keto-$PGF_{1\alpha}$. Aspirin inhibits the thrombosis formation in the rat tail, and then weakens the decreasing effects caused by k-carrageenan on 6-keto-$PGF_{1\alpha}$. Suppression of inflammation by aspirin may be the reason of reducing rat tail thrombosis length [33]. Platelets primarily process PGH_2 to TXA_2 and vascular endothelial cells primarily process PGH_2 to PGI_2. Aspirin selectively inhibits the production of TXA_2 in platelet, while sparing endothelial PGI_2 synthesis [34]. New cyclooxygenase could be produced in endothelial cells, but cannot in anucleate platelets. It was speculated that the different effects of aspirin on platelets and endothelial cells and the newly produced cyclooxygenase from endothelial cells may be the reasons for the raised 6-keto-$PGF_{1\alpha}$ in aspirin group. Under equal molar quantity, AEE produced better effects than single using of eugenol or aspirin on TXB_2 and 6-keto-$PGF_{1\alpha}$. According to these results, AEE might significantly down-regulate TXB_2 and up-regulate 6-keto-$PGF_{1\alpha}$ with the TXB_2/6-keto-$PGF_{1\alpha}$ decreased, indicating that the antithrombotic action of AEE was associated with the regulation of TXB_2 and 6-keto-$PGF_{1\alpha}$.

Analysis of blood biochemical parameters could help veterinarians and breeders assess the general health status of animals [35, 36]. Injection of k-carrageenan disturbed the blood biochemical profile through the increase of AST and TCH and the reduction of TP, ALB, ALP, ALT, Ca and TG in model group. These alterations may be related to the stress caused by acute inflammation. Previous study showed that leukocyte and monocyte counts were significantly increased after k-carrageenan injection, which indicated that the rats suffered from acute and systemic inflammation [23]. Intense inflammation could cause the disorder of liver function, and then result in the changes of biochemical profile [37, 38]. In the present study, the reduction of TP, ALB, ALP and the increasing of AST in model group indicated abnormal liver function. Ca, a key factor in thrombosis formation, may be depleted in thrombosis formation process, which may be the reason for the reduction of Ca in model group. The increase of TCH and the reduction of TG may be related to rat body response [39]. It has been proved that AEE could regulate blood lipids in hyperlipidemic rats [40]. The results of TG and TCH indexes in this experiment were similar as found in previous studies [16, 40]. AEE showed positive effects on changing biochemical characters and possessed the ability to normalize the biochemical profile following inflammation, which may be supported by the prolonged time of drug action [41]. In the present study, the blood biochemical results in eugenol group showed no differences in comparison with CMC-Na group. Several reasons may be for these results. Blood biochemical parameters were drastically changed by k-carrageenan injection, which may mask the changes caused by eugenol. Moreover, the dosage of eugenol used in the experiment or eugenol itself was unable to affect biochemical parameters. Previous studies indicated that administration of 150 mg eugenol for 7 days had no significant effects on clinical biochemical parameters in humans [42].

CMC-Na is a reliable drug carrier that is used in a wide range of applications in the pharmaceutical industry [43, 44]. In this study, CMC-Na as vehicle had influence on 6-keto-$PGF_{1\alpha}$, TXB_2/6-keto-PGF_{1a} ratio, ALB, ALT and LDH. In order to demonstrate the activity of AEE, the comparisons were carried out between CMC-Na and treated groups. Therefore, the effect of CMC-Na was eliminated. Tween 80 is widely applied in emulsifying and dispersing substances in medicinal products. In the present study, Tween 80 was used to prepare eugenol. It had been confirmed that the body had a great tolerance to Tween 80 [45]. The effects of Tween 80 and combination of CMC-Na and Tween 80 were not investigated in this experiment.

AEE on the design of prodrug principle contains ester bond structure that is decomposed easily. Pharmacokinetics studies showed that the plasma concentration of AEE itself was extremely low; indeed it was not detectable in plasma. Therefore, it is speculated that the degradation products of AEE such as salicylic acid and eugenol are responsible for its effects. Salicylic acid and eugenol may play an efficient role and interact in a synergistic manner to prevent thrombosis formation. More studies should be conducted to investigate the action mechanism of AEE on thrombosis prevention. In addition, as a promising chemical compound, AEE should be studied in preclinical experiments to assess its therapeutic effects in various species.

Conclusion

The results obtained in our study showed that AEE had potent antithrombotic effects in rats with k-carrageenan-induced tail thrombosis. Moreover, AEE showed better antithrombotic effect than its precursors under same molar quantity. From the findings, the preventive effect of AEE may come from antiplatelet aggregation, reducing blood and plasma viscosity, balancing TXB_2/6-keto-PGF_{1a} ratio and normalizing blood biochemical parameters. These therapeutic effects of AEE may be related to the synergetic actions of aspirin and eugenol. It may be concluded that AEE was a good candidate for anti-thrombotic agent. These findings provide new insight into the action mechanism of AEE on preventing thrombosis. More studies are necessary to investigate its mechanism of action such as the protective effects of vascular endothelial cells, the way on anti-platelet aggregation and the influences on metabolic profile.

Abbreviations

6-keto-$PGF_{1\alpha}$, 6-keto prostaglandin $F_{1\alpha}$; AA, arachidonic acid; ADP, adenosine diphosphate; AEE, aspirin eugenol ester; ALB, albumin; ALP, alkaline phosphatase; ALT, alanine transaminase; AST, aspartate aminotransferase; BUN, blood urea nitrogen; Ca, calcium; CK, creatine kinase; CMC-Na, sodium carboxymethyl cellulose; CR, creatinine; GGT, gamma glutamyl transpeptidase; GLU, glucose; GPT, glutamic pyruvic transaminase; LDH, lactate dehydrogenase; P, phosphorus; PGI_2, prostacyclin I2; PPP, platelet-poor plasma; PRP, platelet-rich plasma; T-BIL, total bilirubin; TCH, total cholesterol; TG, triglycerides; TP, total protein; TXA_2, thromboxane A2; TXB_2, thromboxane B_2.

Acknowledgments

The work was supported by the National Natural Science Foundation of China (No. 31572573).

Funding

The funders had no role in the design of the study and collection, analysis, and interpretation of data and in writing the manuscript.

Authors' contributions

JYL, YJY and NM designed and supervised the experiments. NM performed platelet aggregation test and ELISA. NM, XWL, IM and XLZ carried out the hemorheological test and blood biochemical analysis. NM, JYL, YJY, DSS and XJK performed data analysis and materials. NM, JYL and YJY prepared the manuscript and reviewed the literature. All authors read and approved the final manuscript.

Competing interests

The authors declare that they have no competing interests.

Consent for publication

Not applicable.

References

1. Kraft W. Geriatrics in canine and feline internal medicine. Eur J Med Res. 1998;3(1–2):31–41.
2. Day MJ. Ageing, immunosenescence and inflammageing in the dog and cat. J Comp Pathol. 2010;142 Suppl 1:S60–9.
3. Barthelemy A, Rannou B, Forterre M, Verwaerde P, Bonnet-Garin JM, Pouzot-Nevoret C, et al. Differences between coagulation and cytokine profiles in dogs of different ages. Vet J. 2015;205(3):410–2.
4. Lunsford KV, Mackin AJ. Thromboembolic therapies in dogs and cats: an evidence-based approach. Vet Clin North Am Small Anim Pract. 2007;37(3):579–609.
5. Wang Y, Andrews M, Yang Y, Lang S, Jin JW, Cameron-Vendrig A, et al. Platelets in thrombosis and hemostasis: old topic with new mechanisms. Cardiovasc Hematol Disord Drug Targets. 2012;12(2):126–32.
6. Sakata C, Kawasaki T, Kato Y, Abe M, Suzuki K, Ohmiya M, et al. ASP6537, a novel highly selective cyclooxygenase-1 inhibitor, exerts potent antithrombotic effect without "aspirin dilemma". Thromb Res. 2013;132(1):56–62.

7. Reggiori G, Occhipinti G, De Gasperi A, Vincent JL, Piagnerelli M. Early alterations of red blood cell rheology in critically ill patients. Crit Care Med. 2009;37(12):3041–6.
8. Goyal VK, Pandey SK, Kakade S, Nirogi R. Evaluation of clinical chemistry analytes from a single mouse using diluted plasma: effective way to reduce the number of animals in toxicity studies. Lab Anim. 2015 doi:10.1177/0023677215620969.
9. Yu C, Qi D, Lian W, Li QZ, Li HJ, Fan HY. Effects of danshensu on platelet aggregation and thrombosis: in vivo arteriovenous shunt and venous thrombosis models in rats. PLoS One. 2014;9(11):e110124.
10. Nansseu JR, Noubiap JJ. Aspirin for primary prevention of cardiovascular disease. Thromb J. 2015;13:38.
11. Ye X, Fu J, Yang Y, Gao Y, Liu L, Chen S. Frequency-risk and duration-risk relationships between aspirin use and gastric cancer: a systematic review and meta-analysis. PLoS One. 2013;8(7):e71522.
12. Yogalakshmi B, Viswanathan P, Anuradha CV. Investigation of antioxidant, anti-inflammatory and DNA-protective properties of eugenol in thioacetamide-induced liver injury in rats. Toxicology. 2010;268(3):204–12.
13. Saeed SA, Simjee RU, Shamim G, Gilani AH. Eugenol: a dual inhibitor of platelet-activating factor and arachidonic acid metabolism. Phytomedicine. 1995;2(1):23–8.
14. Naidu KA. Eugenol–an inhibitor of lipoxygenase-dependent lipid peroxidation. Prostaglandins Leukot Essent Fatty Acids. 1995;53(5):381–3.
15. Capasso R, Pinto L, Vuotto ML, Di Carlo G. Preventive effect of eugenol on PAF and ethanol-induced gastric mucosal damage. Fitoterapia. 2000;71 Suppl 1:S131–7.
16. Li J, Yu Y, Yang Y, Liu X, Zhang J, Li B, et al. A 15-day oral dose toxicity study of aspirin eugenol ester in Wistar rats, vol. 50. 2012. p. 1980–5.
17. Arslan R, Bor Z, Bektas N, Mericli AH, Ozturk Y. Antithrombotic effects of ethanol extract of Crataegus orientalis in the carrageenan-induced mice tail thrombosis model. Thromb Res. 2011;127(3):210–3.
18. Begum R, Sharma M, Pillai KK, Aeri V, Sheliya MA. Inhibitory effect of Careya arborea on inflammatory biomarkers in carrageenan-induced inflammation. Pharm Biol. 2015;53(3):437–445.
19. Yan F, Yan J, Sun W, Yao L, Wang J, Qi Y, et al. Thrombolytic effect of subtilisin QK on carrageenan induced thrombosis model in mice. J Thromb Thrombolysis. 2009;28(4):444–8.
20. Simkhada JR, Cho SS, Mander P, Choi YH, Yoo JC. Purification, biochemical properties and antithrombotic effect of a novel Streptomyces enzyme on carrageenan-induced mice tail thrombosis model. Thromb Res. 2012;129(2):176–82.
21. Arslan R, Bektas N, Bor Z, Sener E. Evaluation of the antithrombotic effects of Crataegus monogyna and Crataegus davisii in the carrageenan-induced tail thrombosis model. Pharm Biol. 2015;53(2):275–9.
22. Majumdar S, Chattopadhyay P, Mukherjee AK. In vivo anticoagulant and thrombolytic activities of a fibrinolytic serine protease (Brevithrombolase) with the k-carrageenan-induced rat tail thrombosis model. Clin Appl Thromb Hemost. 2015 doi:10.1177/1076029615569567.
23. Ma N, Liu XW, Yang YJ, Li JY, Mohamed I, Liu GR, et al. Preventive effect of aspirin eugenol ester on thrombosis in kappa-carrageenan-induced rat tail thrombosis model. PLoS One. 2015;10(7):e133125.
24. Yu S, Yue S, Liu Z, Zhang T, Xiang N, Fu H. Yerba mate (Ilex paraguariensis) improves microcirculation of volunteers with high blood viscosity: a randomized, double-blind, placebo-controlled trial. Exp Gerontol. 2015;62:14–22.
25. Alexy T, Pais E, Wenby RB, Mack WJ, Hodis HN, Kono N, et al. Abnormal blood rheology and chronic low grade inflammation: possible risk factors for accelerated atherosclerosis and coronary artery disease in Lewis negative subjects. Atherosclerosis. 2015;239(1):248–51.
26. Shen Y, Liu X, Yang Y, Li J, Ma N, Li B. In vivo and in vitro metabolism of aspirin eugenol ester in dog by liquid chromatography tandem mass spectrometry. Biomed Chromatogr. 2015;29(1):129–37.
27. Ryu KH, Han HY, Lee SY, Jeon SD, Im G, Lee BY, et al. Ginkgo biloba extract enhances antiplatelet and antithrombotic effects of cilostazol without prolongation of bleeding time. Thromb Res. 2009;124(3):328–34.
28. Nakayama T. Genetic polymorphisms of prostacyclin synthase gene and cardiovascular disease. Int Angiol. 2010;29(2 Suppl):33–42.
29. Kim SF, Huri DA, Snyder SH. Inducible nitric oxide synthase binds, S-nitrosylates, and activates cyclooxygenase-2. Science. 2005;310(5756):1966–70.
30. Raghavendra RH, Naidu KA. Spice active principles as the inhibitors of human platelet aggregation and thromboxane biosynthesis. Prostaglandins Leukot Essent Fatty Acids. 2009;81(1):73–78.
31. Christersson C, Oldgren J, Wallentin L, Siegbahn A. Treatment with an oral direct thrombin inhibitor decreases platelet activity but increases markers of inflammation in patients with myocardial infarction. J Intern Med. 2011;270(3):215–23.
32. Sutcliffe P, Connock M, Gurung T, Freeman K, Johnson S, Ngianga-Bakwin K, et al. Aspirin in primary prevention of cardiovascular disease and cancer: a systematic review of the balance of evidence from reviews of randomized trials. PLoS One. 2013;8(12):e81970.
33. Nantel F, Denis D, Gordon R, Northey A, Cirino M, Metters KM, et al. Distribution and regulation of cyclooxygenase-2 in carrageenan-induced inflammation. Br J Pharmacol. 1999;128(4):853–9.
34. Smith SA. Antithrombotic therapy. Top Companion Anim Med. 2012;27(2):88–94.
35. Orzel D, Zmijewski M, Bronkowska M. Impact of products from ground buckwheat added to balanced diets on biochemical blood markers in Wistar rats. Rocz Panstw Zakl Hig. 2015;66(3):239–44.
36. Bronkowska M, Lozna K, Figurska-Ciura D, Styczynska M, Orzel D, Biernat J, et al. Influence of arsenic on selected biochemical blood parameters in rats fed diet with different fat and protein content. Rocz Panstw Zakl Hig. 2015;66(3):233–7.
37. Liu ZW, Zhang N, Han QY, Zeng JT, Chu YL, Qiu JM, et al. Correlation of serum leptin levels with anthropometric and metabolic parameters and biochemical liver function in Chinese patients with chronic hepatitis C virus infection. World J Gastroenterol. 2005;11(22):3357–62.
38. Kukuk GM, Schaefer SG, Fimmers R, Hadizadeh DR, Ezziddin S, Spengler U, et al. Hepatobiliary magnetic resonance imaging in patients with liver disease: correlation of liver enhancement with biochemical liver function tests. Eur Radiol. 2014;24(10):2482–90.
39. Arya A, Jamil AM, Binti KR, Taha H, Karim KA, Shahid N, et al. Extract of Woodfordia fruticosa flowers ameliorates hyperglycaemia and oxidative stress, and improves beta-cell function in streptozotocin-nicotinamide induced diabetic rat. J Ethnopharmacol. 2015;175:229–240 .
40. Karam I, Ma N, Liu XW, Li SH, Kong XJ, Li JY, et al. Regulation effect of aspirin eugenol ester on blood lipids in Wistar rats with hyperlipidemia. BMC Vet Res. 2015;11:217.
41. Li J, Yu Y, Wang Q, Zhang J, Yang Y, Li B, et al. Synthesis of aspirin eugenol ester and its biological activity. Med Chem Res. 2012;21(7):995–9.
42. Rompelberg CJ, Vogels JT, de Vogel N, Bruijntjes-Rozier GC, Stenhuis WH, Bogaards JJ, et al. Effect of short-term dietary administration of eugenol in humans. Hum Exp Toxicol. 1996;15(2):129–35.
43. Jin Z, Li W, Cao H, Zhang X, Chen G, Wu H, et al. Antimicrobial activity and cytotoxicity of N-2-HACC and characterization of nanoparticles with N-2-HACC and CMC as a vaccine carrier. Chem Eng J. 2013;221:331–41.
44. Abdel-Galil A, Ali HE, Atta A, Balboul MR. Influence of nanostructured TiO2 additives on some physical characteristics of carboxymethyl cellulose (CMC). J Radiat Res Appl Sci. 2014;7(1):36–43.
45. Ema M, Hara H, Matsumoto M, Hirata-Koizumi M, Hirose A, Kamata E. Evaluation of developmental neurotoxicity of polysorbate 80 in rats. Reprod Toxicol. 2008;25(1):89–99.

15

Effects of premedication with oral gabapentin on intraocular pressure changes following tracheal intubation in clinically normal dogs

Alexandra Trbolova[1], Masoud Selk Ghaffari[2*] and Igor Capik[1]

Abstract

Background: Gabapentin is an antiepileptic drug widely approved as an add-on therapy for epilepsy treatment in human and dogs. There is a clinical impression that gabapentin is a suitable drug which attenuates the IOP elevation associated with tracheal intubation in humans. The present study performed to determine the effects of oral gabapentin on intraocular pressure (IOP) changes following tracheal intubation in dogs.

Results: Twenty adult healthy dogs were randomly assigned to treatment ($n = 10$) and control ($n = 10$) groups. Dogs in the treatment group received oral gabapentin (50 mg/kg) 2 h before induction of anesthesia and dogs in the control group received oral gelatin capsule placebo at the same time. The dogs were anesthetized with propofol 6 mg/kg, and anesthesia was maintained with a constant infusion of 0.2 mg/kg/min of propofol for 20 min. IOP were measured immediately before induction and then repeated immediately after induction, as well as 5 min, 10 min and 15 min following tracheal intubation in both groups. IOP was significantly higher immediately after induction, and 5 min after tracheal intubation when compared with IOP reading before induction in the control group. There was no statistically significant change in IOPs immediately after induction, and 5 min after tracheal intubation in comparison to the values before induction in the treatment group.

Conclusions: Based on the findings of this study, preanesthetic oral administration of gabapentin significantly prevents an increase in the IOP associated with tracheal intubation in dogs anesthetized with propofol.

Keywords: Gabapentin, IOP, tracheal intubation, dogs

Background

The sensitivity of maintaining an intraocular pressure within or below reference range throughout sedation or general anesthesia has been the subject of extensive research in humans and animals [1–3].

An appropriate anesthetic protocol for any patient with an ophthalmic problem should include not only drug selection but also a preoperative management plan to provide an optimal postoperative outcome [4]. Abrupt increases in intraocular pressure associated with anesthetic drugs or orotracheal intubation can cause dramatic effects in patients with near-perforating corneal lesions or glaucoma [5]. Hofmeister et al. reported a significant increase in IOP after intubation compared to before induction with propofol in dogs [1].

Gabapentin is an antiepileptic drug widely approved as an add-on therapy for epilepsy treatment in human and dogs [6–9]. There is a clinical impression that gabapentin is a suitable drug which attenuates the IOP elevation associated with tracheal intubation in humans [10].

As far as we know there is no published work on the effects of gabapentin on IOP following orotracheal intubation in dogs. The aim of this study was to determine the effects of oral gabapentin on IOP changes following tracheal intubation in dogs.

* Correspondence: selkghaffari@gmail.com
[2]Department of Clinical Sciences, College of Veterinary Medicine, Karaj Branch, Islamic Azad University, Alborz, Iran
Full list of author information is available at the end of the article

Methods

This study was done with agreement of the Ethic Committee (protocol number: **2048/02–17.**) of the University of Veterinary Medicine and Pharmacy, Kosice, Slovakia, in accordance with Slovakian ethical codes for studies on laboratory animals (All dogs were research animals).

Prior to entering the study, all dogs were determined to be free of disease by means of physical and ocular examination using biomicroscopy, tonometry and indirect ophthalmoscopy. No obvious abnormalities were noted during the ophthalmic examinations.

Twenty adult healthy dogs were included in this study. The dogs were fasted overnight but had free access to water. Dogs were randomly assigned to treatment ($n = 10$) and control ($n = 10$) groups. Dogs in the treatment group received oral gabapentin (50 mg/kg; Teva Pharmaceuticals CR, S.R.O. Praha, Czech Republic; the gabapentin was compounded in order to assure an accurate dose) 2 h before induction of anesthesia and dogs in the control group received oral gelatin capsule placebo at the same time.

After 5 min of preoxygenation, the dogs were anesthetized with propofol (6 mg/kg IV; Fresenius Kabi, GmbH, Graz, Austria; entire calculated dose of propofol was given), and anesthesia was maintained with a constant infusion of 0.2 mg/kg/min of propofol for 20 min.

IOPs were measured immediately before induction (baseline; Tb) and then repeated immediately after induction (T0), as well as 5 min (T5), 10 min (T10) and 15 min (T15) following tracheal intubation in both groups. For all dogs, the same investigator (A.T.) performed all IOP measurements. (A.T.) obtaining IOP blinded to treatment group assignment. During tonometry, the animals were placed in sternal recumbency with head in normal and upright position and the eyelids were not manipulated as measurements were taken.

Before the tonometry, a drop of proparacine hydrochloride (Paracain, Sunways Ltd., Mumbai, India) was applied in both eyes of the dogs immediately. IOP was measured using applanation tonometry with the Tono-Pen AVIA VET (Tono-Pen AVIA, Reichert, NY). The tonometer was factory calibrated before initiation of the study. Only IOP readings with a 5% variance (5% displays on Tono-Pen; we recorded IOP values once we got that one reading with a 5% variance) were recorded.

Cardiorespiratory monitoring was performed by means of assessing hemoglobin saturation (SpO_2), pulse rate, respiration rate, and systolic blood pressure at T_b, T_0, T_5,T_{10}, T_{15} using Mindray- PM - 9000 Vet (Mindray, Hamburg, Germany).

Statistical analysis was performed by using the software package SPSS version 15.0 for Microsoft Windows (SPSS Inc., Chicago, Illinois 60,606, USA). Data were expressed as mean ± SD. Shapiro-Wilk test was used to evaluate whether the data were normally distributed. A 2-way ANOVA was used to compare data within the same group and to assess differences between groups. A p-value of <0.05 was considered statistically significant.

Results

The mean values and SD of IOP and blood pressure in both treatment and control groups are shown in Figs. 1 and 2. All data are expressed as mmHg.

The mean ± SD baseline IOP values (obtained immediately before induction; Tb) for treatment and control groups were 19.5 ± 2.2 and 21.6 ± 2.6, respectively. For baseline IOP values, there was no significant difference between treatment and control groups ($P = 0.05$).

IOP was significantly higher immediately after induction (27.5 ± 3.1; P_0 < 001), and 5 min after tracheal intubation (25.0 ± 2.4; $P_5 = 0.001$) when compared with IOP reading before induction (21.6 ± 2.6) in control group. The systolic blood pressure showed no statistically significant increase after induction (137.5 ± 4.1; $P_0 = 1.00$), also recording values at 5 min after tracheal (131.9 ± 9.4; $P_5 = 1.00$) was still higher than values at before induction (130.6 ± 4.9) but it was not statistically significant.

Comparison between treatment IOP values in the control group revealed significant differences between T0 and T5 ($P = 0.004$) as well as comparison between T5 and T10 ($P = 0.00$).

There was no statistically significant change in IOPs immediately after induction (18.6 ± 1.9; $P_0 = 0.9$), and 5 min after tracheal intubation (17.4 ± 1.8; $P = 0.6$) in comparison to the values before induction (19.5 ± 2.2) in the treatment group. Comparison between treatment IOP values in the treatment group revealed no significant differences ($P \geq 0.9$).

There is a tendency for a systolic blood pressure decreasing effect in treatment group when comparing values with recorded values prior to induction, The mean ± SD values before induction, immediately after

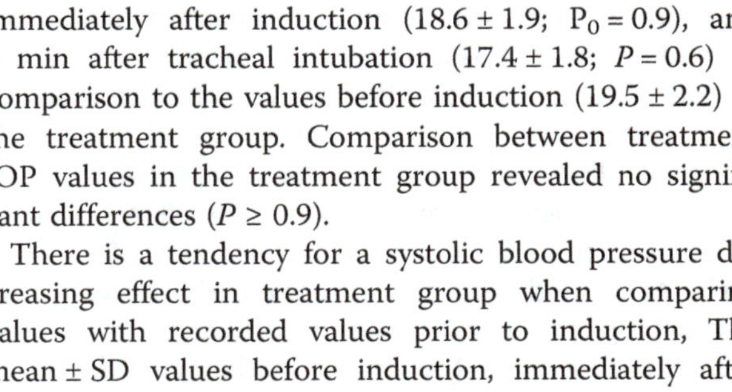

Fig. 1 Mean and SD of intraocular pressure in treatment (10 dogs, received oral gabapentin 2 h before induction of anesthesia) and control (10 dogs, received oral gelatin capsule placebo at the same time) groups at baseline, 0, 5, 10 and 15 min after induction of anesthesia

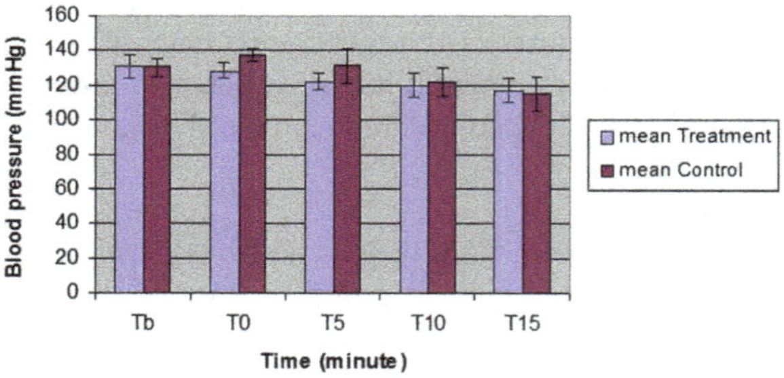

Fig. 2 Mean and SD of blood pressure in both treatment and control groups at baseline, 0, 5, 10 and 15 min after induction of anesthesia

induction and at 5 min after tracheal intubation were 131.0 ± 6.3, 128.5 ± 4.0 ($P = 0.9$), and 122.3 ± 4.6 ($P = 0.2$) respectively.

In both groups, the recorded values for IOP and systolic blood pressure at 15 min after intubation showed statistically significant decrease ($P < 0.05$).

Discussion

This study evaluated the effects of oral gabapentin on IOP changes following tracheal intubation in dogs. At clinically useful doses (10–60 mg/kg), maximum blood levels, reached within 1–3 h after peroral administration [11, 12].

This information helps to explain our results in which oral gabapentin significantly prevent the increase in IOP associated with endotracheal intubation. These findings were similar to a previous study in humans which documented gabapentin as a useful adjuvant in order to prevent an increase in the IOP in response to tracheal intubation [10].

The baseline values of IOP observed prior to treatment in the dogs presented in this study were similar to those reported in normal dogs [13, 14].

The exact mode of action of gabapentin in decreasing IOP in dogs is unclear. Several mechanisms have been proposed to explain gabapentin modulation of IOP in humans. Intraocular blood volume is determined by arterial inflow, venous outflow, and tone of the intraocular vasculature. These variations in intraocular blood volume modify the IOP [4]. It could be suggested that the possible relaxing effects of gabapentin on the ciliary muscle by inhibiting membrane voltage-gated calcium channels, (acting in a manner similar to calcium channel blockers) might lead to the attenuation of the IOP by improving the flow of aqueous humour through the canal of Schlemm [10, 15].

In the present study, post-treatment IOP measurements were compared with baseline and negative control group IOPs. In this investigation, the control group was considered to allow proper evaluation the effects of time, anesthesia, and intubation as variables on IOP readings.

An interesting finding in this study was a significant effect of gabapentin on blood pressure. In the present work, we found a statistically significant decrease in systolic blood pressure 5 min after intubation, when compared with baseline values.

Our findings are in agreement with previous studies in humans which showed that gabapentin attenuated blood pressure increase following tracheal intubation by its inhibitory effects on membrane voltage-gated calcium channels [15, 16].

In fact, the success of an ophthalmic surgery may depend on control of IOP before, during and after the procedure. Anesthetic management should minimize changes, specifically an increase in IOP over the entire anesthetic period.

Maintaining an IOP within or below reference range throughout general anesthesia is essential for certain ocular diseases. For example, corneal lesions that approach full thickness require delicate handling and control of IOP to avoid inadvertent perforation prior to and during surgery. Corneal perforations, particularly those that result in iris prolapse, have a notably worse prognosis for preservation of vision postoperatively [17, 18]. Therefore; exploring safer treatment for abrupt increase of IOP in dogs undergoing ocular surgery is warranted.

Conclusions

Based on the findings of this study, preanesthetic oral administration of gabapentin significantly prevents an increase in the IOP associated with tracheal intubation in dogs anesthetized with propofol. As gabapentin appears to be useful drug in attenuation of increased IOP associated with intubation, its administration can be reliably advised when performing ocular procedures in dogs with deep ulcer or laceration in which increased IOP may result in ocular complications, such as perforation of the globe.

Abbreviations

IOP: Intraocular pressure

Funding

The authors have declared that no funding exists.

Authors' contributions

MSG analyzed the data and drafted the manuscript. AT and IC initiated and carried the study. All authors participated in writing the manuscript and approved the final version.

Consent for publication

Not applicable.

Competing interests
The authors declare that they have no competing interests.

Author details
[1]Clinic of Small Animals, University of Veterinary Medicine and Pharmacy, Kosice, Slovakia. [2]Department of Clinical Sciences, College of Veterinary Medicine, Karaj Branch, Islamic Azad University, Alborz, Iran.

References

1. Hofmeister EH, Williams CO, Braun C. Propofol versus thiopental: effects on peri-induction intraocular pressures in normal dogs. Vet Anesthes Analges. 2008;35:275–81.
2. Almeida DE, Rezende ML, Nunes N. Evaluation of intraocular pressure in association with cardiovascular parameters in normocapnic dogs anesthetized with sevoflurane and desflurane. Vet Ophthalmol. 2004;7:265–59.
3. Selk Ghaffari M, Rezaei MA, Mirani AH, Khorami N. The effects of ketamine-midazolam anesthesia on intraocular pressure in clinically normal dogs. Vet Ophthalmol. 2010;13:9[illegible]–3.
4. Artigas C, Redondo JI, López-Murcia MM. Effects of intravenous administration of dexmedetomidine on intraocular pressure and pupil size in clinically normal dogs. Vet Ophthalmol. 2012;15:79–82.
5. Hofmeister EH, Weinstein WL, Burger D, Brainard BM, Accola PJ, Moore PA. Effects of graded doses of propofol for anesthesia induction on cardiovascular parameters and intraocular pressures in normal dogs. Vet Anesthes Analges. 2009;36:442–8.
6. Bruni J. Gabapentin as adjunctive therapy for partial seizures. Epilepsia. 1999;40:73–4.
7. Herranz JL, Sol JM, Hernández G. Gabapentin used in 559 patients with partial seizures. A multicenter observation study. Spanish Gabapentin work group. Rev Neurol. 2000;30:1141–5.
8. Platt SR, Adams V, Garosi LS, Abramson CJ, Penderis J, De Stefani A, Matiasek L. Treatment with gabapentin of 11 dogs with refractory idiopathic epilepsy. Vet Rec. 2006;159:881–4.
9. Govendir M, Perkins M, Malik R. Improving seizure control in dogs with refractory epilepsy using gabapentin as an adjunctive agent. Aust Vet J. 2005;83:602–8.
10. Kaya FN, Yavascaoglu B, Baykara M, Altun GT, Gülhan N, Ata F. Effect of oral gabapentin on the intraocular pressure and haemodynamic responses induced by tracheal intubation. Acta Anesth Scand. 2008;52:1076–80.
11. Ramsey I. BSAVA Small Animal Formulary, 8th Edition. 2014. p. 173.
12. Vollmer KO, von Hodenberg A, Kölle EU. Pharmacokinetics and metabolism of gabapentin in rat, dog and man. Arzneimittelforschung. 1986;36:830–9.
13. Miller PE, Pickett JP, Majors LJ, Kurzman ID. Clinical comparison of the Mackay-Marg and Tono-pen applanation tonometer in the dog. Prog Vet Comp Ophthalmol. 1991;1:171–6.
14. Gelatt KN, MacKay EO. Distribution of intraocular pressure in dogs. Vet Ophthalmol. 1998;1:109–14.
15. Sarantopoulos C, McCallum B, Kwok WM, Hogan Q. Gabapentin decreases membrane calcium currents in injured as well as in control mammalianprimary afferent neurons. Reg Anesth Pain Med. 2002;27:47–57.
16. Montazeri K, Kashefi P, Honarmand A, Safavi M, Hirmanpour A. Attenuation of the pressor response to direct laryngoscopy and tracheal intubation: oral clonidine vs. oral gabapentin premedication. J Res Med Sci. 2011 77–86.
17. Chmielewski NT, Brooks DE, Smith PJ, et al. Visual outcome and ocular survival following iris prolapse in the horse: a review of 32 cases. Equine Vet J. 1997;29:31–9.
18. Hofmeister EH, Mosunic CB, Torres BT, et al. Effects of ketamine, diazepam, and their combination on intraocular pressures in clinically normal dogs. Am J Vet Res. 2006;67:1136–9.

16

Use of β-caryophyllene to combat bacterial dental plaque formation in dogs

Fábio Alessandro Pieri[1,2], Marina Campos de Castro Souza[2], Ligia Lobato Ramos Vermelho[2], Marina Lobato Ramos Vermelho[2], Pedro Griffo Perciano[2], Fabiano Souza Vargas[3], Andréa Pacheco Batista Borges[2], Valdir Florêncio da Veiga-Junior[3] and Maria Aparecida Scatamburlo Moreira[2*]

Abstract

Background: Periodontal disease is a highly prevalent illness that affects many dogs, reaching up to 85 % prevalence in individuals over the age of 4 years. Currently the drug of choice for combating the formation of dental plaque in these animals, the etiologic agent of the disease, is chlorhexidine, which has several side effects reported. Thus, surveys are conducted throughout the world in order to identify potential substitutes for antimicrobial therapy and prevention of periodontal disease. The objective of the work was to evaluate the antimicrobial activity of β-caryophyllene against bacteria from dog's dental plaque in vitro and in vivo. The minimum inhibitory concentration was evaluated by agar microdilution assay, the induction or inhibition of bacterial adherence by sub-inhibitory concentrations in 96-well plates, and reduction of dental plaque formation in mongrel dogs subjected to topical solution with β-caryophyllene for 15 days.

Results: Results showed minimum inhibitory concentrations above 100 mg/mL for 25 % of the isolates, 100 mg/mL for 3 %, 50 mg/mL for 25 %, 25 mg/mL for 12 %, 12.5 mg/mL for 19 % and 6.25 mg/mL for 16 %. Bacterial adherences of three *Enterococcus* sp., one *Streptococcus* sp., one *Haemophilus* sp., one *Aerococcus* sp., one *Bacillus* sp. and one *Lactococcus* sp. isolates were inhibited by subinhibitory concentration. One *Lactococcus* sp., one *Bacillus* sp. and one *Streptococcus* sp. were stimulated to adhere by concentrations of 0.19, 1.56 and 0.78 mg/mL, respectively. In vivo assay showed reduction in dental plaque formation by β-caryophyllene, with final plaque coverage of 23.3 ± 2.6 % of the total area of the teeth, with significant difference compared with chlorhexidine group (37.5 ± 3.7 % - $p < 0.05$) and negative control group (65.5 ± 2.5 % - $p < 0.001$).

Conclusions: The results showed that β-caryophyllene has antimicrobial activity against the proliferation of dog's dental plaque-forming bacteria representing a suitable alternative to the use of chlorhexidine in prophylaxis and treatment of periodontal disease of dogs.

Keywords: Antimicrobial, Dogs, Dental plaque, Adhesion, Natural phytochemical

Background

Periodontal disease is a highly prevalent illness that affects many dogs, reaching up to 85 % prevalence in individuals over the age of 4 years [1]. It affects the supporting and protective structures of the teeth and its aetiological agent is the bacterial plaque that develops on the tooth surface, and the immune reaction to infection [2]. Tooth brushing is the most suitable procedure for the prevention of periodontal disease through mechanical removal of dental plaque; however, some alternatives can be employed simultaneously to brushing with the intention of increasing the efficiency of plaque removal. Among these alternatives is the administration of antibacterial substances, which, by preventing the proliferation or adhesion of bacteria to the teeth surface, inhibit the development of periodontal disease [3].

In addition, there is evidence that biofilm formation can be stimulated by certain antimicrobials in subinhibitory concentrations, which makes it necessary to investigate a potential stimulus for bacterial adherence

* Correspondence: masm@ufv.br
[2]Departamento de Veterinária, Universidade Federal de Viçosa, Av. P.H. Rolfs, s/n, Câmpus UFV, CEP: 36570-000 Viçosa, Minas Gerais, Brasil
Full list of author information is available at the end of the article

by antimicrobial agents, making its use in therapy impossible [4, 5]. Studies have indicated several classes of antibiotics, including tetracyclines, quinopristina-dalfopristin, erythromycin and enrofloxacin, which stimulate the formation of biofilms by *Staphylococcus epidermidis* and *Escherichia coli* [5, 6]. In contrast, the discovery of therapeutic agents that are capable of inhibiting biofilm formation, even in sub-inhibitory concentrations, would be useful for the prevention of periodontal disease by inhibiting the formation of dental plaque [3].

Chlorhexidine is currently the drug of choice for combating dental plaque bacteria, and is usually commercialised at the concentration of 0.12 % [7]. However, the use of this drug has some side effects, such as darkening of the tooth enamel, loss of taste, burning sensation in the oral cavity and ulceration of the oral mucosa, as well as a bitter taste and the fact that it enables the emergence of resistant bacteria [8]. Therefore, there is a need to search for alternatives to this drug for prophylaxis and treatment of periodontal disease [9].

The β-caryophyllene is a sesquiterpene ($C_{15}H_{24}$ – Fig. 1), identified in the CAS (Chemical Abstract Service) under number 87-44-5; this is found in many plant sources, and shows great potential [10]. Studies have shown low toxicity and high applicability, with this substance being used for several purposes, including local anaesthesia [11], anti-inflammatory action [12, 13], antispasmodic action [14], antimicrobial activity [15], anxiolytic [16], and protection against ischemic injury in neurons [17], among others.

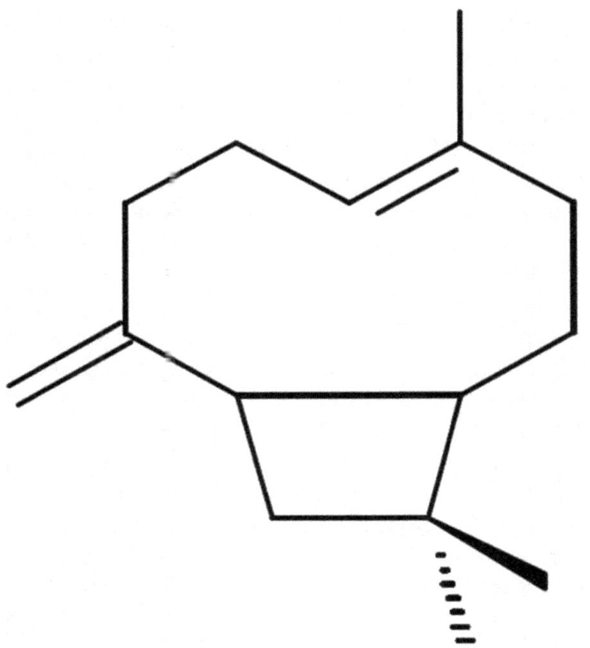

Fig. 1 Chemical structure of β-caryophyllene (4,11,11-trimethyl-8-methylene-bicyclo[7.2.0]undec-4-ene)

Several studies to identify antimicrobial activity have been conducted with plants that have high percentages of β-caryophyllene in their composition, presenting positive results for these extracts against several pathogens: *Thymus kotschyanus* [18], *Spiranthera odoratissima* [19], *Lantana* sp. [20], *Vernonia remotiflorae* V. *brasiliana* [21], *Syzygium cumini* [22], and *Lippia gracillis* [23], among others.

Considering the high prevalence of periodontal disease in dogs, the side effects caused by the drug of choice currently to combat microorganisms of dental plaque, and the described antimicrobial potential of β-caryophyllene, the aim of this work was to evaluate the antimicrobial activity of this phytochemical against dental plaque bacteria on dogs both in vitro and in vivo, and evaluate its ability to interfere in the adherence of bacterial plaque isolates.

Methods

Bacterial isolates

Thirty two bacterial isolates were used from ten different genera, which were obtained from dental plaque of mongrel dogs aged between 1 and 2 years, fed with dry feed ad libitum. The number of isolates within each genus was selected following the same percentage that they represented within the total isolates obtained from dogs in the study performed by Pieri [24]: six *Streptococcus* sp., six *Staphylococcus* sp., six *Enterococcus* sp., three *Lactobacillus* sp., three *Leuconostoc* sp. two *Actinomyces* sp., two *Bacillus* sp., two *Lactococcus* sp., one *Aerococcus* sp., and one *Haemophilus* sp.

Minimum inhibitory concentration (MIC)

The in vitro assay was performed by adaptation of the agar macrodilution technique [25], which was modified for agar microdilution performed in 96-well microtitre plates. The β-caryophyllene (≥98.5 %, Sigma-Aldrich, Saint Louis, MO, USA) was incorporated within agar brain heart infusion (BHI), in serial dilutions of logarithmic base 2, in concentrations ranging between 100 and 6.25 mg/mL. As a positive control, chlorhexidine digluconate was used at concentrations between 20 and 0.015 mg/mL, and bacterial growth control was performed with agar BHI without active principle.

The assay was prepared in triplicate for each isolate, filling corresponding wells with 150 μL of culture medium with different concentrations of β-caryophyllene, 150 μL with chlorhexidine or 150 μL of unsupplemented culture medium. Each well except the last row (non-inoculated as a control of culture medium sterility) was inoculated with 3 μL of the adjusted 3×10^7 UFC/mL and the plates were incubated for 24 h at 37 °C. After incubation, the bacterial growth was evidenced by the addition of 50 μL resazurin solution at 0.01 % as a colorimetric indicator of oxireduction to characterise cell viability. Interpretation of the results was based on the conversion of resazurin in resorufin by microbial metabolism, showing a change of the dye colour from blue to pink when microbial growth occurred. The MIC was based on the lowest concentration of β-caryophyllene and chlorhexidine in which the dye remained blue, indicating the absence of microbial growth.

Stimulation/inhibition of bacterial adherence

The quantification of inhibition or stimulation of the bacterial adherence was performed by a microtiter-plate test for quantification biofilm formation according [26], with modifications performed by [27]. Here, 24 bacterial isolates from dog dental plaque of the following genera were tested: *Actinomyces* sp. (2), *Aerococcus* sp. (1), *Bacillus* sp. (1), *Enterococcus* sp. (6), *Haemophilus* sp. (1), *Lactobacillus* sp. (1), *Lactococcus* sp. (2), *Leuconostoc* sp. (2), *Staphylococcus* sp. (3) and *Streptococcus* sp. (5). From the MIC of β-caryophyllene against each isolate, six descending serial dilutions of logarithmic base 2 were used (final concentrations). The isolates were reactivated in BHI incubated at 37 °C for 24 h and then adjusted to 0.5 McFarland scale (1.5×10^8). For this, 230 μL of each isolate culture was added to the wells of 96 well microtitre plates, and 70 μL of test solution was added to assess the final six different concentrations of each isolate, in triplicate. The positive control of bacterial adherence for each isolate consisted of the addition of 230 μL of adjusted bacterial culture and 70 μL of sterile BHI broth, and the negative control of bacterial adherence was prepared with 300 μL of sterile BHI broth. The plates were incubated at 37 °C for 24 h. After this period, the content was discarded from the plates and these were washed three times with distilled water to remove non-adhered bacteria. Then, 250 μL of methanol was added to each well, which was allowed to stand for 15 min. The methanol was discarded, and the plate was dried for 2 min in laminar flow, following staining with 250 μL of 1 % crystal violet per well for 10 min. The dye was removed from the plate with tap water and then 250 μL of 33 % glacial acetic acid was added. The optical density of each well was measured by a microplate spectrophotometer. With the aid of statistical software Prism 5 (GraphPad Software Inc., La Jolla-CA, USA) the results were analysed by one-way ANOVA comparing treatments to the positive control using the Dunnett's test.

Inhibition of dental plaque formation in dogs

Here, 18 healthy mongrel dogs, aged between 2 and 8 years old, divided randomly in males and females, were divided into three groups: negative control group (treat solution: tween 80, butylated hydroxytoluene, sodium benzoate and distilled water); positive control group (negative control solution with 0.12 % chlorhexidine gluconate – commercial concentration of this drug) and test group (negative control solution with 50 mg/mL of β-caryophyllene added). The dogs were kept during the experimental period, two by two, in masonry kennels (1.50 m × 3.00 m).

At the beginning of the experiment, all animals were subjected to a dental cleaning with dental ultrasound (Profi II AS ceramic, Dabi Atlante, Ribeirão Preto, Brazil) and curettage, for the total exclusion of dental plaque, confirmed with a disclosing solution (0,5 % basic fuchsin solution). The animals in each group were treated with the respective solution twice daily for 15 days. All were fed the same dry food and water ad libitum. At the end of the experimental period, the bacterial dental plaque formed on teeth vestibular surfaces, of canines and pre molars, were observed using 0.5 % basic fuchsin for bacterial identification. These regions were photographed, with digital camera positioned perpendicularly to the imaged surface, distant 30 cm from the animals, and the images were subjected to analysis in graphic software ImageJ 1.44p (National Institute of Health, Bethesda-MD, USA) to obtain the percentage of total tooth surface area with the presence of dental plaque. Vestibular areas of canine and all premolar teeth of each dog were considered for this analysis. Data were subjected to one-way ANOVA and the parametric Tukey test was used to compare treatment means using the Prism 5 software. For this study, $P < 0.05$ was considered significant.

Results and discussion

Minimum inhibitory concentration

The results of the MIC test for β-caryophyllene and chlorhexidine against dental plaque bacterial isolates are shown in Table 1. Overall, 75 % (24/32) of the tested isolates were sensitive to β-caryophyllene at concentrations up to 100 mg/mL. The results of the inhibition of *Streptococcus* sp. should be highlighted, as streptococci are described as the most important in the initial adhesion of dental plaque in humans [28], and all isolates were inhibited by β-caryophyllene. This fact suggests that this compound could also be a potential alternative for dental plaque inhibition in humans, after further studies using strains isolated from human samples. The MIC for 50 % (3/6) of isolates of *Streptococcus* sp. was ≤ 6.25 mg/mL, for 33.3 % (2/6) was between 6.25 and 12.5 mg/mL, and for 16.7 % (1/6) was between 25 and 50 mg/mL. The isolates showed sensitivity to the tested substance with respect to the MIC profile, as shown in Fig. 2.

Relevant findings of antimicrobial activity by β-caryophyllene was described by Huang et al. [15], who found that strains of *Arabidopsis thaliana* flowers that did not have the compound in their chemical composition showed greater growth of bacteria on their stigmas

Table 1 Minimum inhibitory concentrations of β-caryophyllene and chlorhexidine against 32 bacterial isolates obtained from dog dental plaque

Code	Bacterial genus	β-caryophyllene	Chlorhexidine
HQ717206	*Actinomyces* sp.	25 (mg/mL)	≤0.015 mg/mL
HQ717208	*Actinomyces* sp.	12.5 (mg/mL)	≤0.015 mg/mL
HQ717237	*Aerococcus* sp.	25 (mg/mL)	≤0.015 mg/mL
HQ717211	*Bacillus* sp.	50 (mg/mL)	≤0.015 mg/mL
HQ717289	*Bacillus* sp.	>100 (mg/mL)	≤0.015 mg/mL
HQ717176	*Enterococcus* sp.	50 (mg/mL)	≤0.015 mg/mL
HQ717205	*Enterococcus* sp.	50 (mg/mL)	≤0.015 mg/mL
HQ717227	*Enterococcus* sp.	50 (mg/mL)	≤0.015 mg/mL
HQ717268	*Enterococcus* sp.	12,5 (mg/mL)	≤0.015 mg/mL
HQ717302	*Enterococcus* sp.	12.5 (mg/mL)	≤0.015 mg/mL
HQ717350	*Enterococcus* sp.	25 (mg/mL)	≤0.015 mg/mL
HQ717319	*Haemophilus* sp.	100 (mg/mL)	≤0.015 mg/mL
HQ717266	*Lactobacillus* sp.	12.5 (mg/mL)	≤0.015 mg/mL
HQ717270	*Lactobacillus* sp.	50 (mg/mL)	≤0.015 mg/mL
HQ717278	*Lactobacillus* sp.	50 (mg/mL)	≤0.015 mg/mL
HQ717330	*Lactococcus* sp.	6.25 (mg/mL)	≤0.015 mg/mL
HQ717335	*Lactococcus* sp.	6.25 (mg/mL)	≤0.015 mg/mL
HQ717296	*Leuconostoc* sp.	50 (mg/mL)	≤0.015 mg/mL
HQ717308	*Leuconostoc* sp.	>100 (mg/mL)	≤0.015 mg/mL
HQ717331	*Leuconostoc* sp.	>100 (mg/mL)	≤0.015 mg/mL
HQ717182	*Staphylococcus* sp.	25 (mg/mL)	≤0.015 mg/mL
HQ717223	*Staphylococcus* sp.	>100 (mg/mL)	≤0.015 mg/mL
HQ717224	*Staphylococcus* sp.	>100 (mg/mL)	≤0.015 mg/mL
HQ717232	*Staphylococcus* sp.	>100 (mg/mL)	≤0.015 mg/mL
HQ717306	*Staphylococcus*sp.	>100 (mg/mL)	≤0.015 mg/mL
HQ717309	*Staphylococcus* sp.	>100 (mg/mL)	≤0.015 mg/mL
HQ717228	*Streptococcus* sp.	50 (mg/mL)	≤0.015 mg/mL
HQ717229	*Streptococcus* sp.	6.25 (mg/mL)	≤0.015 mg/mL
HQ717242	*Streptococcus* sp.	6.25 (mg/mL)	≤0.015 mg/mL
HQ717243	*Streptococcus* sp.	6.25 (mg/mL)	≤0.015 mg/mL
HQ717249	*Streptococcus* sp.	12.5 (mg/mL)	≤0.015 mg/mL
HQ717305	*Streptococcus* sp.	12.5 (mg/mL)	≤0.015 mg/mL

Codes presented are the respective numbers of deposit of the 16S rRNA sequences of each isolate in GenBank

compared with the wild type that showed β-caryophyllene in its composition.

In vitro studies showed natural products that are present as the major compound β-caryophyllene, with significant antimicrobial activity, suggesting that the substance possibly participated in this activity. Da Costa et al. [20] studied the antibacterial activity of extract of *Lantana camara*, composed 31.5 % byβ-caryophyllene. The results showed significant antimicrobial activity, especially against *Proteus vulgaris* (ATCC 13315) and *Escherichia coli* (ATCC 25922). Maia et al. [21] presented the antibacterial activity of the essential oils of *Vernonia remotiflora* and *V. braziliana*, both with more than 40 % β-caryophyllene, with a broad spectrum of antibacterial activity, inhibiting the growth of several tested Gram-negative and Gram-positive bacteria, including *S. aureus* and *Pseudomonas aeruginosa*.

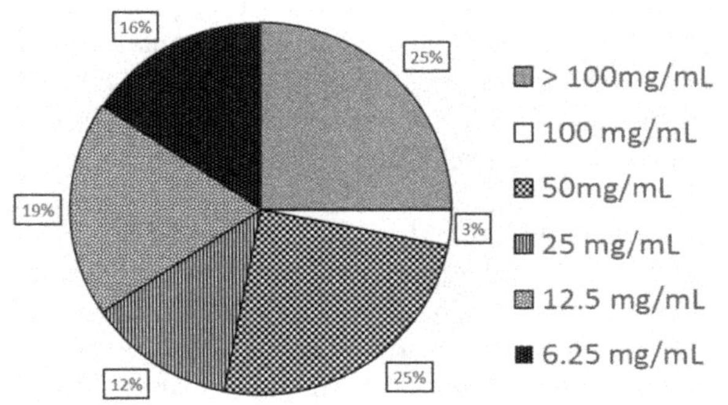

Fig. 2 Distribution of sensitivity of 32 dental plaque bacterial isolates obtained from dogs classified based on minimum inhibitory concentrations of β-caryophyllene

Ghosh et al. [29] evaluated the activity of essential oils of *Alpinia nigra* (47.7 to 49 % of β-caryophyllene) against Gram-positive and Gram-negative bacteria. The lowest MIC was found against *Yersinia enterocolitica* (1.56 μL/mL). In the present study, *Staphylococcus* isolates had relatively high MICs (one was 25 mg/mL and five were resistant up to 100 mg/mL) compared to the isolate of *S. aureus* in the study of Ghosh et al. [29], which showed MICs ranging between 3.12 and 6.25 μL/mL depending on the essential oil of *A. nigra* analysed. This difference in susceptibility of bacteria of the same genus may have occurred by synergistic action of β-caryophyllene with other substances present in the tested oil [30], or due to the intrinsic resistance of wild isolates of the present study to this phytotherapic was higher when compared to that strain tested by Ghosh et al. [29].

Souza et al. [30] investigated the antibacterial activity of β-caryophyllene against cariogenic bacteria in humans, *Streptococcus mutans*, *S. mitis*, *S. sobrinus*, *S. sanguinis*, and *Lactobacillus casei*, and showed MICs of 200, 150, 180, 200 and 150 μg/mL, respectively. These concentrations were lower than those found in the present study, indicating a higher susceptibility of bacteria in human dental plaque than those isolated from dogs, making it an even more promising compound for use in dental therapy in humans.

Corroborating this promising employment in human dental therapy, Mussi [31] conducted tests of MIC with one oil from *Copaifera officinalis* (with 50.78 % β-caryophyllene) against bacteria that cause severe periodontal disease in humans: *Fusobacterium nucleatum* and *Porphyromonas gingivalis*. The solution of copaiba was active against *F. nucleatum* from the concentration

100 μL/mL, while the MIC against *P. gingivalis* was 2 μL/mL. However, for *P. gingivalis* the nature of the antimicrobial activity was bacteriostatic at all concentrations tested, while for *F. nucleatum* the MIC was also the minimum bactericidal concentration (MBC).

Stimulation/inhibition of bacterial adherence

Table 2 lists the isolates that showed some inhibition or stimulation in its adherence capability by some sub-inhibitory concentration of β-caryophyllene, with statistical significance ($P < 0.05$) when compared with the control. Within the 24 isolates tested, eight (33.33 %) showed an altered ability to form biofilms enough to be detected by statistical analysis. An isolate of *Lactococcus* sp. suffered inhibition of its adherence by concentrations of 1.56 mg/mL % and 3.12 mg/mL ($P < 0.05$), while concerning the challenge with 0.19 mg/mL of β-caryophyllene, the activity was the stimulus to the adherence of the same isolate ($P < 0.05$). One *Streptococcus* sp. and one *Bacillus* sp. presented similar results, being inhibited to adhere by some concentrations and stimulated by other one (Table 2).

It can be seen in Table 2 that the eight isolates that showed statistical differences in the adherence to microtitre plate orifices were from six different genera, *Streptococcus* sp. (1/5), *Haemophilus* sp. (1/1), *Aerococcus* sp. (1/1), *Lactococcus* sp. (1/2), *Bacillus* sp. (1/1) and *Enterococcus* sp. (3/6). As more than one isolate of each genus were tested for *Streptococcus*, *Enterococcus* and *Lactococcus*, it can be stated, at least to these genera, that the susceptibility to

Table 2 Stimulation/Inhibition of bacterial adherence in microtiter plates by subinhibitory concentrations of β-caryophyllene

Code	Bacterial genus	Subinhibitory concentration (mg/mL)	Action on bacterial adherence	Control OD mean (SE)	Treated OD mean (SE)
HQ717249	*Streptococcus* sp.	6.25	Inhibition	0.306 (0.018)	0.093 (0.011)
		3.12	Inhibition	0.306 (0.018)	0.106 (0.009)
		1.56	Inhibition	0.306 (0.018)	0.117 (0.013)
		0.78	Stimulus	0.306 (0.018)	0.578 (0.021)
HQ717319	*Haemophilus* sp.	50.00	Inhibition	0.125 (0.001)	0.076 (0.001)
		25.00	Inhibition	0.125 (0.001)	0.071 (0.001)
		12.50	Inhibition	0.125 (0.001)	0.087 (0.004)
		6.25	Inhibition	0.125 (0.001)	0.089 (0.003)
HQ717330	*Lactococcus* sp.	3.12	Inhibition	1.072 (0.050)	0.203 (0.065)
		1.56	Inhibition	1.072 (0.050)	0.458 (0.080)
		0.19	Stimulus	1.072 (0.050)	1.590 (0.157)
HQ717350	*Enterococcus sp.*	12.50	Inhibition	0.209 (0.005)	0.076 (0.001)
HQ717176	*Enterococcus sp.*	25.00	Inhibition	0.114 (0.003)	0.075 (0.001)
		12.50	Inhibition	0.114 (0.003)	0.073 (0.005)
		6.25	Inhibition	0.114 (0.003)	0.065 (0.001)
		1.56	Inhibition	0.114 (0.003)	0.073 (0.003)
HQ717227	*Enterococcus* sp.	25.00	Inhibition	0.676 (0.061)	0.094 (0.017)
		12.50	Inhibition	0.676 (0.061)	0.075 (0.007)
		6.25	Inhibition	0.676 (0.061)	0.068 (0,001)
		3.12	Inhibition	0.676 (0.061)	0.083 (0.005)
		1.56	Inhibition	0.676 (0.061)	0.122 (0.017)
HQ717211	*Bacillus* sp.	25.00	Inhibition	0.398 (0.008)	0.088 (0.013)
		12.50	Inhibition	0.398 (0.008)	0.077 (0.009)
		6.25	Inhibition	0.398 (0.008)	0.112 (0.031)
		3.12	Inhibition	0.398 (0.008)	0.168 (0.019)
		1.56	Stimulus	0.398 (0.008)	0.517 (0.055)
HQ717237	*Aerococcus* sp.	12.50	Inhibition	0.119 (0.005)	0.082 (0.002)
		1.56	Inhibition	0.119 (0.005)	0.071 (0.001)

Codes presented are the respective numbers of deposit of the 16S rRNA sequences of each isolate in GenBank. Means (±SE) of optical density are related to measurement under 550 nm absorbance (OD_{550}). All of the presented results showed a significant difference between the test treatment and the control of isolates natural adherence without any treatment ($P < 0.05$)

changes in adherence capability is characterised in strain level. This fact was presented before [6], with different *E. coli* strains presenting different interference levels in biofilm formation when challenged by enrofloxacin.

Pieri et al. [3] studied the effects of *Copaifera officinalis* oil, which is described in the work of Mussi [31] as containing more than 50 % β-caryophyllene, on the adhesion of the bacteria *Streptococcus mutans*, the main involved in the initial formation of dental plaque in humans. Analysis of the inhibition of adherence assays showed superiority of the test group compared with the negative control and positive control with chlorhexidine. In the present study, an isolate of the same genus had its adhesiveness inhibited by sub-inhibitory concentrations of β-caryophyllene between 1.56 and 6.25 mg/mL and stimulated to adhere at 0.78 mg/mL. However, other isolates of *Streptococcus* sp. were also tested, but presented no significant change in their ability to adhere, which supports the individuality of each strain with respect to variation in adherence capability by the tested compound.

Mussi [31] conducted tests to evaluate the co-aggregation and self-aggregation (processes related to microbial adherence in dental plaque of the advanced periodontal disease) by the periodontal pathogens *Fusobacterium nucleatum* and *Porphyromonas gingivalis* challenged with sub-inhibitory concentrations of *Copaifera officinalis* oil, composed of 50.78 % of β-caryophyllene. When *F. nucleatum* was treated, a reduction in the self-aggregation process was observed when compared to untreated cells. *P. gingivalis* was not able to self-aggregate under the tested conditions. The solution of *C. officinalis* tested also inhibited co-aggregation between these two bacterial species, which is an important event in the progression of periodontal disease in humans, again demonstrating the great employment potential of β-caryophyllene in human dentistry.

It's significant to highlight that in the present work we used aerobes as target strains. This kind of bacteria are not involved in the etiology of periodontal disease, but are critical to early stages in development of dental biofilm, creating from its installation, a favorable environment for the development of anaerobes, which actively participate in the development of the disease [32]. Thus the results of this study point to a relevant activity of β-caryophyllene on aerobes, presenting relevant potential in use to combat dental plaque formation in its early stages. The use in combating plaque formation could promote a prevention of the disease through a reduction of the environmental conditions that promote the development of periodontal pathogens in the biofilm. However, further studies should be conducted evaluating the direct antimicrobial effect on the anaerobic periodontal pathogens, which may point beyond the preventive potential, the possibility of use β-caryophyllene in the treatment of disease.

Inhibition of dental plaque formation in dogs

The results obtained in the in vivo assay are shown in Fig. 3. The results indicated the coverage area of teeth with plaque (mean ± SE) to be 23.3 ± 2.6 % for β-caryophyllene test solution, 37.5 ± 3.7 % for the positive control solution and 65.56 ± 2.5 % coverage for the negative control solution. The test and positive control groups were statistically lower on average than the negative control ($P < 0.001$) dental plaque presence and were different ($P < 0.05$) with regard to inhibiting dental plaque formation, with better results for β-caryophyllene. These results indicate that β-caryophyllene is a potential natural alternative to the use of chlorhexidine in reducing dental plaque in dogs, resulting in a patent application of pharmaceutical formulations containing β-caryophyllene for use in the treatment and prophylaxis of canine periodontal disease [33].

A similar assay was performed by Pieri et al. [3] using one *Copaifera officinalis* oil with good results in the inhibition of dental plaque formation when compared to negative control. In their work, chlorhexidine reduced the formation of dental plaque to a final coverage of 28.5 % of the analysed area of teeth, while in the present work, the group treated with the same substance presented 37.5 % plaque coverage. This difference could be happen due to different susceptibility to chlorhexidine of the dogs' dental microbiota in the different works, or the different treatment periods, which was 8 days in the previous work and 15 days in the current study. However, it is interesting to highlight that the level of final plaque coverage of groups treated with *C. officinalis* [3] and β-caryophyllene (present work) were very close. As this oil is frequently associated with high concentrations of β-

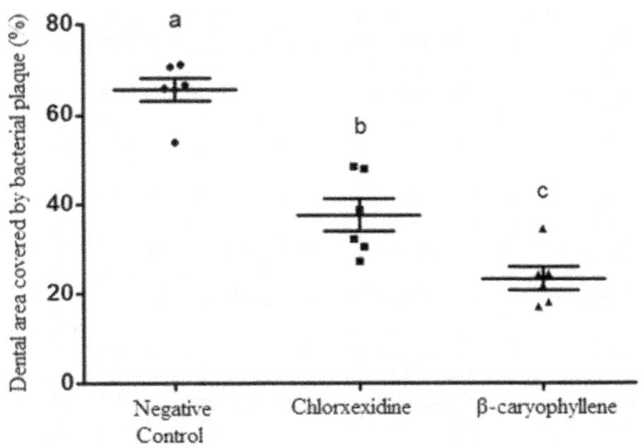

Fig. 3 Dental plaque coverage on teeth surfaces in eighteen dogs (six per group), after 15 days of treatment with different solutions. Results are expressed by percentage of total area of vestibular surface of canines and premolars teeth that was covered by plaque. Results were submitted to ANOVA and means were compared by tukey test. Different letters (**a**, **b** and **c**) indicate statistical significant difference ($P < 0.05$). central bars: mean; marginal bars: standard error

caryophyllene, the activity of *C. officinalis* oil used in that work against dogs' dental plaque [3] could be due to the presence of this compound.

Conclusions

With the data obtained it can be concluded that β-caryophyllene has antimicrobial activity against dental plaque bacteria of dogs, and this activity is reflected in the reduction of this on the teeth surfaces of dogs. Therefore, after other clinical trials with a larger number of dogs and different breeds, β-caryophyllene could be indicated as an alternative to the use of chlorhexidine in the treatment and prophylaxis of periodontal disease in these animals.

Abbreviations

ANOVA: Analysis of variance; ATCC: American type culture collection; BHI: Brain heart infusion; CEUA: Ethics Committee on Animal Use; COBEA: Brazilian College for Animal Experimentation; MBC: Minimum bactericidal concentration; MIC: Minimum inhibitory concentration; SE: Standard error

Acknowledgements

The authors thank the Fundação de Amparo à Pesquisa do Estado de Minas Gerais (FAPEMIG), Coordenação de Aperfeiçoamento de Pessoal de Nível Superior (CAPES) and Conselho Nacional de Desenvolvimento Científico e Tecnológico (CNPq) for financial support. Our acknowledgements also go to the Veterinarians Camila Corsini, Elisa Bourguignon, Letícia Correa, Lívia Alvarenga, Clara Ochoa and Raul Dornas for conducting the initial dental cleaning in vivo and Natalia Fernandes and Gustavo Pereira for the care of the animals during the experimental period.

Authors' contribution

FAP contributed to conception and design of the study, acquisition, analysis and interpretation of data. MCCS contributed to acquisition, analysis and interpretation of data. LLRV, MLRV and PGP contributed to acquisition of data. FSV, APBB and VFVJ contributed to analysis and interpretation of data. MASM contributed to conception and design of the study, analysis and interpretation of data. All authors revised the manuscript critically for important intellectual content, have given final approval of the version to be submitted and are accountable for all aspects of the work in ensuring that questions related to the accuracy or integrity of any part of the work are appropriately investigated and resolved.

Authors' information

FAP is graduated in Veterinary Medicine and PhD in Veterinary Medicine from the Universidade Federal de Viçosa (UFV), Brazil, working with phytopharmacology applied to Veterinary Dentistry Microbiology. Is currently professor of Microbiology to the graduation courses of Dentistry, Pharmacy and Medicine at Universidade Federal de Juiz de Fora (UFJF), Brazil. MCCS, LLRV and MLRV are graduated in Veterinary Medicine from UFV; PGP is graduated in Veterinary Medicine from Universidade Federal do Espírito Santo (UFES), Brazil. FSV is graduated in Pharmacy and PhD in Biotechnology from the Universidade Federal do Amazonas (UFAM); APBB is Graduated in Veterinary Medicine from UFV and PhD in animal science from Universidade Federal de Minas Gerais (UFMG). She is currently professor of animal surgery in veterinary college at UFV. VFVJ is graduated in chemistry and PhD in the same area from Universidade Federal do Rio de Janeiro (UFRJ). He currently is professor in Chemistry college at UFAM, working with organic chemistry and natural products. MASM is graduated in veterinary medicine from UFV and PhD in Agricultural Microbiology from UFV. He is currently professor of veterinary microbiology and bacterial diseases of veterinary college at UFV.

Competing interests

The authors declare that they have no competing interests.

Author details

Departamento de Ciências Básicas da Vida, Universidade Federal de Juiz de Fora, Rua Israel Pinheiro, 2000, Bairro Universitário, CEP: 35020-220 Governador Valadares, Minas Gerais, Brasil. [2]Departamento de Veterinária, Universidade Federal de Viçosa, Av. P.H. Rolfs, s/n, Câmpus UFV, CEP: 36570-000 Viçosa, Minas Gerais, Brasil. [3]Instituto de Ciências Exatas, Universidade Federal do Amazonas, Av. Rodrigo Otávio, 6200, Coroado, CEP: 69.080-005 Manaus, Amazonas, Brasil.

References

1. Kyllar M, Witter K. Prevalence of dental disorders in pet dogs. Vet Med. 2005; 50(11):496–505.
2. Niemiec BA. Periodontal disease. Top Companion Anim Med. 2008;23(2):72–80.
3. Pieri FA, Mussi MC, Fiorini JE, Schneedorf JM. Clinical and microbiological effects of copaiba oil (Copaifera officinalis) on dental plaque forming bacteria in dogs]. Arquivo Brasileiro de Medicina Veterinaria e Zootecnia. 2010;62(3):578–85.
4. Hoffman LR, D'Argenio DA, MacCoss MJ, Zhang Z, Jones RA, Miller SI. Aminoglycoside antibiotics induce bacterial biofilm formation. Nature. 2005; 436(7054):1171–5.
5. Melchior MB, Vaarkamp H, Fink-Gremmels J. Biofilms: a role in recurrent mastitis infections? Vet J. 2006;171(3):398–407.
6. Costa JCM, Espeschit IDF, Pieri FA, Benjamin LDA, Moreira MAS. Increased production of biofilms by Escherichia coli in the presence of enrofloxacin. Vet Microbiol. 2012;160(3–4):488–90.
7. Hennet P. Effectiveness of a dental gel to reduce plaque in beagle dogs. J Vet Dent. 2002;19(1):11–4.
8. Dantas E, Xavier C, Segundo G, Paiva M, Lima K. Dental staining by chlorhexidine: case report. Odontologia Clin Cientif. 2007;6:175–8.
9. Pieri FA, Silva VO, Vargas FS, Veiga Junior VF, Moreira MAS. Antimicrobial activity of Copaifera langsdorffii oil and evaluation of its most bioactive fraction against bacteria of dog's dental plaque. Pakistan Vet J. 2014;34(2):165–9.
10. CAS. Chemical Book. Columbus: Chemical Abstract Service; 2010.
11. Ghelardini C, Galeotti N, Di Cesare ML, Mazzant G, Bartolini A. Local anaesthetic activity of β-caryophyllene. Farmaco. 2001;56(5–7):387–9.
12. Abbas MA, Taha MO, Zihlif MA, Disi AM. β-Caryophyllene causes regression of endometrial implants in a rat model of endometriosis without affecting fertility. Eur J Pharmacol. 2013;702(1–3):12–9.
13. Cho JY, Chang HJ, Lee SK, Kim HJ, Hwang JK, Chun HS. Amelioration of dextran sulfate sodium-induced colitis in mice by oral administration of β-caryophyllene, a sesquiterpene. Life Sci. 2007;80(10):932–9.
14. Leonhardt V, Leal-Cardoso JH, Lahlou S, Albuquerque AAC, Porto RS, Celedônio NR, et al. Antispasmodic effects of essential oil of Pterodon polygalaeflorus and its main constituent β-caryophyllene on rat isolated ileum. Fundam Clin Pharmacol. 2010;24(6):749–58.
15. Huang M, Sanchez-Moreiras AM, Abel C, Sohrab R, Lee S, Gershenzon J, et al. The major volatile organic compound emitted from Arabidopsis thaliana flowers, the sesquiterpene (E)-β-caryophyllene, is a defense against a bacterial pathogen. New Phytologist. 2012;193(4):997–1008.
16. Galdino PM, Nascimento MVM, Florentino IF, Lino RC, Fajemiroye JO, Chaibub BA, et al. The anxiolytic-like effect of an essential oil derived from Spiranthera odoratissima A. St. Hil. leaves and its major component, β-caryophyllene, in male mice. Prog Neuropsychopharmacol Biol Psychiatry. 2012;38(2):276–84.
17. Chang HJ, Kim JM, Lee JC, Kim WK, Chun HS. Protective effect of β-caryophyllene, a natural bicyclic sesquiterpene, against cerebral ischemic injury. J Med Food. 2013;16(6):471–80.
18. Rasooli I, Mirmostafa SA. Bacterial susceptibility to and chemical composition of essential oils from Thymus kotschyanus and Thymus persicus. J Agric Food Chem. 2003;51(8):2200–5. doi:10.1021/jf0261755.
19. Chaibub BA, Oliveira TB, Fiuza TS, Bara MTF, Tresvenzol LMF, Paula JR. Chemical composition of the essential oil and evaluation of the antimicrobial activity of essential oil, crude ethanol extract and fractions of

Spiranthera odoratissima A. St.-Hil. Leaves. Revista Brasileira de Plantas Medicinais. 2013;15(2):2[illegible]5–9.

20. Da Costa JGM, De Sousa EO, Rodrigues FFG, De Lima SG, Braz-Filho R. Chemical composition, evaluation of antibacterial activity and toxicity of the essential oils from Lantana camara L. and Lantana sp. Braz J Pharmacog. 2009;19(3):710–4.
21. Maia AIV, Torres MCM, Pessoa ODL, De Menezes JESA, Costa SMO, Nogueira VLR, et al. Volatile leaf oils of Vernonia Brasiliana and Vernonia remotiflora: chemical composition and biological activity. Quimica Nova. 2010;33(3):584–6.
22. Machado RRP, Jardim DF, Souza AR, Scio E, Fabri RL, Carpanez AG, et al. The effect of essential oil of Syzygium cumini on the development of granulomatous inflammation in mice. Braz J Pharmacog. 2013;23(3):488–96.
23. Bitu V, Botelho MA, da Costa JGM, Rodrigues FFG, Veras HNH, Martins KT, et al. Phythochemical screening and antimicrobial activity phytochemical of essential oil of Lippia gracillis. Revista Brasileira de Farmacognosia. 2012; 22(1):69–75. doi:10.1590/S0102-695X2011005000173.
24. Pieri FA. Atividade antimicrobiana do óleo de copaíba (Copaifera langsdorffii) e seus constituintes, e avaliação do bioproduto obtido na inibição de bactérias da placa dental de cães. Viçosa-MG: Universidade Federal de Viçosa; 201[illegible].
25. CLSI. Methods for Dilution Antimicrobial Susceptibility Tests for Bacteria That Grow Aerobically; Approved Standard. 9th edition. CLSI document M07-A9. 9th ed. Waine: Clinical and Laboratory Standards Institute; 2012.
26. Stepanović S, Vuković D, Dakić I, Savić B, Švabić-Vlahović M. A modified microtiter-plate test for quantification of staphylococcal biofilm formation. J Microbiol Methods. 2000;40(2):175–9.
27. Costa JCM, Espeschit I[illegible], Pieri FA, Carvalho IA, Moreira MAS. Sensitivity profile of planktonic and sessile cells of escherichia coli to antimicrobial used in the treatment of bovine mastitis. Arquivo Brasileiro de Medicina Veterinaria e Zootecnia. 2014;66(1):129–36.
28. Katsura H, Tsukiyama [illegible], Suzuki A, Kobayashi M. In vitro antimicrobial activities of bakuchiol against oral microorganisms. Antimicrob Agents Chemother. 2001;45(1[illegible]):3009–13.
29. Ghosh S, Ozek T, Tabanca N, Ali A, ur Rehman J, Khan IA, et al. Chemical composition and bioactivity studies of Alpinia nigra essential oils. Ind Crops Prod. 2014;53:111–9.
30. Souza AB, Martins CHG, Souza MGM, Furtado NAJC, Heleno VCG, De Sousa JPB, et al. Antimicrobial activity of terpenoids from Copaifera langsdorffii Desf. against cariogenic bacteria. Phytother Res. 2011;25(2):215–20.
31. Mussi MCM. Análise da atividade antimicrobiana dos óleos de copaíba (Copaifera officinalis) e de melaleuca (Melaleuca alternifólia) sobre Fusobacterium nucleatum e Porphyromonas gingivalis: determinação das concentrações inibitórias e bactericidas mínimas e efeito de concentrações subinibitórias sobre a agregação. Bauru-SP: Universidade de São Paulo; 2011.
32. Davis IJ, Wallis C, Deusch O, Colyer A, Millella L, Loman N, et al. A cross-sectional survey of bacterial species in plaque from client owned dogs with healthy gingiva, gingivitis or mild periodontitis. PLoS One. 2013;8(12), e83158.
33. Moreira MAS, Pieri FA, Silva VO, Veiga Junior VF, Vargas FS, Inventors. Formulação farmacêutica contendo beta-cariofileno e uso no tratamento e profilaxia da doença periodontal canina. Rio de Janeiro: Instituto Nacional da Propriedade Intelectual; 2013.

17

Systematic review of antiepileptic drugs safety and effectiveness in feline epilepsy

Marios Charalambous[1*], Akos Pakozdy[2], Sofie F. M. Bhatti[1] and Holger A. Volk[3]

Abstract

Background: Understanding the efficacy and safety profile of antiepileptic drugs (AEDs) in feline epilepsy is a crucial consideration for managing this important brain disease. However, there is a lack of information about the treatment of feline epilepsy and therefore a systematic review was constructed to assess current evidence for the AEDs' efficacy and tolerability in cats. The methods and materials of our former systematic reviews in canine epilepsy were mostly mirrored for the current systematic review in cats. Databases of PubMed, CAB Direct and Google scholar were searched to detect peer-reviewed studies reporting efficacy and/or adverse effects of AEDs in cats. The studies were assessed with regards to their quality of evidence, i.e. study design, study population, diagnostic criteria and overall risk of bias and the outcome measures reported, i.e. prevalence and 95% confidence interval of the successful and affected population in each study and in total.

Results: Forty studies describing clinical outcomes of AEDs' efficacy and safety were included. Only two studies were classified as "blinded randomised controlled trials". The majority of the studies offered high overall risk of bias and described low feline populations with unclear diagnostic criteria and short treatment or follow-up periods. Individual AED assessments of efficacy and safety profile showed that phenobarbital might currently be considered as the first choice AED followed by levetiracetam and imepitoin. Only imepitoin's safety profile was supported by strong level of evidence. Imepitoin's efficacy as well as remaining AEDs' efficacy and safety profile were supported by weak level of evidence.

Conclusions: This systematic review reflects an evidence-based assessment of the published data on the AEDs' efficacy and safety for feline epilepsy. Currently, phenobarbital is likely to be the first-line for feline epileptic patients followed by levetiracetam and imepitoin. It is essential that clinicians evaluate both AEDs' effectiveness and tolerability before tailoring AED to the individual patient. Further studies in feline epilepsy treatment are by far crucial in order to establish definite guidelines for AEDs' efficacy and safety.

Keywords: comprehensive review, epilepsy, feline, antiepileptic drugs, efficacy, adverse effects

Background

There is a paucity of literature about feline epilepsy compared to canine epilepsy, however epileptic seizures are a common neurological manifestation in cats with an estimated prevalence in a referral hospital population of 0.5-3.5% [1, 2]. Idiopathic epilepsy (IE) has not been studied in cats as thoroughly as in dogs but between 21-59% of cats presenting with recurrent seizures can be diagnosed with IE [3–5].

Treatment between canine and feline epileptic patients is rather different mainly due to the divergent safety profile between the two species [6, 7] but it is acceptable that in both species the effectiveness of an AED may outweigh its adverse effects, and therefore both the efficacy and safety profile should be considered before choosing the most appropriate AED(s) for patients [8].

Systematic reviews are powerful and objective tools to evaluate AEDs' efficacy as well as severity and incidence of AEDs' safety profile described in literature [9–12]. Guidelines with regards to AEDs' efficacy and safety have been established in canine epilepsy [13, 14] based on previous systematic reviews and meta-analysis [8, 15]. However, such guidelines lack in feline epilepsy. The

* Correspondence: marios.charalambous@ugent.be
[1]Small Animal Department, Faculty of Veterinary Medicine, Ghent University, Merelbeke, Belgium
Full list of author information is available at the end of the article

goal of this systematic review was to summarize and assess the results of the current studies regarding AEDs' efficacy and safety in cats and provide evidence on the treatment of feline epilepsy.

Methods

The methodology followed in this study was based on previous similar studies published by the authors [8, 15].

Search strategy

Studies evaluating or describing the effectiveness and safety of an AED in cats were searched. As it was described in our previous systematic reviews [8, 15], studies were assessed based on four inclusion criteria adapted for feline patients, i.e. type of study (any peer-reviewed study), case definition (cats that were investigated and diagnosed with confirmed or presumed idiopathic epilepsy), treatment (cats treated with antiepileptic drugs only) and outcome (description of efficacy or safety outcomes after treatment). Final electronic searches were carried out on 21 June 2017 with no date or language restrictions and the same databases were searched with the same search strategies as it was described before [8, 15], i.e. Pub Med, CAB Abstracts, Google Scholar and searching of articles, proceedings and textbooks to identify reference lists of published papers and proceedings of relevant scientific conferences such as the annual American College of Veterinary Internal Medicine forum and the European College of Veterinary Neurology Symposium. The search terms used for the electronic databases were also the same as in our two previous systematic reviews on canine [8, 15] but adapted for feline subjects, i.e. the terms 'dog' and 'canine' were replaced by the terms 'cat' and 'feline', respectively.

Study Selection

The same two-stage screening process that was recruited in our previous systematic reviews [8, 15] was used; in summary, at stage 1, papers' titles and abstracts were only evaluated and at stage 2, full-length papers were evaluated based on the inclusion criteria 2, 3 and 4 to exclude the ones irrelevant to our outcomes.

Assessment of quality of evidence

As in our previous systematic reviews [8, 15], studies were categorised based on their study design, i.e. "blinded randomised clinical trials" (bRCTs), "blinded randomised experimental laboratory animal studies" (bRELAS), "non-blinded RCTs" (nbRCTs), "non-blinded randomised ELAS" (nbRELAS), "non-randomised clinical trials" (NRCTs), "non-randomised ELAS" (NRELAS), "uncontrolled clinical trials" (UCTs), "uncontrolled ELAS" (UELAS), "case series and case reports [16, 17]". In addition, the same three-part system of evidence quality evaluation to characterize weaknesses and strengths of each study within each group was used as it was described in our previous systematic reviews [8, 15], i.e. "(a) study group sizes, (b) subject enrolment quality and (c) overall risk of bias based on Cochrane [18] and Syrcle's [19] 'risk of bias' assessment tool in order to provide an indicator of confidence associated with the findings of each study". All in all, bRCTs or bRELAS with large population, clear and thorough diagnostic criteria and low overall risk of bias were considered as studies with the highest quality of evidence. Lastly, the treatment or follow-up period was reported for each study and was considered short or long if it was less or more than 6 months, respectively.

Study group sizes

The same system that was reported in our previous systematic reviews [8, 15] was used to evaluate the population size in each study, i.e. "(a) >50 subjects per group ('good' number), (b) 20–50 subjects ('moderate' number), (c) 10–19 subjects ('small' number) and (d) <10 subjects ('very small' number)".

Assessment of subject enrolment quality

Information with regards to the investigations used for the diagnosis of IE were reviewed to assess the quality of subject definition in each study as 'well characterized', 'fairly characterized', 'poorly characterized' or 'unclear.' As far as the ELAS are concerned, that included investigations for describing non-epileptic healthy animals, two categories were described, i.e. 'clearly characterized' and 'unclear'. The systems used were adapted for feline patients from our previous systematic reviews [8, 15]. The main difference is that for the "well characterized" category, tests for infectious diseases (including feline leukemia virus, feline immunodeficiency virus, feline infectious peritonitis, toxoplasmosis) were also included but these were desirable but not mandatory.

Assessment of overall risk of bias and level of the studies' evidence

The same methodology followed in our previous systematic review was used [8], i.e. "the studies were assessed based on the 'risk of bias' components and were categorised as presenting 'high', 'low' or 'unclear' risk for each component. The components were the random sequence generation, allocation concealment, blinding of participants, personnel and outcome assessment, completeness of outcome data, selective reporting of outcomes, random housing and baseline characteristics of cats (only for ELAS) and other sources of bias".

Assessment of outcome measures

The outcome measure was the assessment of the effectiveness and tolerability of AED(s) administered in cats.

AEDs' effectiveness

The assessment of the effectiveness was performed based on our previous canine systematic review [15]. In addition, the 95% confidence interval (CI) of the successful population in each study was also calculated and assessed as previously [15]; in summary, in each study, the cats with ≥50% reduction in seizure frequency were considered as successful cases and if the 95% CI of successfully treated cases was within ranges greater than 50%, then it was assumed that the majority of the study population was successfully treated.

AEDs' safety

The adverse effects were categorised by organ system, i.e. neurological, gastro-intestinal, etc. and types, i.e. type I (dose-dependent) and type II (idiosyncratic or dose-independent). The assessment of the safety was performed based on our previous systematic review [8]; in summary, the prevalence of the affected population in each study (i.e. number of cats that experienced adverse effects divided by the total size of the study population) and proportion of specific adverse effects for each individual AED (i.e. number of studies that reported a specific adverse effect divided by the total number of the studies for this AED) were evaluated. A further outcome measure was also added which was the proportion of specific adverse effects for each AED based on the total affected population (i.e. number of subjects that developed a specific adverse effect divided by the total population size from all the studies). In addition, the 95% CI of the affected population in each study was also calculated and assessed as previously [8]. If the 95% CI of the affected cases was within ranges greater than 50%, then it was considered that the majority of the study population showed adverse effects.

Results

Description of studies

By 21 June 2017, a total number of 684 unique citations were found; 676 articles and eight major conference abstracts from manual and electronic searches. One hundred seventy six items fulfilled stage 1 screening criteria, of which, 40 final studies (published between 1973 and 2017) also fulfilled stage 2 selection criteria and were therefore chosen for thorough evaluation. The process is also shown via a flow diagram (Additional file 1). One study included three different trials [20] and another study included both a trial and a retrospective part [21]. The included studies represented 2/40 (5%) bRELAS, 1/40 (2.5%) nbRCT, 2/40 (5%) nbRELAS, 5/40 (12.5%) UCTs, 11/40 (27.5%) UELAS, 12/40 (30%) retrospective case series and 7/40 (17.5%) case reports (Table 1). Overall, the 40 selected studies described 10 different AEDs. AEDs were usually given orally in all but three studies, where medication was given intraperitoneally or via transdermal application.

Signalment and baseline characteristics of study subjects

Baseline characteristics, i.e. breed, age and sex, of feline population were reported to some degree in all the studies. Signalment was reported in all the clinical studies, with various breeds, both sexes and a wide range of ages at study entry (range 0.25-19 years) being reported. The most common reported breed was domestic shorthaired cats followed by Birmans, domestic longhaired cats, Siamese, Burmese, Bengals, Himalayan and Maine Coon. Males were more commonly affected compared to females, though these results were not statistically examined in order to specifically report the prevalence of IE on the grounds of sex.

Disease characterization and subject enrolment quality

In approximately half of the studies (19/40, 48%), the inclusion criteria for diagnosing IE (clinical studies) or healthy cats (ELAS) were not well described (Table 1). Three case reports, each one described an otherwise healthy cat that was suspected with structural epilepsy due to an anesthesia-related hypoxic event [22] or post-tramatic/vascular event [23, 24]. However, these studies were included in our review for evaluating the AED safety profile, as their aim was to describe an AED-related adverse effect that was unrelated to the cause of the epilepsy.

Study group sizes

Many studies (36/40, 90%) assessed small or very small study size groups (Table 1).

Methodological quality of included studies

Many studies (96%) showed high or unclear risk of bias (Table 1).

AEDs efficacy and safety profile

As in our previous systematic reviews [8, 15], details of studies' data, characteristics and outcomes are summarized in the manuscript with further details captured in Additional file 2: Table S1, Tables 2, 3 and 4 and Figs. 1, 2, 3 and 4.

Phenobarbital

Eight studies [4, 25–31] assessed the efficacy of phenobarbital as a monotherapy agent or in combination with other AEDs (two studies), providing a total size of 137 cats. Based on the 95% CI, in all the studies but three

Table 1 Details of study design, risk of bias, disease characterization and study group size

	Study design	Risk of bias						Disease definitions (characterization)	Study groups size
		Blinding of outcome assessment	Randomization	allocation concealment	Incomplete outcome data	Selective reporting	other sources of bias		
Engel et al. [20] study 1	bRELAS	low	low	high	low	high	high; company funding	well	very small
Engel et al. [20] study 2		low	low	high	low	high	high; company funding	well	very small
Lowrie et al. [26]	nbRCT	high	low	high	high	low	unclear	poorly	good
Sawchuk et al. [47]	nbRELAS	high	low	low	low	high	unclear	clear	small
Carnes et al. [42]		high	low	high	low	high	unclear	clear	small
Engel et al. [20] study 3	UCT	high	high	high	low	high	high; company funding	well	very small
Dewey et al. [41]		high	high	high	low	high	high; conference abstract	unclear	very small
Ukai et al. [51]		high	high	high	high	high	unclear	well	very small
Volk et al. [36]		high	high	high	low	low	high; conference abstract	well	very small
Bailey et al. [40]		high	high	high	high	high	unclear	fairly	small
Roye et al. [48]	UELAS	high	high	high	low	high	unclear	unclear	very small
Barnard et al. [43]		high	high	high	low	high	unclear; conference abstract	clear	very small
Solomon et al. [34]		high	high	high	low	high	unclear	unclear	very small
Hasegawa et al. [50]		high	high	high	low	high	unclear	unclear	very small
Pellegrini et al. [53]		high	high	high	low	high	unclear	unclear	very small
Cochrane, Black et al. [32]		high	high	high	low	high	unclear	clear	very small
Cochrane, Parent et al. [33]		high	high	high	low	high	unclear	clear	very small
Boothe et al. [21]		high	high	high	low	high	low	clear	very small
Cautela et al. [52]		high	high	high	low	high	high; conference abstract	clear	very small
Gasper et al. [35]		high	high	high	high	high	unclear	clear	small
Dreimann [55]		high	high	high	low	high	High; abstract; dissertation	unclear	small
Schwartz-Porsche and Kaiser [44]	retrospective case series	NA						unclear	moderate
Brewer et al. [49]								unclear	very small
Center et al. [45]								unclear	small
Hughes et al. [46]								clear	very small

Table 1 Details of study design, risk of bias, disease characterization and study group size *(Continued)*

	Study design	Risk of bias						Disease definitions (characterization)	Study groups size
		Blinding of outcome assessment	Randomization	allocation concealment	Incomplete outcome data	Selective reporting	other sources of bias		
Wagner [38]								unclear	moderate
Boothe et al. [21]								unclear	small
Volk et al. [28]								well	small
Schriefl et al. [4]								fairly	small
Bertolani et al. [37]								unclear	very small
Pakozdy et al. [27]								fairly	moderate
Finnerty et al. [25]								well	small
Wahle et al. [31]								well	small
Ducote et al. [23]	Case reports	NA						NA	very small
Zoran et al. [54]								clear	very small
Lieser and Schwedes 2016								NA	very small
Boydell [29]								well	very small
Baho et al. [22]								NA	very small
Klang et al. [39]								well	very small
Cuff et al. [30]								well	very small

Sample size; >50 subjects per group ('good' number), 20–50 subjects ('moderate' number), 10–19 subjects ('small' number) and (d) <10 subjects ('very small' number)

Table 2 Details of feline population size, seizure frequency, treatment time, doses of AED(s), seizure frequency reduction after AED initiation, 95% CI for the successful and affected cases and evidence statements for each study

References	Wagner [38]	Volk et al. [36]	Boothe et al. [21]	Boothe et al. [21] (retrospective part)	Bertolani et al. [37]	Volk et al. [28]	Klang et sl. [39]	Carnes et al. [42]	Bailey et al. [40]	Lowrie et al. [26]	Dewey et al. [41]	Cuff et al. [30]	Barnard et al. [43]
AED evaluated	Potassium Bromide							LEV					
2nd AED	-	-	-	PB (12)	-	-	PB	-	PB (12)		PB (4)	PB	-
3rd AED	-	-	-	-	-	-	LEV	-	-		-	-	
4th AED	-	-	-	-	-	-	Gabapentin	-	-		-	-	-
No of cats	26	9	7	17	7	5	1	10 (non-epileptic cats)	12 (10 completed the efficacy analysis)	34 (28 completed the efficacy analysis)	4 (3 had presumed IE)	1	7 (non-epileptic cats)
Age of cats at seizure onset (years)	NA	mean 4.1	NA	mean 8.6	median 3; mean 3.2; range 1-8	NA	4	NA	median 2; range 0.25-16	median 16; range 10-19	NA	10	NA
Period of treatment or follow-up (months)	range 1.75-14	mean 13.63	2	mean 12.5	median 8; mean 18; range 1-96	NA	0.75	1 day	median 9; mean 12; range 6-24	3	Minimum 3 months	2	0.06
Dose of AED(s) (mg/kg)	NA	mean 16.5 PO BID	15 PO BID	12 PO BID	NA	NA	PBr 100 (total dose) PO BID; PB: 30 (total dose) PO BID; LEV: 50 (total dose) PO TID; gabapentin 100 (total dose) PO TID	20 mg/kg PO or IV SID (only one single dose)	PB: median 3.02; range 0.75-4.9 PO BID; LEV: median 23.6; range 17.2-34.7 PO TID	median 62.5; range 60-93.75 PO SID	20 mg/kg PO TID	PB: 4.5 PO BID; LEV 50 PO TID	500 mg PO single dose (extended release)
Serum levels of AED(s)	NA	mean 1.15 mg/ml	mean 1.1 mg/ml	PBr: mean 1.5 mg/ml. PB: range, 13-47 μg/ml	NA	NA	NA	median 26.77; mean 25.54; range 13.22-37.11 μg/ml	PB: median 29; range 5.6-75 μg/ml; LEV: median 25.5 μg/ml	NA	PB: mean 35.8 μg/ml; LEV: mean, 16.5; range: 6.9–24.3 μg/ml	NA	89.7 +/−25.7 μg/ml
Pre-treatment SF (seizures/month or year)	NA	mean 4/month (recorder over a period of 6-12 months)	NA	NA	NA	NA	NA	NA	median 2.1; range 0.8-42.4/month (recorder over a period of median 4.5; range 0.3-46 months)	65/month	NA	continuous	NA
Post-treatment SF (seizures/month or year)	NA	0.52/month	NA	NA	NA	NA	NA	NA	median 0.42; range 0-1.25/month	NA	NA	0 (recorded over a period of 2 months)	NA

Table 2 Details of feline population size, seizure frequency, treatment time, doses of AED(s), seizure frequency reduction after AED initiation, 95% CI for the successful and affected cases and evidence statements for each study *(Continued)*

References	Wagner [38]	Volk et al. [36]	Boothe et al. [21]	Boothe et al. [21] (retrospective part)	Bertolani et al. [37]	Volk et al. [28]	Klang et sl. [39]	Carnes et al. [42]	Bailey et al. [40]	Lowrie et al. [26]	Dewey et al. [41]	Cuff et al. [30]	Barnard et al. [43]
No of cats that were failures	NA	1/9 (11%)	NA	-	NA	0	NA	NA	0%	0/28 (0%)	1/4 (25%)	-	NA
No of cats with >0% - <50% reduction in SF	NA	-	NA	8/15 (53%)	NA	0	NA	NA	3/10 (30%)	0/28 (0%)	3/4 (75%)	-	NA
No of cats with ≥50% - <100% reduction in SF	NA	3/9 (33%)	NA	-	NA	0	NA	NA	4/10 (40%)	14/28 (50%)	0	-	NA
No of cats with 100% reduction in SF	NA	5/9 (56%)	NA	7/15 (47%) (available for 15 cats only and 3/7 were receiving also PB)	NA	5/5 (100%)	NA	NA	3/10 (30%)	14/28 (50%)	0	1/1 (100%)	NA
95% CI of successfully treated cases	NA	56-98%	NA	25-70%	NA	100%	NA	NA	40%-90%	100%	0%	100%	NA
Prevalence of adverse effects	11/26 (42%)	6/9 (67%)	0%	8/17 (47%)	NA	4/5 (80%)	NA	10/10 (100%)	2/12 (17%)	5/34 (18%)	2/4 (50%)	NA	0%
95% CI of cases that developed adverse effects	26-61%	35-88%	0%	26%-70%	NA	38-96%	NA	100%	4-45%	6-30%	15-85%	NA	0%
Body system affected and adverse effects	Respiratory (cough(11), dyspnea(2))	Respiratory (cough(6)), dermatological (dermatitis/ bromoderma(1))	NA	Respiratory (cough (6)), GI (vomiting (1)), Neurological (sedation/ataxia (2)), weight gain (1), PD (1)	Respiratory (cough(7), dyspnea(2), tachypnea (2))	Respiratory (cough, dyspnea)	Respiratory (cough, tachypnea)	GI (hypersalivation)	Neurological (sedation(1)), GI (anorexia(2))	Neurological (sedation (4), ataxia (2), GI (anorexia (3)), PD (1)	ClinPath (increased ALP(2))	NA	NA
Most common adverse effects	Cough	Cough	NA	Cough	Cough	Cough	NA	hypersalivation (after PO administration only)	anorexia	sedation, anorexia	increased ALP	NA	NA
Adverse effect type	II	II	NA	I & II	II	II	II	I	I	I	I	NA	NA

Table 2 Details of feline population size, seizure frequency, treatment time, doses of AED(s), seizure frequency reduction after AED initiation, 95% CI for the successful and affected cases and evidence statements for each study *(Continued)*

References	Wagner [38]	Volk et al. [36]	Boothe et al. [21]	Boothe et al. [21] (retrospective part)	Bertolani et al. [37]	Volk et al. [28]	Klang et sl. [39]	Carnes et al. [42]	Bailey et al. [40]	Lowrie et al. [26]	Dewey et al. [41]	Cuff et al. [30]	Barnard et al. [43]
Proportion of specific adverse effects for each AED based on all study reports	Type I: sedation, ataxia, vomiting, weight gain and PD (1/7; 14%) Type II: cough (6/7; 86%), dyspnea (3/7; 43%), tachypnea (2/7; 29%), dermatitis/bromoderma (1/7; 14%) One study reported that there were no adverse effects.							Type I: sedation (2/5; 40%), anorexia (2/5; 40%), ataxia (1/5; 20%), hypersalivation (1/5; 20%), elevated serum ALP (1/5; 20%) and PD (1/5; 20%)					
Proportion of specific adverse effects for each AED based on the total affected population	Cough (35/72; 49%), dyspnea (9/72; 12%), tachypnea (3/72; 4%), sedation (2/72; 3%), ataxia (2/72; 3%), dermatitis/bromoderma (1/72; 1%), vomiting (1/72; 1%), weight gain (1/72; 1%) and PD (1/72; 1%)							Hypersalivation (10/67; 15%), sedation (5/67; 7%), anorexia (5/67; 7%), ataxia (2/67; 3%), elevated serum ALP (2/67; 3%) and PD (1/67; 1%)					
Overall level of evidence supporting the efficacy and safety profile of an AED	Weak level of evidence for potassium bromide's efficacy and safety profile							Weak level of evidence for levetiracetam's efficacy and safety profile					

AED(s) anti-epileptic drug(s), *BID* bis in die (twice daily), *CI* confidence interval, *GI* gastrointestinal, *IE* idiopathic epilepsy, *LEV* Levetiracetam, *m* month(s), *NA* Not Available, *PB* phenobarbital, *PD* polydipsia, *PU* polyuria, *PP* polyphagia, *PBr* potassium bromide, *PO* per os, *SID* semel in die (once daily), *TID* ter in die (three times daily), *w* week(s), *y* year(s)

Table 3 Details of feline population size, seizure frequency, treatment time, doses of AED(s), seizure frequency reduction after AED initiation, 95% CI for the successful and affected cases and evidence statements for each study

References	Engel et al. [20] (ELAS 1)	Engel et al. [20] (ELAS 2)	Engel et al. [20] (Clinical trial)	Center et al. [45]	Hughes et al. [46]	Schwarz-Porsche & Kaiser, [44]	Sawchuk et al. [47]	Schwarz-Porsche & Kaiser, [44]	Roye et al., [48]	Schwarz-Porsche & Kaiser [44]
AED evaluated	Imepitoin			Diazepam			Primidone		Phenytoin	
2nd AED	-					-	-	-	-	Diazepam
3rd AED	-					-	-	-	-	-
4th AED	-					-	-	-	-	-
No of cats	6	6	8 (7 were evaluated for the safety profile)	11 (non-epileptic cats)	5 (non-epileptic cats)	NA	11	6	4 (non-epileptic cats)	2
Age of cats at seizure onset (years)	NA	NA	median 4; mean 6.3; range 1-15	NA	range 1-12	range 0.2-9	NA	range 0.2-9	NA	range 0.2-9
Period of treatment or follow-up (months)	1	1	at least 2 (for the seizure-freedom cases the period was mean 4; range 2-7.5)	0.5	0.25-0.5	6	3	range 5-108	0.8	>3-9
Dose of AED(s) (mg/kg)	30 PO BID	40 & 80 PO BID	median 30; mean 27.92 PO BID	1.25-2 PO SID or BID	0.23-0.82 PO SID	0.5-2 PO (divided in 3 daily doses)	20 mg/kg PO BID	40-50 PO (divided in three daily doses)	10 PO and intramuscularly SID	1.5 PO SID
Serum levels of AED(s)	NA	NA	NA	NA	NA	NA	4.1 μg/mL	NA	25-35 μg/mL	6.5-17 μg/mL
Pre-treatment SF (seizures/month or year)	NA	NA	Median 20; mean 57.71; range 2-200		NA	NA	NA	NA	NA	NA
Post-treatment SF (seizures/month or year)	NA	NA	Median 1.5; mean 19.43; range 0-100	NA	NA	NA	NA	NA	NA	NA
No of cats that were failures	NA	NA	3/8 (37%)	NA	NA	-	NA	2/6 (33%)	NA	1/2 (50%)
No of cats with >0% - <50% reduction in SF	NA	NA	-	NA	NA	20%	NA	-	NA	-
No of cats with ≥50% - <100% reduction in SF	NA	NA	1/8 (13%)	NA	NA	40%	NA	2/6 (33%)	NA	-
No of cats with 100% reduction in SF	NA	NA	4/8 (50%)	NA	NA	40%	NA	2/6 (33%)	NA	1/2 (50%)
95% CI of successfully treated cases	NA	NA	30-86%	NA	NA	NA	NA	30-90%	NA	9-90%
Prevalence of adverse effects	0 % (apart from intermittent/rare vomiting)	0 % (apart from intermittent/rare vomiting, hypersalivation and slightly decreased appetite)	5/7 (71%)	NA	NA	0%	11/11 (100%)	1/6 (17%)	4/4 (100%)	2/2 (100%)
	NA	NA	36-92%	NA	NA	0%	100%	3-56%	100%	100%

Table 3 Details of feline population size, seizure frequency, treatment time, doses of AED(s), seizure frequency reduction after AED initiation, 95% CI for the successful and affected cases and evidence statements for each study *(Continued)*

References	Engel et al. [20] (ELAS 1)	Engel et al. [20] (ELAS 2)	Engel et al. [20] (Clinical trial)	Center et al. [45]	Hughes et al. [46]	Schwarz-Porsche & Kaiser, [44]	Sawchuk et al. [47]	Schwarz-Porsche & Kaiser, [44]	Roye et al., [48]	Schwarz-Porsche & Kaiser [44]
95% CI of cases that developed adverse effects										
Body system affected and adverse effects	NA	NA	Neurological (sedation (2), ataxia (1)), GI (anorexia (2), PP (1), vomit (2), hypersalivation (1)), PD (1), decreased drinking (1)	Neurological (sedation(5), ataxia(5)), GI (acute hepatic necrosis(11), anorexia (5))	GI (acute hepatic necrosis)	NA	Neurological (sedation, ataxia)	Neurological (sedation), GI (anorexia, weight loss)	Neurological (sedation, ataxia) GI (anorexia)	GI (anorexia), ClinPath (increased liver enzymes)
Most common adverse effects	Intermitent vomit	Intermittent vomit	Sedation, vomit, decreased appetite	NA	NA	NA	NA	NA	NA	NA
Adverse effect type	I	I	I	I & II	II	NA	I	NA	I	I
Proportion of specific adverse effects for each AED based on all study reports	Type I: sedation (1/3; 33%) and ataxia (1/3; 33%), GI signs, i.e. anorexia (1/3; 33%), PP (1/3; 33%), vomiting (1/3; 33%), hypersalivation (1/3; 33%), and PD (1/3; 33%) or decreased water consumption (1/3; 33%)			Type I: sedation and ataxia Type II: acute hepatic necrosis One study reported no adverse effects			Type I: sedation (2/2; 100%), ataxia (1/2; 50%), anorexia (1/2; 50%) and weight loss (1/2; 50%)		Type I: anorexia (2/2; 100%), sedation (1/2; 50%), ataxia (1/2; 50%), increased liver enzymes (1/2; 50%)	
Proportion of specific adverse effects for each AED based on the total affected population	Sedation (2/19; 11%), anorexia (2/19; 11%), vomiting (2/19; 11%), ataxia (1/19; 5%), PP (1/19; 5%), hypersalivation (1/19; 5%), PD (1/19; 5%) and decreased drinking (1/19; 5%)			NA			Sedation (12/17; 71%), ataxia (11/17; 65%), anorexia (1/17; 6%) and weight loss (1/17; 6%)		Anorexia (6/6; 100%), sedation (4/6; 67%) ataxia (4/6; 67%) and increased liver enzymes (2/6; 33%)	
	Weak and good level of evidence for imepitoin's efficacy and safety profile, respectively			Weak level of evidence for diazepam's efficacy and safety profile			Weak level of evidence for primidone's efficacy and safety profile		Weak level of evidence for phenytoin's efficacy and safety profile	

AED(s), anti-epileptic drug(s); BID, bis in die (twice daily); CI, confidence interval; GI, gastrointestinal; IE, idiopathic epilepsy; LEV, Levetiracetam; m, month(s); NA, Not Available; PB, phenobarbital; PD, polydipsia; PU, polyuria; PP, polyphagia; PBr, potassium bromide; PO, per os; SID, semel in die (once daily); TID, ter in die (three times daily); w, week(s); year(s); y

Table 4 Details of feline population size, seizure frequency, treatment time, doses of AED(s), seizure frequency reduction after AED initiation, 95% CI for the successful and affected cases and evidence statements for each study

References	Hasegawa et al. [50]	Brewer et al. [49]	Ukai et al. [51]	Cautela et al. [52]	Pellegrini et al., [53]	Zoran et al., [54]	Dreimann [55]
AED evaluated	Zonisamide			Pregabalin	Valproic acid		
2nd AED	-	PB (5)	-		-	-	-
3rd AED	-	-	-		-	-	-
4th AED	-	-	-		-	-	-
No of cats	6 (non-epileptic cats)	5	8	6 (non-epileptic cats)	8 (non-epileptic cats)	1 (non-epileptic cat)	6 (non-epileptic cats)
Age of cats at seizure onset (years)	NA	NA	median 8.75; range 6.75 -11.5	NA	NA	NA	NA
Period of treatment or follow-up (months)	2.1	3	0.75	NA	0.12-0.25	NA	0.5
Dose of AED(s) (mg/kg)	20 PO SID	mean 11.54; range 6.14-17 PO SID	2.5 PO BID for a week, then 5 PO BID	4 PO (one dose only)	range 25- 130 intraperitoneally TID	< 111 PO at once	40 PO and IV BID
Serum levels of AED(s)	median 52.9; mean 56.9 μg/mL	Zonisamide: mean 19.44; range 8.8-38.6 mcg/ml; PB: NA	median 5.9 (2.1–8.3) for a week, then 13.45 (11.9–24.4)	range 2.8-8.2 μg/mL	<5 μg/ml	3.4 μg/ml	50-150 μg/ml
Pre-treatment SF (seizures/ month or year)	NA	NA	NA	NA	NA	NA	NA
Post-treatment SF (seizures/ month or year)	NA	NA	NA	NA	NA	NA	NA
No of cats that were failures	NA	0	NA	NA	NA	NA	NA
No of cats with >0% - <50% reduction in SF	NA	2/5 (40%)	NA	NA	NA	NA	NA
No of cats with ≥50% - <100% reduction in SF	NA	3/5 (60%)	NA	NA	NA	NA	NA
No of cats with 100% reduction in SF	NA	0	NA	NA	NA	NA	NA
95% CI of successfully treated cases	NA	23%-88%	NA	NA	NA	NA	NA
Prevalence of adverse effects	3/6 (50%)	2/5 (40%)	0%	4/6 (67%)	>4/8 (>50%)	NA	6/6 (100%)
95% CI of cases that developed adverse effects	19-81%	12%-77%	0%	30-90%	NA	NA	100%
Body system affected and adverse effects	Neurological (sedation, ataxia) GI (vomiting, diarrhea, anorexia)	Neurological (sedation (1)), GI (anorexia (1))	0%	Neurological (sedation)	Neurological (sedation, ataxia, drowsiness, head tremor), GI (anorexia)	Neurological (hyperactivity), dermatological (alopecia)	Neurological (sedation), GI (vomiting, anorexia)
Most common adverse effects	NA	NA	NA	NA	Sedation, drowsiness, head tremor, anorexia	NA	NA

Table 4 Details of feline population size, seizure frequency, treatment time, doses of AED(s), seizure frequency reduction after AED initiation, 95% CI for the successful and affected cases and evidence statements for each study *(Continued)*

References	Hasegawa et al. [50]	Brewer et al. [49]	Ukai et al. [51]	Cautela et al. [52]	Pellegrini et al., [53]	Zoran et al., [54]	Dreimann [55]
Adverse effect type	I	I		I	I	I & II	I
Proportion of specific adverse effects for each AED based on all study reports	Type I: sedation (2/3; 67%), anorexia (2/3; 67%), ataxia (1/3; 33%), vomiting (1/3; 33%) and diarhoea (1/3; 33%)			Type I: sedation	Type I: sedation (2/3; 67%), anorexia (2/3; 67%), ataxia (1/3; 33%), drowsiness (1/3; 33%), head tremor (1/3; 33%), hyperactivity (1/3; 33%) and vomiting (1/3; 33%) Type II: alopecia (1/3; 33%)		
Proportion of specific adverse effects for each AED based on the total affected population	Sedation (4/19; 21%), anorexia (4/19; 21%), ataxia (3/19; 16%), vomiting (3/19; 16%) and diarrhea (3/19; 16%)			NA	Sedation (>10/15; 67%), anorexia (>10/15; 67%), ataxia (>4/15; 27%), drowsiness (>4/15; 17%), head tremor (>4/15; 17%), vomiting (6/15; 40%), hyperactivity (1/15; 7%) and alopecia (1/15; 7%)		
Overall level of evidence supporting the efficacy and safety profile of an AED	Weak level of evidence for zonisamide's efficacy and safety profile			Absent and weak level of evidence for pregabalin's efficacy and safety profile	Absent and weak evidence for valproic acid's safety profile and efficacy respectively		

AED(s), anti-epileptic drug(s); BID, bis in die (twice daily); CI, confidence interval; GI, gastrointestinal; IE, idiopathic epilepsy; LEV, Levetiracetam; m, month(s); NA, Not Available; PB, phenobarbital; PD, polydipsia; PU, polyuria; PP, polyphagia; PBr, potassium bromide; PO, per os; SID, semel in die (once daily); TID, ter in die (three times daily); w, week(s); year(s); y

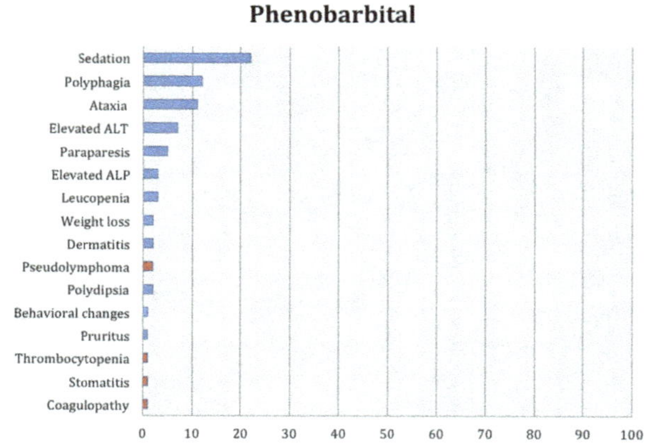

Fig. 1 Proportion of specific adverse effects for phenobarbital. Each adverse effect represents the percentage of cats that were affected by this with regards to the overall combined population for phenobarbital. The blue and red bars indicate type I and II adverse effects, respectively

[4, 26, 31] (63%), the majority of the study population was treated successfully. In one of these studies though [26], phenobarbital was only used to treat a specific type of epileptic seizures in cats, i.e. feline auditory reactive seizures (FARS), which might have biased the results for the drug's overall efficacy to control seizures.

Twelve studies [22–28, 31–35] evaluated the safety profile of phenobarbital, providing a total size of 147 cats. Three studies documented type I adverse effects, including dermatological and neurological signs, clinic-pathological abnormalities, polyphagia [36], polydipsia (PD) and weight loss (Additional file 2: Table S1). Four studies reported type II adverse effects including clinic-pathological abnormalities and lympho-reticular and gastrointestinal signs (GI) signs (Additional file 2: Table S1). Three studies reported that there were no adverse effects. Based on the 95% CI, in all studies but two [27, 34] (83%), the majority of reported population did not show adverse effects. The most common adverse effect was sedation and the least common were behavioral changes, pruritus, thrombocytopenia, ulcerative stomatitis and coagulopathy (Additional file 2: Table S1, Fig. 1).

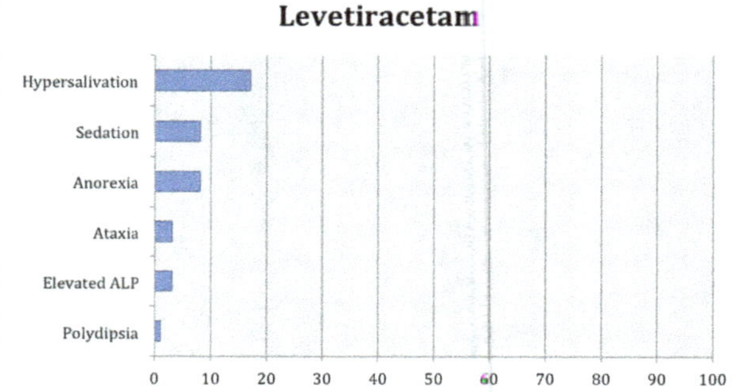

Fig. 3 Proportion of adverse effects for levetiracetam. Each adverse effect represents the percentage of cats that were affected by this with regards to the overall combined population for levetiracetam. The blue bars indicate type I adverse effects

The treatment or follow-up period was reported adequately in 14/15 (93%) studies (Additional file 2: Table S1). From these, in 9/14 (60%) the follow-up time was short (<6 months). Dose and serum levels were provided adequately in 13/15 (87%) and 11/15 (73%) studies respectively (Additional file 2: Table S1). The phenobarbital maintenance doses and serum levels were higher than the normal reference range [6] in 8/13 (62%) and 4/11 (36%) studies respectively. In all, type I and II adverse effects did not follow a dose or serum levels dependent pattern. In summary, the level of evidence for phenobarbital's efficacy and safety profile was weak.

Potassium Bromide

Three studies [21, 28, 36] assessed potassium bromide's efficacy as a monotherapy agent or in combination to phenobarbital (one study), providing a total group size

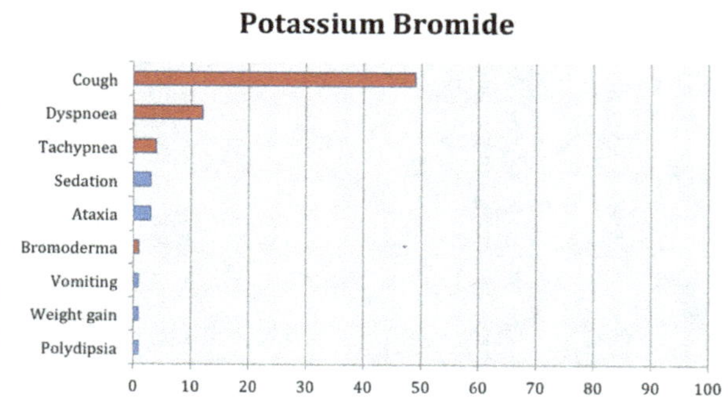

Fig. 2 Proportion of specific adverse effects for potassium bromide. Each adverse effect represents the percentage of cats that were affected by this with regards to the overall combined population for potassium bromide. The blue and red bars indicate type I and II adverse effects, respectively

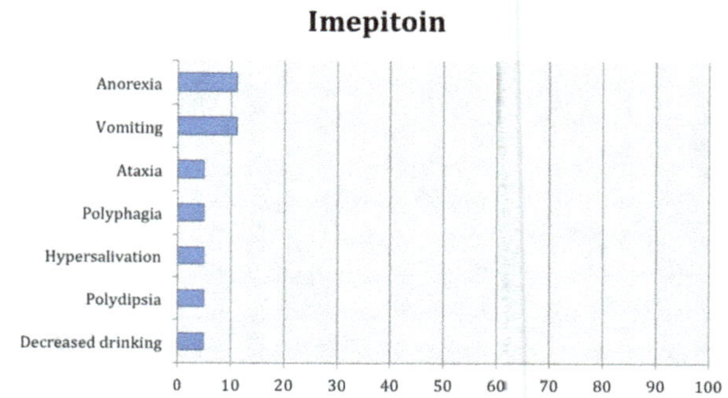

Fig. 4 Proportion of specific adverse effects for imepitoin. Each adverse effect represents the percentage of cats that were affected by this with regards to the overall combined population for imepitoin. The blue bars indicate type I adverse effects

of 29 cats. Based on the 95% CI, in all the studies but one [21] (66%), the majority of the study population was treated successfully.

Six studies [21, 28, 36–39] evaluated the safety profile of potassium bromide, providing a total size of 72 cats. One of these studies included both a UCT and retrospective case series part [21]. One study documented type I adverse effects, such as neurological, GI signs and PD. Five studies reported type II adverse effects, such as respiratory and dermatological signs (Table 2). One study reported that there were no adverse effects. Applying the 95% CI, in all the studies (100%), the majority of the cases reported did not have adverse effects. The most common adverse effect was cough and least common were dermatitis/bromoderma, vomiting, weight gain and PD (Table 2, Fig. 2).

Treatment or follow-up time was reported adequately in 6/7 (86%) (Table 2). From these, in 2/6 (33%) the period was short (<6 months). The dose and serum levels were documented adequately in 4/7 (57%) and 3/7 (43%) studies (Table 2). There was no adequate information to relate specific range values of dose and serum levels with the development of type I or II adverse effects. In summary the level of evidence for potassium bromide's efficacy and safety profile was weak.

Levetiracetam

Four studies [26, 30, 40, 41] assessed the efficacy of levetiracetam as a monotherapy agent or in combination to phenobarbital (three studies), providing a total group size of 43 cats. Based on the 95% CI, in two of the studies [26, 30] (50%) the majority of the study population was treated successfully.

Five studies [26, 40–43] reported the safety profile of levetiracetam, providing a total group size of 67 cats. Only type I adverse effects were reported in all evaluated studies, including neurological and GI signs and clinicopathological abnormalities (Table 2). Based on the 95% CI, in all of the studies but one [42] (75%), the majority had no adverse effects reported. One study reported no adverse effects [43]. The most common adverse effect was hypersalivation and the least common was PD (Table 2, Fig. 3).

The treatment or follow-up time was reported adequately in all the studies (Table 2), but was short (<6 months) in 5/6 (83%). The dose and serum levels were reported adequately in 6/6 (100%) and 4/6 (66%) studies respectively (Table 2). The levetiracetam maintenance doses reported were higher than normal in 2/6 (33%) studies. In all, type I adverse effects did not follow a dose or serum levels dependent pattern. The level of evidence for levetiracetam's efficacy and safety profile was weak.

Imepitoin

One study [20] assessed the efficacy of imepitoin as monotherapy agent in 8 cats. With such a small population size studied the 95% CI could not demonstrate that the majority of cases were managed successfully.

Three studies, which were included as part of one report [20], reported the safety profile of imepitoin, providing a total study size of 19 cats. In one study, only type I adverse effects were reported including neurological, GI signs and PD or decreased water consumption. In the two other studies though, no such effects were reported but intermittent vomiting, hypersalivation and slightly decreased appetite (Table 3). Applying the 95% CI to all study data (100%), the majority of cases did not experience adverse effects. There was an equal distribution among all the adverse effects (Table 3, Fig. 4).

The treatment or follow-up time was reported adequately in all studies (Table 3). In all studies (100%) the period was short (<6 months). The dose and serum levels was provided adequately in 3/3 (100%) and 0/3 (0%) studies, respectively (Table 3). Higher imepitoin maintenance doses, i.e. 40 or 80 mg/kg PO BID, were associated with higher incidence of adverse effects. The level of evidence for imepitoin's efficacy was weak but the level of evidence for safety profile was strong.

Diazepam

One study [44] assessed the efficacy of diazepam as monotherapy. The study reported that the majority of the cases was managed successfully, but the 95% CI could not be calculated.

Three studies [44–46] reported the safety profile of diazepam, providing a total size of 16 cats. One study documented type I adverse effects, i.e. neurological signs (Table 3). Two studies documented type II adverse effects, i.e. GI signs (Table 3). One study reported that there were no adverse effects. Since all the studies, but one [44], selectively included cats that manifested adverse effects, the 95% CI and adverse effects prevalence could not be calculated (Table 3).

The treatment or follow-up time was reported adequately in 3/3 (100%), but was considered short in all (Table 3). The dose and serum levels were reported adequately in 3/3 (100%) and 0/3 (0%) studies respectively (Table 3). In all, type I and II adverse effects did not follow a dose or serum levels dependent pattern. The level of evidence for diazepam's efficacy and safety profile was weak.

Primidone

One study [44] assessed the efficacy of primidone as a monotherapy agent in 6 cats. Applying the 95% CI to such a small study population showed that the majority was not managed successfully.

Two studies [44, 47] reported the safety profile of primidone, providing a total group size of 17 cats. The studies reported type I adverse effects, such as GI and neurological signs and weight loss. No type II adverse effects were reported (Table 3). Applying the 95% CI to one study [44] (50%), the majority of cases did not have adverse effects reported. The most common adverse effect was sedation and the least common were anorexia and weight loss (Table 3).

The treatment or follow-up period was reported adequately in 2/2 (100%) (Table 3). From these, in 1/2 (50%) the period was short (<6 months). The dose and serum levels was reported adequately in 2/2 (100%) and 1/2 (50%) studies respectively (Table 3). There was inadequate information to relate specific range values of dose and serum levels with the development of type I or II adverse effects. The level of evidence for primidone's efficacy and safety profile was weak.

Phenytoin

One study [44] evaluated the efficacy of phenytoin as an adjunct to diazepam in 2 cats.

Two studies [44, 48] reported the safety profile of phenytoin, providing a total size of 6 cats. The studies documented type I adverse effects, such as GI and neurological signs and clinic-pathological abnormalities. No type II adverse effects were documented (Table 3). Based on the 95% CI, in all the studies (100%), the majority of the study population experienced adverse effects. The most common adverse effect was anorexia and the least common was increased serum liver enzymes (Table 3).

The treatment or follow-up period was reported adequately in 2/2 (100%) (Table 3). From these, in 1/2 (50%) the period was short (<6 months). The dose and serum levels were reported adequately in 2/2 (100%) studies (Table 3). There was inadequate information to relate specific range values of dose and serum levels with the development of type I or II adverse effects. The level of evidence for phenytoin's efficacy and safety profile was weak.

Zonisamide

One study [49] assessed the efficacy of zonisamide as an adjunct to phenobarbital in 5 cats. Applying the 95% CI to such a small study population showed that the majority was not managed successfully.

Three studies [49–51] reported the safety profile of zonisamide in 19 cats. The studies documented type I adverse effects, such as GI and neurological signs (Table 4). Based on the 95% CI, in all studies (100%), the majority of the study population did not have adverse effects. One study reported no adverse effects [51]

The treatment or follow-up time was reported adequately but was considered short in all studies (Table 4). The dose and serum levels were also reported adequately in all studies (Table 4). There was inadequate information to relate specific range values of dose and serum levels with the development of type I or II adverse effects. In summary, the level of evidence for zonisamide's efficacy and safety profile was weak.

Pregabalin

There were no original studies evaluating the efficacy of pregabalin in cats except for experts' opinion. One study [52] reported the safety profile of pregabalin in 6 cats. The study documented type I adverse effects, i.e. neurological signs. No type II adverse effects were documented (Table 4). Applying the 95% CI to the studied population, the majority did not experience adverse effects.

The treatment or follow-up time was inadequately reported (Table 4). The dose and serum levels was reported adequately (Table 4). There was inadequate information to relate specific range values of dose and serum levels with the development of type I or II adverse effects. There was no evidence for pregabalin's efficacy and an overall weak level of evidence for pregabalin's safety profile.

Valproic acid

There were no original studies evaluating the efficacy of valproic acid in cats except for experts' opinion. Three studies [53–55] reported the safety profile of valproic acid, giving a combined sample size of 15 cats. Three studies documented type I adverse effects, such as GI and neurological signs. One study documented type II adverse effects, i.e. dermatological signs (Table 4). There was inadequate information to calculate the 95% CI but one study [55] showed that the whole population had adverse effects. The most common adverse effects were sedation ataxia, drowsiness, head tremor and anorexia and the least common were hyperactivity and alopecia.

The treatment or follow-up time was reported adequately in 2/3 (67%) studies and was considered short. The dose and serum levels were reported adequately in 3/3 (100%) (Table 4). There was inadequate information to relate specific range values of dose and serum levels with the development of type I or II adverse effects. There was no evidence for valproic acid's efficacy and weak level of evidence for safety profile.

Discussion

To the authors' knowledge, this is the first systematic review of AEDs' efficacy and safety in cats. The authors were based on the PRISMA (Preferred Reporting Items for Systematic Reviews and Meta-Analyses) statement to report this systematic review [56]. The systematic review found that the level of evidence in feline epilepsy treatment is weak to absent, in particular for AEDs' efficacy. The results showed that phenobarbital was considered the most effective AED followed by levetiracetam and potassium bromide then imepitoin and diazepam and lastly zonisamide, primidone and phenytoin (Fig. 5). All supported by weak level of evidence. There was insufficient evidence for the efficacy of pregabalin and valproic acid. As far as the safety profile of all the AEDs is concerned, imepitoin was considered the safest AED, followed by levetiracetam and phenobarbital, then zonisamide and pregabalin followed by primidone, phenytoin and valproic acid and lastly potassium bromide and diazepam (Fig. 6). All supported by weak level of evidence apart from imepitoin, which was supported by good level of evidence. Although this systematic review focused on evaluating the use of AEDs in feline patients, it would be an omission not to mention that other substances have been proposed for managing seizures in cats [57, 58], with taurine as the most representative example. In a feline case report, administration of 300 mg taurine subcutaneously twice a day for two days followed by 100 mg taurine orally once a day for one month resulted in reduction in seizure frequency, supported by clinical and electroencephalographic observations. Abrupt cessation led to a rise of frequency [57]. Further clinical studies are crucial to support taurine's potential efficacy in feline epilepsy.

The AEDs' adverse effects were categorised as type I (predictable or dose-dependent) or type II (idiosyncratic/unpredictable or dose-independent) which are usually considered as non-immunological reactions [59]. It was challenging to detect a correlation between the AED dose or serum concentration and the type of adverse effects in feline patients. This could be attributed either to the possibility that, in feline patients, adverse effects might not follow a dose or serum related pattern or to the fact that there was inadequate information to allow us assessing any potential correlation between the incidence of adverse effects and the AEDs' dose or serum concentrations. Severe type II adverse effects were reported mainly in cats being treated with potassium bromide or diazepam. Type II adverse effects are non-dose dependent, unpredictable, usually rare and caused by a cytotoxin, a drug or its metabolite [59]. Idiosyncratic reactions are most likely secondary to an individual difference in rate of formation and detoxification of reactive metabolites [59]. However, in the case of potassium bromide and, in particular, diazepam in feline patients, the incidence of these type II effects was high and in case of diazepam, they were considered life-threatening. This can give rise to evidence that the type II adverse effects of these two drugs in cats are species-related rather than individual-related.

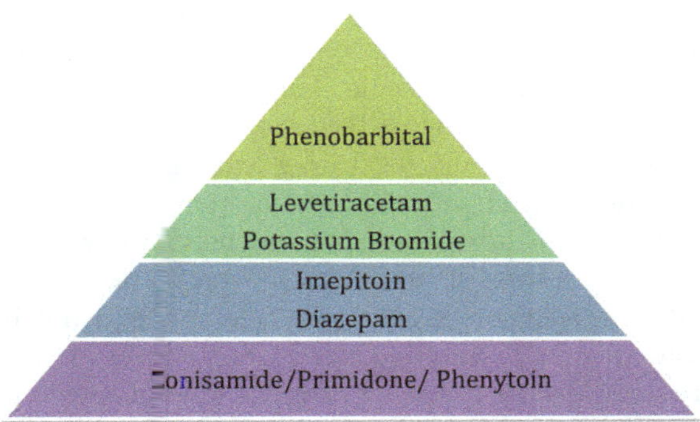

Fig. 5 Pyramid of AEDs' efficacy hierarchy based on the quality of evidence and outcomes assessment

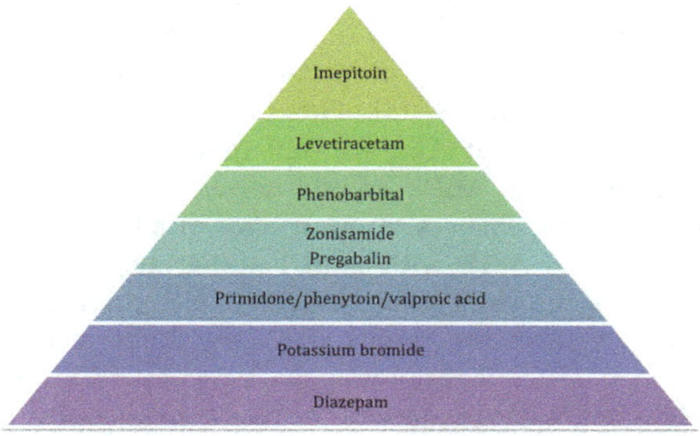

Fig. 6 Pyramid of AEDs' safety hierarchy based on the quality of evidence and outcomes assessment

In canine epilepsy, the majority of studies lacked a high level of evidence [8, 15]. However, in feline epilepsy, almost none of the studies provided high quality of evidence. The studies manifested high overall risk of bias. In addition, only 47% and 2% of all studies had well clinically defined groups and assessed a sufficient number of cats, respectively. The 95% CI, that was used as an indicator of the 'real' population of successful (AED efficacy) or affected (AED safety) cases, revealed a wide range of values mainly due to the inadequate feline population in the studies. Therefore, conclusions drawn based on the 95% CI results should be interpreted with caution. In addition, there were no bRCTs evaluating any AEDs in cats but two bRELAS assessing imepitoin's safety profile. The follow up time was rather limited and short (<6months) to assess adequately long-term efficacy and tolerability. In all, due to the lack of studies with overall low risk of bias, insufficient disease characterisations and small group sizes, clear suggestions concerning AEDs' efficacy and safety are difficult.

In contrast to canine epilepsy, many studies evaluated the efficacy and safety of an AED as monotherapy (with the exception of levetiracetam), making it easier to determine whether an AED's adverse effects and efficacy were attributed mainly to its administration. However, certain evaluated factors might have influenced our assessment of AEDs' efficacy and safety profile similar to the ones described in our previous systematic reviews for canine patients [8, 15]. These included the dosages used of a particular AED (i.e. different among studies), the frequency of AEDs' administration (i.e. factor that could alter the chances of occurrence of adverse effects particularly in AEDs with short half-life due to fluctuations of serum drug levels; although this characteristic might not affect the results [60]), the duration of the study (i.e. insufficient duration, as it was found in many studies, might have reduced the chance for the most frequent adverse effects to occur or for adequately evaluate an AED's efficacy). Lastly, a few AEDs have been used more often in feline epilepsy and been in the market for longer period compared to others. Therefore, more evidence is available which could influence the conclusions with regards to their efficacy and safety. A characteristic example is phenobarbital for which, compared to other AEDs, there are more reports of not only its efficacy but also its adverse effects.

As it was found in the previous canine systematic reviews and meta-analysis [8, 15], some characteristics may have also adversely affected the evaluation of the included studies. Similarly, multiple factors could have influenced our results such as signalment differed between studies, heterogeneity in treatment methods among studies, variation in study publication dates, publication bias, several introduced biases detected, lack of high quality evidence studies (i.e. bRCTs and bRELAS), lack of well characterized diagnostic procedures and enrolment of relatively small study population.

Implications for research

Systematic reviews are a good step towards clinical evidence medicine, however the evaluation and comparison among AEDs through a meta-analysis could provide far further information and aid clinician's decision to choose the most appropriate AED for every patient. A meta-analysis was not feasible here due to the variations in baseline characteristics of the cats involved, the significant differences between study designs, the several sources of identified bias and mainly due to the lack of comparison group studies. Although the 95% CI and the prevalence of successfully treated cases and adverse effects in each study provide a general indicator of each AED's efficacy and safety profile, respectively, and can lead to indirect comparisons between AEDs, comparison group studies are essential as they allow thorough statistics to be performed for direct and thus more reliable comparisons. Therefore, further comparison groups and blinded randomized studies are essential for feline epilepsy treatment that would allow a meta-analysis towards this goal.

Lastly, a further problem that was found during the studies evaluation was the lack of reported information. This led to difficulties in performing statistical analysis for AEDs' comparisons. Therefore, it is essential that future trials should provide precise information and scientists have open access to trials' data. It would be crucial that journals enforce authors to report their results based on guidelines such as STROBE (Strengthening the Reporting of Observational studies in Epidemiology), ARRIVE (Animal Research: Reporting of In Vivo Experiments) and CONSORT (Consolidated Standards of Reporting Trials).

Implications for clinical practice

Current evidence did not allow comparisons among AEDs, and therefore it would be rather inaccurate to make definite statements on which one should be considered as a first or second choice in terms of both efficacy and safety profile. However, if clinicians focus on AED's efficacy, phenobarbital can be used as first-choice monotherapy and if they focus on AED's safety, imepitoin or levetiracetam can be used. It is important to report that, similarly to canine epilepsy [8], phenobarbital should not be overstated as an AED with high incidence of detrimental adverse effects and therefore, in healthy cats with no pre-existing liver disease, phenobarbital might be the most appropriate choice. Levetiracetam or imepitoin can also be considered as a safe alternative for monotherapy, especially in cats that develop unexpected adverse effects to phenobarbital. For certain epilepsy phenotypes, such as myoclonic epilepsy in elderly cats, levetiracetam monotherapy can be considered. Levetiracetam, imepitoin or phenorbarbital and, to a quite lesser degree, zonisamide might be considered as add-on medication when first line treatment chosen is not sufficient to control seizures. Potassium bromide can be used as adjunctive AEDs only as a last resort and after a signed owner's consent form in cases manifesting resistance to >2 AEDs and should be closely monitored for type II adverse effects. Diazepam might not be an appropriate choice due to the inadequate evidence supporting its efficacy and the possibility of severe and potentially life-threatening type II adverse effects. It is also important to note that the recommendations made are on the basis of the evidence provided in the available literature and local drug legislation need to be considered prior of prescribing medications.

In general, as it was found in our previous systematic review [8], most of the AED adverse effects documented were inconsistent, fairly tolerable and not life-threatening and ceased once doses and serum levels were decreased or following drug withdrawal. Exceptions included specific type II adverse effects and specific antiepileptic drugs (in particular diazepam and to a lesser degree potassium bromide). It is essential that clinicians assess both the benefits (i.e. value for money, dosing regimen, efficacy) and risks (i.e. safety and tolerability, and impact of adverse effects on the cat's and owner's quality of life) before choosing a specific AED.

Conclusion

This systematic review provides an evidence-based assessment of the data on the AEDs' efficacy and adverse effects for feline epilepsy. Factors that need to be considered when evaluating these results are: i) drugs that have been used and been on the market for longer periods provided more evidence, ii) the vast majority of the studies offered overall high risk of bias and included small number of cats with unclear or fair disease characterization criteria and short-term follow-up. Individual AED assessments of efficacy and safety profile showed that phenobarbital can be used as the first-choice AED followed by imepitoin and levetiracetam. Further studies in feline epilepsy treatment are by far essential in order to establish definite guidelines for AEDs' efficacy and safety.

Abbreviations

AED(s): anti-epileptic drug(s); BID: bis in die (twice daily); bELAS: blinded experimental laboratory animal studies; bRCTs: blinded randomised clinical trials; CI: confidence interval; CTs: clinical trials; GI: gastrointestinal; IE: idiopathic epilepsy; LEV: levetiracetam; m: month(s); MRI: magnetic resonance imaging; NA: Not Available; nbELAS: non-blinded experimental laboratory animal studies; nbRCTs: non-blinded randomised clinical trials; NRELAS: non-randomised experimental laboratory studies; NRCTs: non-randomised clinical trials; PB: phenobarbital; PBr: potassium bromide; PD: polydipsia; PO: per os; PP: polyphagia; PU: polyuria; SID: semel in die (once daily); TID: ter in die (three times daily); UCTs: uncontrolled clinical trials; UELAS: uncontrolled experimental laboratory studies; w: week(s)

Acknowledgements

Not applicable.

Funding

Not applicable.

Authors' contributions

MC and SB collected the data. MC screened and evaluated the data and drafted the manuscript. AP and HV helped to draft the manuscript and participated in its design. All authors read and approved the final manuscript.

Consent for publication

Not applicable

Competing interests

HV is a member of the editorial board of the journal.

Author details

[1]Small Animal Department, Faculty of Veterinary Medicine, Ghent University, Merelbeke, Belgium. [2]Clinical Unit of Internal Medicine Small Animals, University of Veterinary Medicine, Vienna, Austria. [3]Department of Clinical Science and Services, Royal Veterinary College, Hawkshead Lane, Brookmans Park, UK.

References

1. Schwartz-Porsche D. Epidemiological, clinical and pharmacokinetic studies in spontaneously epileptic dogs and cats. In: *The 4th Annual American College of Veterinary Internal Medicine Forum: 1986. Washington, DC*: JVIM; 1986. p. 61–3.
2. Pakozdy A, Leschnik M, Sarchahi AA, Tichy AG, Thalhammer JG. Clinical comparison of primary versus secondary epilepsy in 125 cats. J Feline Med Surg. 2010;**12**(12):910–6.
3. Cizinauskas S, Fatzer R, Schenkel M, Gandini G, Jaggy A. Can idiopathic epilepsy be confirmed in cats? Journal of Veterinary Internal Medicine. 2003;17:246.
4. Schriefl S, Steinberg TA, Matiasek K, Ossig A, Fenske N, Fischer A. Etiologic classification of seizures, signalment, clinical signs, and outcome in cats with seizure disorders: 91 cases (2000-2004). J Am Vet Med Assoc. 2008;233(10):1591–7.
5. Quesnel AD, Parent JM, McDonell W, Percy D, Lumsden JH. Diagnostic evaluation of cats with seizure disorders: 30 cases (1991-1993). J Am Vet Med Assoc. 1997;210(1):65–71.
6. Bailey KS, Dewey CW. THE SEIZURING CAT Diagnostic work-up and therapy. Journal of Feline Medicine and Surgery. 2009;11(5):385–94.
7. Pakozdy A, Halasz P, Klang A. Epilepsy in cats: theory and practice. J Vet Intern Med. 2014;28(2):255–63.
8. Charalambous M, Shivapour SK, Brodbelt DC, Volk HA. Antiepileptic drugs' tolerability and safety–a systematic review and meta-analysis of adverse effects in dogs. BMC Vet Res. 2016;12:79.
9. Papanikolaou PN, Ioannidis JP. Availability of large-scale evidence on specific harms from systematic reviews of randomized trials. The American journal of medicine. 2004;117(8):582–9.
10. Ross SD. Drug-related adverse events: a readers' guide to assessing literature reviews and meta-analyses. Archives of internal medicine. 2001;161(8):1041–6.
11. Chou R, Helfand M. Challenges in systematic reviews that assess treatment harms. Annals of internal medicine. 2005;142(12 Pt 2):1090–9.
12. Berlin JA, Colditz GA. The role of meta-analysis in the regulatory process for foods, drugs, and devices. Jama. 1999;281(9):830–4.
13. Bhatti SF, De Risio L, Munana K, Penderis J, Stein VM, Tipold A, Berendt M, Farquhar RG, Fischer A, Long S, et al. International Veterinary Epilepsy Task Force consensus proposal: medical treatment of canine epilepsy in Europe. BMC Vet Res. 2015;11:176.
14. Podell M, Volk HA, Berendt M, Loscher W, Munana K, Patterson EE, Platt SR. 2015 ACVIM Small Animal Consensus Statement on Seizure Management in Dogs. J Vet Intern Med. 2016;30(2):477–90.
15. Charalambous M, Brodbelt D, Volk HA. Treatment in canine epilepsy–a systematic review. BMC Vet Res. 2014;10:257.
16. Guyatt GH, Oxman AD, Vist GE, Kunz R, Falck-Ytter Y, Schunemann H, Grp GW. GRADE: what is "quality of evidence" and why is it important to clinicians? Brit Med J. 2008;336(7651):995–999b.
17. Holmes MA. Philosophical foundations of evidence-based medicine for veterinary clinicians. Javma-J Am Vet Med A. 2009;235(9):1035–9.
18. Higgins J. A., C. SJ: In: Higgins JPT, Green S, eds. Cochrane Handbook for Systematic Reviews of Interventions Version 5.1.0. Part 2: General methods for Cochrane reviews, Chapter 8: Assessing risk of bias in included studies, Table 8.5.d: Criteria for judging risk of bias in the 'Risk of bias' assessment tool. In: *The Cochrane Collaboration*. edn.; 2011.
19. Hooijmans CR, Rovers MM, de Vries RB, Leenaars M, Ritskes-Hoitinga M, Langendam MW. SYRCLE's risk of bias tool for animal studies. BMC Med Res Methodol. 2014;14:43.
20. Engel O, von Klopmann T, Maiolini A, Freundt-Revilla J, Tipold A. Imepitoin is well tolerated in healthy and epileptic cats. BMC Vet Res. 2017;13(172):1–7.
21. Boothe DM, George KL, Couch P. Disposition and clinical use of bromide in cats. J Am Vet Med Assoc. 2002;221(8):1131–5.
22. Baho MJ, Hostutler R, Fenner W, Corn S. Suspected phenobarbital-induced pseudolymphoma in a cat. J Am Vet Med Assoc. 2011;238(3):353–5.

23. Ducote JM, Coates JR, Dewey CW, Kennis RA. Suspected hypersensitivity to phenobarbital in a cat. J Feline Med Surg. 1999;1(2):123–6.
24. Lieser J, Schwedes CS. Pseudolymphoma in a cat on phenobarbital treatment. J Small Anim Pract. 2017;
25. Finnerty KE, Barnes Heller HL, Mercier MN, Giovanella CJ, Lau VW, Rylander H. Evaluation of therapeutic phenobarbital concentrations and application of a classification system for seizures in cats: 30 cases (2004-2013). J Am Vet Med Assoc. 2014;244(2):195–9.
26. Lowrie M, Thomson S, Bessant C, Sparkes A, Harvey RJ, Garosi L. Levetiracetam in the management of feline audiogenic reflex seizures: a randomised, controlled, open-label study. J Feline Med Surg. 2017;19(2):200–6.
27. Pakozdy A, Sarchahi AA, Leschnik M, Tichy AG, Halasz P, Thalhammer JG. Treatment and long-term follow-up of cats with suspected primary epilepsy. J Feline Med Surg. 2012;15(4):267–73.
28. Volk H, Coleing JAL, Platt S, Chandler K. Clinical presentation and response to treatment of cats with epilepsy. Birmingham: *BSAVA congress*; 2007.
29. Boydell P. Rub epilepsy in a cat. Vet Rec. 2010;166(10):308.
30. Cuff DE, Bush WW, Stecker MM, Williams DC. Use of continuous electroencephalography for diagnosis and monitoring of treatment of nonconvulsive status epilepticus in a cat. J Am Vet Med Assoc. 2014;244(6):708–14.
31. Wahle AM, Bruhschwein A, Matiasek K, Putschbach K, Wagner E, Mueller RS, Fischer A. Clinical characterization of epilepsy of unknown cause in cats. J Vet Intern Med. 2014;28(1):182–8.
32. Cochrane SM, Black WD, Parent JM, Allen DG, Lumsden JH. Pharmacokinetics of phenobarbital in the cat following intravenous and oral administration. Can J Vet Res. 1990;54(1):132–8.
33. Cochrane SM, Parent JM, Black WD, Allen DG, Lumsden JH. Pharmacokinetics of phenobarbital in the cat following multiple oral administration. Can J Vet Res. 1990;54(3):309–12.
34. Solomon GE, Hilgartner MW, Kutt H. Phenobarbital-induced coagulation defects in cats. Neurology. 1974;24(10):920–4.
35. Gasper JAD, Heller HLB, Robertson M, Trepanier LA. Therapeutic serum phenobarbital concentrations obtained using chronic transdermal administration of phenobarbital in healthy cats. Journal of Feline Medicine and Surgery. 2015;17(4):359–63.
36. Volk HA, Chandler KE, Cappello R, Cherubini GB: New insights into efficacy and side effects of potassium bromide in epileptic cats. In: *24th American College of Veterinary Internal Medicine: 2006; Louisville, KY*: Journal of Veterinary Internal Medicine; 2006.
37. Bertolani C, Hernandez J, Gomes E, Cauzinille L, Poujade A, Gabriel A. Bromide-associated lower airway disease: a retrospective study of seven cats. J Feline Med Surg. 2012;14(8):591–7.
38. Wagner S. Lower airway disease in cats on bromide therapy for seizures. In: *19th American College of Veterinary Internal Medicine: 2001. Denver, CO*: Journal of Veterinary Internal Medicine; 2001.
39. Klang A, Schmidt P, Pakozdy A, Kneissl S, Schwendenwein I, Hirt R. Histopathological pulmonary changes in a cat with potassium bromide-induced lower airway disease. *Wiener Tierärztliche Monatsschrift – Veterinary Medicine Austria*. 2012;99:34–7.
40. Bailey KS, Dewey CW, Boothe DM, Barone G, Kortz GD. Levetiracetam as an adjunct to phenobarbital treatment in cats with suspected idiopathic epilepsy. J Am Vet Med Assoc. 2008;232(6):867–72.
41. Dewey CW, Barone G, Boothe DM, Smith K, O'Connor JH. The use of oral levetiracetam as an add-on anticonulsant drug in cats receiving phenobarbital. In: *ACVIM forum*, vol. 19. Baltimore, MD: Journal of Veterinary Internal Medicine; 2005. p. 458.
42. Carnes MB, Axlund TW, Boothe DM. Pharmacokinetics of levetiracetam after oral and intravenous administration of a single dose to clinically normal cats. Am J Vet Res. 2011;72(9):1247–52.
43. Barnard LR, Barnes Heller HL. Pharmacokinetic analysis of single dose extended release levetiracetam per os in healthy cats. In: *Journal of Veterinary Internal Medicine: 2017. Maryland: National Harbor*, 2017. p. 1225–361.
44. Schwartz-Porsche D, Kaiser E. Feline epilepsy. Probl Vet Med. 1989;1(4):628–49.
45. Center SA, Elston TH, Rowland PH, Rosen DK, Reitz BL, Brunt JE, Rodan I, House J, Bank S, Lynch LR, et al. Fulminant hepatic failure associated with oral administration of diazepam in 11 cats. J Am Vet Med Assoc. 1996;209(3):618–25.
46. Hughes D, Moreau ER, Overall LK, Van Winkle JT. Acute heptic necrosis and liver failure associated with benzodiazepine thereapy in six cats, 1986-1995. The Journal of Veterinary Emergency and Critical Care. 1996;6(1):13–12o.
47. Sawchuk AS, Parker JA, Neff-Davis C, Davis EL. Primidone in the cat. Journal of the American Animal Hospital Association. 1985;21:647–50.
48. Roye DB, Serrano EE, Hammer RH, Wilder BJ. Plasma kinetics of diphenylhydantoin in dogs and cats. Am J Vet Res. 1973;34(7):947–50.
49. Brewer DM, Cerda-Gonzalez S, Dewey CW. Zonisamide therapy for refractory seizures in five cats with presumptive idiopathic epilepsy. In: *ACVIM forum: 2010; California*: Journal of Veterinary Internal Medicine; 2010. p. 660–795.
50. Hasegawa D, Kobayashi M, Kuwabara T, Ohmura T, Fujita M, Orima H. Pharmacokinetics and toxicity of zonisamide in cats. J Feline Med Surg. 2008;10(4):418–21.
51. Ukai M, Hamamoto Y, Yu Y, Fujiwara-Igarashi A, Fujita M, Hasegawa D. Efficacy of zonisamide on interictal electroencephalography in familial spontaneous epileptic cats. Journal of Feline Medicine and Surgery. 2017;
52. Cautela MA, Dewey CW, Schwark WS, Cerda-Gonzalez S, Badgley BL. Pharmacokinetics of oral pregabalin in cats after single dose administration. In: *ACVIM forum: 2010. Anaheim, CA*: Journal of Veterinary Internal Medicine; 2010. p. 739–40.
53. Pellegrini A, Gloor P, Sherwin AL. Effect of valproate sodium on generalized penicillin epilepsy in the cat. Epilepsia. 1978;19(4):351–60.
54. Zoran DL, Boeckh A, Boothe DM. Hyperactivity and alopecia associated with ingestion of valproic acid in a cat. J Am Vet Med Assoc. 2001;218(10):1587–1589, 1580.
55. Dreimann E. Pharmakokinetik und klinische Nebenwirkungen der Antiepileptika Carbamazepin und Valproinsäure bei der Katze: Freie Universität Berlin; 1992.
56. Moher D, Liberati A, Tetzlaff J, Altman DG, Group P. Preferred reporting items for systematic reviews and meta-analyses the PRISMA statement. BMJ. 2009;339:b2535.
57. van Gelder NM, Koyama I, Jasper HH. Taurine treatment of spontaneous chronic epilepsy in a cat. Epilepsia. 1977;18(1):45–54.
58. Wada JA, Osawa T, Wake A, Corcoran ME. Effects of taurine on kindled amygdaloid seizures in rats, cats, and photosensitive baboons. Epilepsia. 1975;16(2):229–34.
59. Zaccara G, Franciotta D, Perucca E. Idiosyncratic adverse reactions to antiepileptic drugs. Epilepsia. 2007;48(7):1223–44.
60. Zaccara G, Gangemi PF, Cincotta M. Central nervous system adverse effects of new antiepileptic drugs. A meta-analysis of placebo-controlled studies. Seizure. 2008;17(5):405–21.

18

Haemodynamic changes during propofol induction in dogs: new findings and approach of monitoring

Andrea Cattai[1], Roberto Rabozzi[2*], Heidi Ferasin[3], Maurizio Isola[1] and Paolo Franci[1]

Abstract

Background: Propofol is one of the most widely used injectable anaesthetic agents in veterinary practice. Cardiovascular effects related to propofol use in dogs remain less well defined. The main objective of this study was to evaluate the haemodynamic changes during induction of general anaesthesia with propofol in healthy dogs, by a beat-to-beat continuous monitoring. All dogs were premedicated with intramuscular acepromazine (0.015 mg/kg) and methadone (0.15 mg/kg). Transthoracic echocardiography was used to measure the velocity time integral (VTI) of the left ventricular outflow tract. A syringe driver, programmed to deliver propofol 5 mg/kg over 30 s followed by a continuous infusion of 25 mg/kg/h, was used to induce and maintain anaesthesia. From the initiation of propofol administration, heart rate (HR) and mean invasive arterial blood pressure (MAP) were recorded every 5 s for 300 s, while aortic blood flow was continuously recorded and stored for 300 S. *maximum* cardiovascular depression was defined the lowest MAP (MAP_Tpeak) recorded during the monitored interval. VTI and VTI*HR were calculated at 0, 30, 90, 120, 150 and 300 s post administration of propofol, and at MAP_Tpeak. Haemodynamic effects of propofol in relation to plasma and biophase concentrations were also evaluated by pharmacokinetics simulation.

Results: The median (range) HR was significantly higher ($p = 0.006$) at the moment of maximum hemodynamic depression (Tpeak) [105(70–148) bpm] compared with pre-induction values (T0) [65(50–120) bpm]. The median (range) MAP was significantly lower ($p < 0.001$) at Tpeak [61(51–69) mmHg] compared with T0 [88(72–97) mmHg]. The median (range) VTI and VTI*HR were similar at the two time points [11.9(8.1–17.3) vs 13,3(9,4-16,5) cm, and 1172(806–1554) vs 1002(630–1159) cm*bpm, respectively].

Conclusions: Induction of anaesthesia with propofol causes a drop of arterial pressure in healthy dogs, however cardiac output is well maintained by compensatory chronotropic response. The magnitude of MAP_Tpeak may be strictly related with propofol plasma concentration.

Keywords: Propofol, Haemodynamic effects, Baroreflex, Anaesthesia, Transthoracic echocardiography, Dog

Background

Induction of anaesthesia in dogs can be accomplished by using propofol (2,6-di-isopropylphenol), one of the most widely used injectable anaesthetic agents in veterinary practice. Cardiovascular effects related to propofol use have been subjected to intense research, often using the dog as a research model and with conflicting results. Blood pressure (BP) decrease is a common finding when propofol is used to induce anaesthesia in dogs [1–7]. Several mechanisms have been suggested as possible contributory causes of cardiovascular effects of propofol at clinically relevant concentrations: decrease in left ventricular preload produced by direct venous vasodilatation [8, 9]; reduction in systemic vascular resistance by arterial relaxation, most likely due to inhibition of sympathetic nervous system activity [2, 10] and negative inotropic effect [11–13].

The heart rate response to propofol administration in dogs remains less well defined. After different doses of propofol administered intravenous (IV) in dogs, either a

* Correspondence: rob.rabozzi@gmail.com
[2]CVRS – Policlinico Veterinario Roma Sud, Rome, Italy
Full list of author information is available at the end of the article

significant increase of heart rate (HR) [1, 2] or no significant chronotropic effects [3–5, 7] have been reported. Propofol has also shown conflicting results on attenuation of baroreflex function in other species, either demonstrating no effect or attenuation related to propofol blood concentration [14–18].

One of the difficulties in monitoring hemodynamic changes during induction of general anaesthesia is the ability to record the rapidly occurring cardiovascular variations in a subject which moves from being fully conscious to being anaesthetised. Beat-to-beat monitoring of the cardiac stroke volume is crucial to accomplish this task. In this respect, transthoracic echocardiography has some advantages over other methods of cardiovascular monitoring, being a non-invasive technique that allows quantitative assessment of left ventricular function. Cardiac ultrasound machines are also widely available in the veterinary field and, therefore, it does not normally incur further financial expenses. Its use to monitor haemodynamic changes during anaesthesia has been reported [19, 20]. Doppler echocardiography can be used as a method to monitor velocity time integral (VTI) variations of the aortic blood flow during and after administration of drugs in dogs [21], which is commonly used to evaluate stroke volume (SV) variation on the same subject [21–26]. Pulsed Doppler echocardiographic assessment of cardiac output (CO) is a validated non-invasive method in humans [27, 28].

The aim of the present study was to investigate the haemodynamic changes produced by propofol, administered intravenously over 30 s in healthy dogs, through the use of continuous monitoring of electrocardiograph (ECG), invasive BP and trans-aortic flow over 300 s. Haemodynamic effects of propofol in relation to plasma and biophase concentrations were also evaluated by pharmacokinetics simulation.

Methods

The study was approved by the Ethic Committee of the University of Padua (Prot. N. 89,556).

Animals

Dogs admitted to the Ospedale Veterinario Roma Sud for various scheduled procedures were eligible for enrolment in the study. All animals underwent a physical examination and blood test analysis. Dogs were excluded from the study if owner consent was not granted, if the subject was assigned to American Society of Anesthesiology (ASA) physical status classification more than I, if they were < 1 year of age, or had a temperament that precluded use of a standard anaesthetic technique.

Study protocol

Dogs were premedicated with acepromazine 0.015 mg/kg (Fatro S.p.A., Ozzano dell'Emilia, Italy) and methadone 0.15 mg/kg (Dechra, Bladel, Netherlands) mixed in the same syringe and administered intramuscularly. After 40 min, two over-the-needle catheters were aseptically inserted, one into a cephalic vein and another one in a dorsal pedal artery. Cardiovascular and respiratory variables were monitored by a multiparameter monitor (Datex Ohmeda AS/3, GE Healthcare). Dogs were positioned in a right lateral recumbent position and continuous ECG monitoring and invasive BP monitoring was started. Hair was clipped over the xiphoid area. Transthoracic echocardiography was used to measure the VTI of the left ventricular outflow tract, with a phased array PA240 probe (Esaote MyLab 70 CV). Sweep speed during recordings was set to 240 Hz (180–300 Hz). Optimised subcostal standard view of the left ventricular inflow and outflow tracts was used for data acquisition. Two-dimensional cine loops and Doppler tracings were recorded and stored on the internal hard drive of the echocardiograph and off-line analysed. The system was set to store raw DICOM data.

In order to induce anaesthesia a 50 ml syringe loaded with propofol (Esteve, Milano, Italy) was mounted on a syringe driver (Graseby 3500, Smiths Medical, England), which was programmed to intravenously deliver 5 mg/kg over 30 s, followed by a continuous infusion of 25 mg/kg/h to induce and maintain anaesthesia. At 2 min from initiation of the infusion the dog was assessed the first time to determine if endotracheal intubation was possible. When weakened palpebral reflex, rostromedial rotation of the eyeball, reduction in jaw tone and lack of tongue withdrawal were obtained, endotracheal intubation was facilitated and the dog was connected to a circle breathing system for 100% oxygen delivery. If a dog became apnoeic (no spontaneous ventilation for 30 s) or hypercapnic, it was manually ventilated until it was able to spontaneously maintain normocapnia (35– 50 mmHg).

Trans-aortic flow was continuously recorded for 300 s, after the beginning of the infusion. Heart rate and systolic, diastolic and mean arterial blood pressure (MAP) were also recorded every 5 s for 300 s, using an electronic spread sheet throughout available via a commercial software (Monitor Software version 6.1, University of Hong Kong). Data were downloaded onto a laptop computer connected to the anaesthesia monitor by a serial port adaptor. Aortic velocity time integral was obtained from digital still images as a mean of 10 consecutive measurements, which were obtained during spontaneous breathing. Only high-quality images were used for data analysis. All measurements were made off-line by an investigator (RR). Maximum cardiovascular depression was defined the lowest MAP (MAP_Tpeak) recorded during the monitored interval (Tpeak). VTI and VTI*HR (minute distance) were calculated at 0, 30, 90, 120, 150 and 300 s post administration of propofol, and at Tpeak.

A pharmacokinetics (PK) simulation of the anaesthetic protocol used in this study was carried out, running on a personal computer the Computer Control Infusion Pump V.2.0E software, programmed with a validated PK model [29] and a specific K_{e0} [30]. During the simulation this software provided data of the predicted propofol plasma concentration, and the related estimated effect-site concentration every 5 s.

Statistical analysis

Continuous variables were checked for normal distribution by visual inspection of the bar graph, frequency of distribution and performing the Shapiro–Wilk normality test. Variables that were normally distributed were reported as the mean and standard deviation, whereas non-normally distributed variables were expressed as the median (range). Friedman Test was used to analyse differences within subjects and Dunn's post hoc test was applied. The significant level was set at 5%. According to a priori power analysis (Power = 80%, α = 0.05), based on previously reported data on HR and MAP variations in dogs treated with a similar anaesthesia protocol [7], ≥4 subjects needed to detect significant effects. Statistical analysis was performed using MedCalc Software version 12.6.1.0 and Dell Statistica Software version 13.1.

Results

Eight mixed breed dogs (2 males and 6 females) were included in this study. Median age and median body weight were 54 months (18–120 months) and 17 kg (6–35 kg), respectively. The median intubation time after the start of the propofol infusion was 140 (130–180) seconds. Neither apnoea, nor other anaesthetic-related adverse effects were observed.

The changes in haemodynamic variables, at different time points after the bolus of propofol, are shown in Table 1 and Figs 1, 2, 3 and 4. There was a significant increase in the HR at Tpeak ($p < 0.01$), 120 and 150 s ($p < 0.05$), compared to the baseline. There was a significant decrease in the MAP at Tpeak ($p < 0.001$), 90 and 300 s ($p < 0.05$), and in the VTI at 120, 150 and 300 s ($p < 0.05$).

Based on the pharmacokinetics simulation, the estimated peak plasma concentration ($6.24\mu gml^{-1}$) of propofol (Cmax) was reached after 30 s and at the time of equilibration between plasma and biophase (five and a half minutes) was $5.68\mu gml^{-1}$.

Discussion

In this study a bolus of 5 mg/kg of propofol, administered over 30 s IV, caused a rapid drop in arterial BP, however cardiac output was well maintained by a significant rise in HR.

The reduction in arterial BP, following propofol administration, can be due to any mechanism acting on both cardiac output and systemic vascular resistance. CO is expressed as the product of SV and HR. SV depends on three primary factors (preload, afterload, and myocardial contractility), all of which are interrelated. The direct negative inotropic effect of propofol seems to be relatively small when it is used within clinical concentrations [13, 31]. Most likely, the decrease in BP arises primarily as a result of the vasodilatory effect of propofol. This could be due to both, a reduction of sympathetic tone and a direct effect on smooth muscle. Induction of anaesthesia with propofol in dogs has been demonstrated to result in a dose-dependent decrease of systemic vascular resistance [2].

Arterial baroreflex function is an important short-term neural control system for maintaining cardiovascular stability. Attenuation of this reflex by propofol, due to a central or peripheral effect on sympathetic nervous activity, has been reported in humans [17, 18]. Sato et al. [18] reported that an estimated blood propofol concentration of 5 $\mu g\ ml^{-1}$ would result in baroreflex inhibition. Running the pharmacokinetics simulation of the protocol of administration used in our study, this concentration was already achieved and exceeded at the end of the 30 s bolus of propofol. Other studies, in humans and other species, have shown no or only slight effects on baroreflex sensitivity

Table 1 Haemodynamic variables in dogs ($n = 8$) receiving a bolus of 5 mg/kg of propofol, administered over 30 s IV, at different time points

	Pre-induction	30 s	Tpeak 55 (50–60) sec	90 s	120 s	150 s	300 s
HR	65 (50–120)	76 (50–130)	105 (70–148))**	87 (54–162)	91 (55–154)*	106 (50-146)*	82 (53–135)
MAP	88 (72–92)	88 (71–99)	61 (51–69)***	70 (50-79)*	71 (59-82)	76 (49–90)	68 (61–88)*
VTI	13.3 (9.4–16.5)	12.2 (8–18)	11.9 (8.1–17.3)	11.5 (8.5–13.5)	11.8 (7.9–13.3)*	11.6 (7.7–14.3)*	10.9 (7.5–14.7)*
VTI*HR	1002 (63[illegible]-1159)	899 (537–1705)	1172 (806–1554)	952 (629–1377)	1053 (678–1262)	1082 (593–1516)	950 (616–1254)

Tpeak, moment of maximum haemodynamic depression; HR, heart rate (beats minute-1); MAP, mean arterial pressure (mmHg); VTI, velocity time integral (centimetres)
Data expressed as median (range)
Values significantly different from pre-induction
*$0.01 < p < 0.05$
**$0.001 < p < 0.01$
***$p < 0.001$

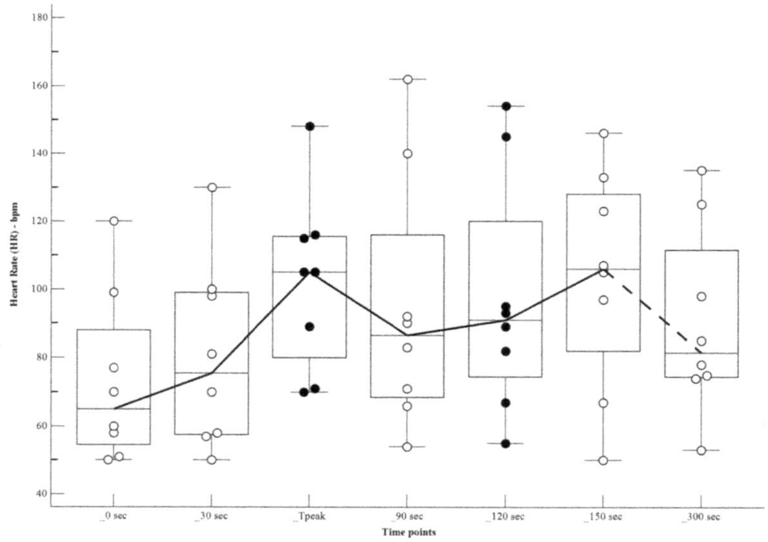

Fig. 1 Values of heart rate (beats minute^{-1}) in dogs ($n = 8$) receiving a bolus of propofol at different time points. The central box represents the values from the lower to upper quartile. The middle line represents the median. Time points non-significantly different (empty circles) and significantly different (full circles) from the baseline

[14–16]. Our results in dogs seem to be in agreement with the latter. The continuous recording of arterial BP in this study allowed identification of the time of maximal hemodynamic depression as occurring after about one minute [55 (50–60) sec] from the start of propofol administration. Based on the pharmacokinetics simulation, the Cmax of propofol was reached close to MAP_Tpeak, while the peak of the estimated propofol biophase concentration occurred about four and a half minutes later. In humans, the maximal BP depression is reached about 2.5 min after the administration of a bolus of propofol to induce anaesthesia [16, 32]. This delay is similar to the time to peak propofol effect-site concentration that is reported for adult patients [32, 33]. This remarkable difference suggests that the mechanism mainly involved in causing the decrease of BP may be different between the two species. Looking at the time to peak effect in humans, which is quite close to the peak of cardiovascular

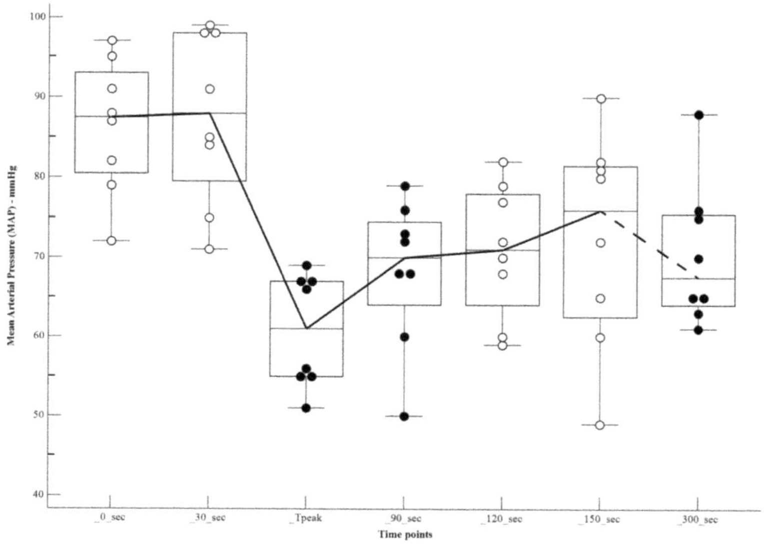

Fig. 2 Values of mean arterial pressure (mmHg) in dogs ($n = 8$) receiving a bolus of propofol at different time points. The central box represents the values from the lower to upper quartile. The middle line represents the median. Time points non-significantly different (empty circles) and significantly different (full circles) from the baseline

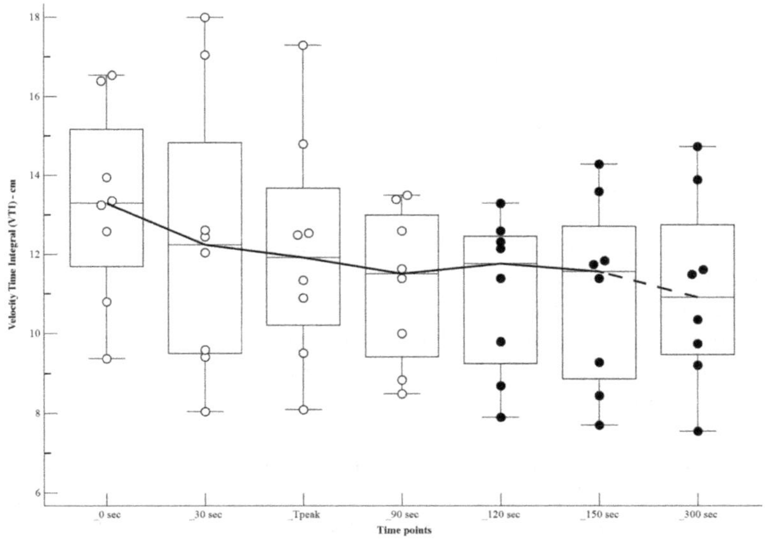

Fig. 3 Values of velocity time integral (centimetres) in dogs ($n = 8$) receiving a bolus of propofol at different time points. The central box represents the values from the lower to upper quartile. The middle line represents the median. Time points non-significantly different (empty circles) and significantly different (full circles) from the baseline

depression, it is likely that a drop in BP in this species occurs mainly by a centrally mediated mechanism. Based on findings of our study in dogs the MAP_Tpeak happens much earlier than the peak effect after a bolus of propofol. This would suggest that haemodynamic depression may not be mainly mediated by a central mechanism but could rather be a peripheral interaction within the vascular bed.

The study setting presented in this work offers an acceptable solution when studying rapidly occurring hemodynamic events in a clinical environment. These studies have to accomplish with two substantial requirements, a continuous beat-to-beat monitoring, enable recording instantaneous variations of hemodynamic variables and an ethically acceptable way of doing it. Both transthoracic echocardiography and invasive blood pressure measurement could provide the above-mentioned tasks, allowing us to collect data before and over the entire induction time. Moreover, adequate equipment and clinical competence to run this type of

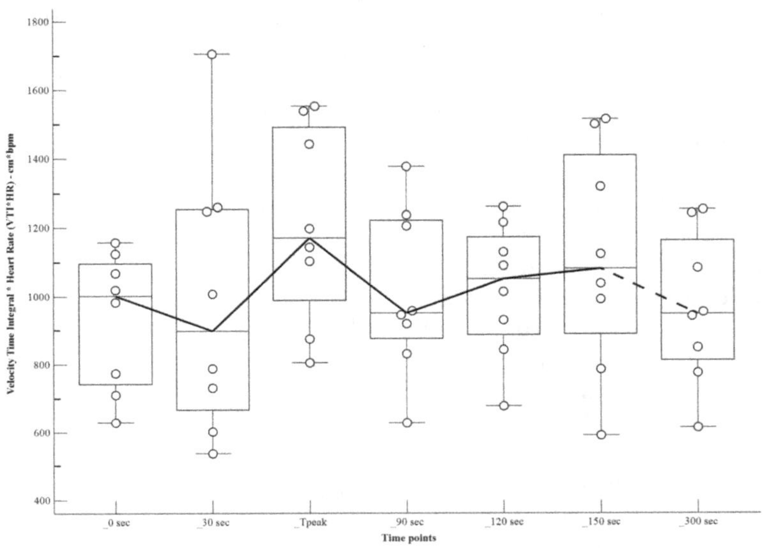

Fig. 4 Values of velocity time integral*heart rate (centimetres*beats minute^{-1}) in dogs ($n = 8$) receiving a bolus of propofol at different time points. The central box represents the values from the lower to upper quartile. The middle line represents the median. Time points non-significantly different (empty circles) and significantly different (full circles) from the baseline

cardiac scanning and images interpretation are commonly available in the vast majority of the veterinary hospitals.

A significant increase in heart rate after propofol administration was previously reported, but in chronically instrumented dogs [1, 2]. Other authors found a non-statistically-significant increase in heart rate after BP drop following induction with similar dose of propofol [4, 5, 7], however, cardiovascular variables were not measured immediately after injection of propofol and continuous monitoring methods were not used.

Without actual determinations of plasma propofol concentrations the predictions of the pharmacokinetics simulation could be imprecise, as related to the predictive performance of the Beths PK model (median bias of the predictions −3.05%, median inaccuracy 27.15% in their validation study). In addition, the effect-site equilibration constant used to describe the delay equilibration between the plasma concentration and the drug effect, could not be the most accurate. The value of K_{e0} can be determined from complex studies combining blood concentrations with frequent measurements of drug effect, unfortunately, in the dog, it has been little studied.

Considering that the reduction in blood pressure following a bolus of propofol is closely related to blood plasma drug concentration, a different speed of injection of the bolus may well have produced different degrees of variation in blood pressure within this group of dogs, especially as this finding has already been demonstrated in sheep [34].

This study has some limitations. The use of acepromazine and methadone as a premedication before propofol induction may have had some impact on the cardiovascular system. Acepromazine is an α1-adrenergic receptor antagonist that induces dose-dependent negative haemodynamic changes in dogs: a low dose of 0.05 mg/kg (three times the dose used in this study) administered IV has been shown to potentiate isoflurane-induced vasodilation without altering CO [35]. However, the same dose administered intramuscularly was shown to reduce BP at 5 and 15 min and HR at 5 min, compared with baseline values [36]. Methadone alone could cause dose-dependent sedation and a decrease in HR [37], an effect most likely attributable to a centrally mediated increase in vagal tone [38]. Nevertheless, premedication facilitated arterial catheter placement, reduced the pre-operative stress and excitement in dogs which itself would have had a greater haemodynamic influence, due to sympathetic stimulation, and allowed to use properly the Beths PK model for propofol.

In this study the minute distance, used as analogue of CO, did not change significantly at MAP_Tpeak (mild increase). However, considering the fairly small number of subject, it is possible that a significant effect was not detected. Despite this limitation of the study, our finding is consistent with previous results in premedicated [7] or unpremedicated [2, 3] dogs, in which CO remained essentially unchanged from the pre-induction value after administration of a similar or higher dose of propofol (4 to 15 mg/kg). Nevertheless, neither SV nor CO was directly measured throughout this study. The CO can be calculated by multiplying the cross-sectional area of the aorta * VTI * HR, however, comparing different values on the same subject, the first can be omitted in the calculation. In order to measure SV variation, the left ventricular outflow tract (LVOT) VTI was monitored. LVOT-VTI, or 'stroke distance', is commonly used as SV surrogate to measure variation of the left ventricular ejection on the same subject in human clinical studies [24–27]. Its use is reported also in animals [21–23]. VTI*HR, or 'minute distance', is directly related to cardiac output and has often been used as a useful alternative measure to evaluate the CO, particularly when more invasive methods are not available [21, 27, 39–41].

In this study, neither apnoea, nor other anaesthetic-related adverse effects were observed during induction and in the following minutes, despite these reported to be possible after propofol administration in other studies [42, 43]. Observing HR trend at the different time points a second peak at 150 s can be notice. This could be a consequence of a sympathetic stimulation, due to endotracheal intubation [32].

Conclusions

In conclusion, this study has found that in healthy premedicated dogs, a bolus of propofol administered IV over 30 s causes a transitory drop in blood pressure, however the cardiac output was well maintained due to a raise in heart rate. We have also found that MAP_Tpeak happens closely to predicted Cmax and, therefore, their magnitude may be strictly related. To investigate how other drugs commonly used as part of canine anaesthetic protocols (such as alpha2-agonists or short-acting opioids) can affect reflex heart rate response following propofol administration, and how a reduction of the magnitude of Cmax can mitigate MAP_Tpeak, may be an interesting field of research.

Abbreviations

BP: Blood pressure; Cmax: Estimated peak plasma concentration of propofol; CO: Cardiac output; HR: Heart rate; IV: Intravenous; LVOT: Left ventricular outflow tract; MAP: Mean invasive arterial blood pressure; MAP_Tpeak: Lowest MAP recorded; PK: Pharmacokinetic; SV: Stroke volume Tpeak: Moment of maximum hemodynamic depression; VTI: Velocity time integral

Acknowledgements

The authors thank Barbara Contiero for technical assistance.

Funding

This research did not receive any specific grant from funding agencies in the public, commercial, or not-for-profit sectors.

Authors' contributions

AC and RR designed the study, acquired and analyzed the data. HF, MI and PF contributed to the interpretation of data, drafting and revision of the manuscript. All authors participated in writing the manuscript and approved the final version.

Consent for publication

Not applicable

Competing interests

The authors declare that they have no competing interests.

Author details

[1]Department of Animal Medicine, Production and Health, Agripolis, Università degli Studi di Padova, Padua, Italy. [2]CVRS – Policlinico Veterinario Roma Sud, Rome, Italy. [3]Specialist Veterinary Cardiology Consultancy, Lymington Bottom, Four Marks, Hampshire, UK.

References

1. Mayer N, Legat K, Weinstabl C, Zimpfer M. Effects of propofol on the function of normal, collateral-dependent, and ischemic myocardium. Anesth Analg. 1993;76:33–9.
2. Wouters PF, Van de Velde M, Marcus M, Deruyter HA, Van Aken H. Hemodynamic changes during induction of anesthesia with eltanolone and propofol in dogs. Anesth Analg. 1995;81:125–31.
3. Quandt JE, Robinson EP, Rivers WJ, Raffe MR. Cardiorespiratory and anesthetic effects of propofol and thiopental in dogs. Am J Vet Re. 1998;59: 1137–43.
4. Musk GC, Pang DS, Beths T, Flaherty DA. Target-controlled infusion of propofol in dogs--evaluation of four targets for induction of anaesthesia. Vet Rec. 2005;157:766–70.
5. Sams L, Braun C, Allman D, Hofmeister E. A comparison of the effects of propofol and etomidate on the induction of anesthesia and on cardiopulmonary parameters in dogs. Vet Anaesth Analg. 2008;35:488–94.
6. Silva A, Ribeiro LM, Bressan N, Oliveira P, Ferreira DA, Antunes LM. Dogs mean arterial pressure and heart rate responses during high propofol plasma concentrations estimated by a pharmacokinetic model. Res Vet Sci. 2011;91:278–80.
7. Henao-Guerrero N, Riccó CH. Comparison of the cardiorespiratory effects of a combination of ketamine and propofol, propofol alone, or a combination of ketamine and diazepam before and after induction of anesthesia in dogs sedated with acepromazine and oxymorphone. Am J Vet Re. 2014;75:231–9.
8. Goodchild CS, Serrao JM. Cardiovascular effects of Propofol in the anesthetized dog. Br J Anaest. 1989;63:87–92.
9. Pagel PS, Hettrick DA, Kersten JR, Lowe D, Warltier DC. Cardiovascular effects of propofol in dogs with dilated cardiomyopathy. Anesthesiology. 1998;88:180–9.
10. Claeys MA, Gepts E, Camu F. Haemodynamic changes during anaesthesia induced and maintained with propofol. Br J Anaesth. 1988;60:3–9.
11. Pagel PS, Warltier DC. Negative inotropic effects of propofol as evaluated by the regional preload recruitable stroke work relationship in chronically instrumented dogs. Anesthesiology. 1993;78:100–8.
12. Nagashima Y, Furukawa Y, Chiba S. Propofol decreases contractility of isolated blood-perfused left ventricular muscle in the dog. J Anesth. 2000; 14:45–7.
13. Fujinaka W, Shimizu J, Iribe G, Imaoka T, Oshima Y, Kiyooka T, Morita K, Mohri S. Efects of propofol on left ventricular mechanoenergetics in the excised cross-circulated canine heart. Acta Med Okayama. 2012;66:435–42.
14. Cullen PM, Turtle M, Prys-Roberts C, Way WL, Dye J. Effect of propofol anesthesia on baroreflex activity in humans. Anesth Analg. 1987;66:1115–20.
15. Blake DW, Jover B, Mcgrath BP. Haemodynamic and heart rate reflex responses to propofol in the rabbit: Comparison with althesin. Br J Anaesth. 1988;61:194–9.
16. Sellgren J, Biber B, Henriksson B, Martner J, Pontén J. The effects of propofol, methohexitone and isoflurane on the baroreceptor reflex in the cat. Acta Anaesthesiol Scand. 1992;36:784–90.
17. Ebert TJ, Muzi M, Berens R, Goff D, Kampine JP. Sympathetic response to induction of anesthesia in humans with propofol or etomidate. Anesthesiology. 1992;76:725–33.
18. Sato M, Tanaka M, Umehara S, Nishikawa T. Baroreflex control of heart rate during and after propofol infusion in humans. Br J Anaesth. 2005;94:577–81.
19. Saeian K, Wann LS, Sagar KB. Doppler echocardiographic evaluation of left ventricular function. Echocardiography. 1990;7:21–5.
20. Yang HS, Song BG, Kim JY, Kim SN, Kim TY. Impact of propofol anesthesia induction on cardiac function in low-risk patients as measured by intraoperative Doppler tissue imaging. J Am Soc Echocardiogr. 2013;26:727–35.
21. Sohn S, Kim HS, Han JJ. Doppler flow velocity measurement to assess changes in Inotropy and Afterload : a study in healthy dogs. Echocardiography. 2002;19:207–13.
22. Young LE, Blissitt KJ, Clutton RE, Molony V. Haemodynamic effects of a sixty minute infusion of dopamine hydrochloride in horses anaesthetised with halothane. Equine Vet J. 1998;30:310–6.
23. Slama M, Masson H, Teboul J, Arnout M, Susic D, Frohlich E, Andrejak M. Respiratory variations of aortic VTI: a new index of hypovolemia and fluid responsiveness. Am J Physiol Heart Circ Physiol. 2002;283:1729–33.
24. Thomas DE, Yousef ZR, Fraser AG. A critical comparison of echocardiographic measurements used for optimizing cardiac resynchronization therapy: stroke distance is best. Eur J Heart Fail. 2009;11:779–88.
25. Pereira de Souza Neto E, Grousson S, Duflo DFC, Joly H, Convert J, Mottolese C, Dailler F, Cannesson M. Predicting fluid responsiveness in mechanically ventilated children under general anaesthesia using dynamic parameters and transthoracic echocardiography. Br J Anaesth. 2011;106:856–64.
26. Navaratnam M, Punn R, Ramamoorthy T, Tacy TA. LVOT-VTI is a useful Indicator of low ventricular function in young patients. Pediatr Cardiol. 2017; 38:1148–54.
27. Richardson JR, Ferguson J, Hiscox J, Rawles J. Non-invasive assessment ofcardiac output in children. J Accid Emerg Med. 1998;15:304–7.
28. Lewis JF, Kuo LC, Nelson JG, Limacher MC, Quinones MA. Pulsed Doppler echocardiographic determination of stroke volume and cardiac output: clinical validation of two new methods using the apical window. Circulation. 1984;70:425–31.
29. Beths T, Reid J, Monteiro AM, Nolan AM. Evaluation and optimisation of a target controlled infusion system for administering propofol to dogs as part of a total intravenous anaesthetic technique during dental surgery. Vet Rec. 2001;148:198–203.
30. Brás S, Bressan N, Ribeiro L, Ferreira DA, Antunes L, Nunes CS. A step towards effect-site target-controlled infusion with propofol in dogs: a k(e0) for propofol. J Vet Pharmacol Ther. 2009;32:182–8.
31. Ismail EF, Kim SJ, Salem R, Crystal GJ. Direct effects of Propofol on myocardial contractility in in situ canine hearts. Anesthesiology. 1992;77:964–72.
32. Billard V, Moulla F, Bourgain JL, Megnigbeto A, Stanski DR. Hemodynamic response to induction and intubation. Anesthesiology. 1994;81:1384–93.
33. Struys MM, Coppens MJ, De Neve N, Mortier EP, Doufas AG, Van Bocxlaer JF, Shafer SL. Influence of administration rate on propofol plasma-effect site equilibration. Anesthesiology. 2007;107:386–96.
34. Zheng D, Upton RN, Martinez AM, Grant C, Ludbrook GL. The influence of the bolus injection rate of Propofol on its cardiovascular effects and peak blood concentrations in sheep. Anesth Analg. 1998;86:1109–15.
35. Sinclair MD, Dyson DH. The impact of acepromazine on the efficacy of crystalloid, dextran or ephedrine treatment in hypotensive dogs under isoflurane anesthesia. Vet Anaesth Analg. 2012;39:563–73.
36. Grasso SC, Ko JC, Weil AB, Paranjape V, Constable PD. Hemodynamic influence of acepromazine or dexmedetomidine premedication in isoflurane-anesthetized dogs. J Am Vet Med Assoc. 2015;246:754–64.
37. Menegheti TM, Wagatsuma JT, Pacheco AD, Perez B, Pacheco CM, Abimussi CJ, dos Santos PP, de Souza Oliva VN. Electrocardiographic evaluation of the degree of sedation and the isolated use of methadone in healthy dogs. Vet Anaesth Analg. 2014;41:97–104.
38. Stanley TH, Liu WS, Webster LR, Johansen RK. Haemodynamic effects of intravenous methadone anaesthesia in dogs. Can Anaesth Soc J. 1980;27:52–7.

39. Weiner Z, Farmakides G, Schulman H, Casale A, Itskovitz-Eldor J. Central and peripheral haemodynamic changes in post-term fetuses: correlation with oligohydramnios and abnormal fetal heart rate pattern. Br J Obstet Gynaecol. 1996;103:541–6.
40. Grow MP, Singh A, Fleming NW, Young N, Watnik M. Cardiac output monitoring during off-pump coronary artery bypass grafting. J Cardiothorac Vasc Anesth. 2004;18:43–6.
41. Goldberg DJ, French B, Szwast AL, McBride MG, Marino BS, Mirarchi N, Hanna BD, Wernovsky G, Paridon SM, Rychik J. Impact of sildenafil on echocardiographic indices of myocardial performance after the fontan operation. Pediatr Cardiol. 2012;33:689–96.
42. Smith JA, Gaynor JS, Bednarski RM, Muir WW. Adverse effects of administration of propofol with various preanesthetic regimens in dogs. J Am Vet Med Assoc. 1993;202:1111–5.
43. Cattai A, Rabozzi R, Natale V, Franci P. The incidence of spontaneous movements (myoclonus) in dogs undergoing total intravenous anaesthesia with propofol. Vet Anaesth Analg. 2015;42:93–8.

Phase II study of the oral selective inhibitor of nuclear export (SINE) KPT-335 (verdinexor) in dogs with lymphoma

Abbey R. Sadowski[1†], Heather L. Gardner[2†], Antonella Borgatti[3], Heather Wilson[4], David M. Vail[5], Joshua Lachowicz[6], Christina Manley[7], Avenelle Turner[8], Mary K. Klein[9], Angharad Waite[10], Alexandra Sahora[11] and Cheryl A. London[1,12*]

Abstract

Background: Chemotherapeutic options for the treatment of canine lymphoma have not changed in several decades necessitating the identification of new therapeutics to improve patient outcome. KPT-335 (verdinexor) is a novel orally bioavailable selective inhibitor of nuclear export (SINE) that exhibited anti-tumor activity against non-Hodgkin lymphoma in a prior phase I study. The objective of this phase II study was to expand upon the initial findings and assess the activity and safety in a larger population of dogs with lymphoma.

Results: Fifty-eight dogs with naïve or progressive B-cell and T-cell lymphoma were enrolled in this clinical trial. KPT-335 was administered orally in one of three dosing groups, based on the previously established biologically active dose of 1.5 mg/kg three times weekly. Treatment with single-agent, orally administered KPT-335 resulted in an objective response rate (ORR) of 37%, of which dogs with T-cell lymphoma had an ORR of 71%. KPT-335 was well tolerated in all dose groups with grade 1–2 anorexia being the most common adverse event. Anorexia was responsive to symptomatic and supportive medications, including prednisone.

Conclusions: These data demonstrate that KPT-335 has biologic activity in canine lymphoma, and support continued evaluation of SINE compounds such as KPT-335 in combination with standard chemotherapeutics in canine lymphoma.

Keywords: Non-Hodgkin lymphoma, Nuclear export, Clinical trial, Anti-tumor agent

Background

The transport of specific proteins between the nucleus to the cytoplasm is critical for the normal function of tumor suppressor proteins (TSP) and growth regulatory proteins (GRP). Neoplastic cells utilize the process of nucleo-cytoplasmic transport to export known TSP and GRP outside of the nucleus, inactivating these pathways and overcoming the normal cell cycle and genomic instability checkpoints [1, 2]. Nuclear export of proteins depends on the activity of transport proteins called exportins. Exportin-1, also known as XPO1, is the main mediator of nuclear export. XPO1 inhibition forces the nuclear retention of key TSP and GRP such as p53, p21, pRB, FOXO and NF-κB [3, 4].

XPO1 is overexpressed in many hematologic and nonhematologic malignancies in humans and is associated with a poor prognosis in aggressive diseases [3]. Several small molecule inhibitors targeting XPO1 have been investigated, including KPT-251, KPT-276 and KPT-330 [5]. A phase I study of orally administered KPT-330 showed safety and feasibility of long-term treatment in a variety of patients with advanced solid tumors. Out of 157 patients, 27 patients (17%) achieved stable disease for four months or longer [6]. Given the safety profile and cytotoxic effects of KPT-330 on rapidly proliferating leukemia cells in animal models and patient samples, several studies have investigated the efficacy and safety of KPT-330

* Correspondence: Cheryl.London@tufts.edu
†Abbey R. Sadowski and Heather L. Gardner contributed equally to this work.
[1]Cummings School, Tufts University, Foster Hospital for Small Animals, 200 Westboro Rd, N. Grafton, MA 01536, USA
[12]Department of Veterinary Biosciences, College of Veterinary Medicine, The Ohio State University, Columbus, OH, USA
Full list of author information is available at the end of the article

in refractory or relapsed acute myeloid leukemia and non-Hodgkin's lymphoma [7, 8]. KPT-330 was efficacious in refractory or relapsed AML patients, with a greater than 50% decrease in bone marrow blasts and significant improvement in overall survival in responders vs. nonresponders (9.7 months vs 2.7 months) [9]. Similarly, a phase I trial of people with relapsed or refractory lymphoma showed an objective response rate of 31% (22/71 patients) [10]. Therefore, XPO1 is an attractive target for patients with aggressive hematologic cancers.

KPT-335 is an orally bioavailable selective inhibitor of nuclear export (SINE) that transiently binds to XPO1 in a slowly reversible manner [3, 4]. KPT-335 was recently shown to be safe and biologically active in a phase I study of dogs with spontaneous cancer [11]. The maximum tolerated dose was found to be 1.75 mg/kg administered twice weekly, with biologic activity observed at 1 mg/kg. Clinical benefit was seen in 9/14 dogs with Non-Hodgkin's lymphoma leading to a dose expansion study of 6 dogs given KPT-335 at 1.5 mg/kg on Monday/Wednesday/Friday. Clinical benefit was demonstrated in 4 out of the 6 dogs [11].

The primary objective of this phase II study was to build upon the phase I study findings, and describe the safety and anti-tumor activity of oral KPT-335 in dogs with naïve lymphoma, or after a single relapse. These data will provide information on the best use of SINE compounds in future clinical studies.

Methods

Clinical trial eligibility

This clinical trial was approved by the Animal Clinical Investigation (ACI) Animal Care and Use Committee (ACUC); IACUC or equivalent approval was obtained at all participating study sites. Written informed consent was obtained from each pet owner prior to study entry. KPT-335 was administered to dogs with newly diagnosed or first relapse B-cell or T-cell non-Hodgkin's lymphoma (NHL). Dogs were administered KPT-335 orally until disease progression or intolerance to the drug. To be eligible for the study, each dog must have had a cytologic or histologic diagnosis of B or T cell lymphoma and met all the inclusion criteria and none of the exclusion criteria. Eligibility criteria included: at least 1 year of age, at least one measurable peripherally located tumor-infiltrated lymph node, adequate organ function, dogs with naïve lymphoma or experiencing first relapse on study entry, completion of any prior chemotherapy at least 14 days prior to study entry and no evidence of central nervous system involvement or concomitant serious systemic disorder as determined by the supervising clinician.

KPT-335 formulation

KPT-335 was prepared as whole tablets of 2.5, 10 and 50 mg strengths of active ingredient (KABS – St-Hubert Quebec, Canada), using pharmaceutical grade excipients.

Study design

This was a phase II open-label field study of the safety and anti-tumor activity of KPT-335 in client owned dogs with lymphoma. Analysis of dogs for tumor response was performed by caliper measurement of the longest diameter of a maximum of five lesions. Tumor response was determined using the VCOG peripheral nodal lymphoma response criteria [12]. A partial response (PR) was identified if the target lesions demonstrated at least a 30% decrease in the mean sum of the longest diameter. A complete response (CR) was defined as complete disappearance of disease, evaluated by caliper measurements. Progressive disease was defined by at least a 20% increase in the mean sum of the longest diameter, using the smallest sum since initiation of the clinical trial as a reference, or any new lesion. Dogs were assessed as having stable disease (SD) if they did not meet the criteria for PR or PD. Assessment of hematologic and biochemical toxicities was performed at screening and every 7 days until day 28, and then every 2 weeks until study discontinuation. Time to progression (TTP) was defined as the period of time from the first date of treatment to the date that the dog developed progressive disease because of clinical or radiographic progressive disease or death from any cause, including euthanasia. Duration of Response (DOR) was defined as the period of time between the first of two evaluations demonstrating an objective response until the date of progression or death. Disease Control Rate (DCR) was defined as the number of patients with confirmed complete or partial responses, OR stable disease, as a percentage of all patients treated with KPT-335 in this protocol. Objective Response Rate (ORR) was defined as the number of patients with confirmed complete or partial responses as a percentage of all evaluable patients treated with KPT-335 in this protocol.

Dogs were initially treated with 1.5 mg/kg KPT-335 orally three times weekly (Monday, Wednesday, Friday) (Group 1) based on previous data showing safety and clinical benefit in dogs at this dose [11]. Two additional dosing groups were implemented at a decreased dose of 1.25 mg/kg PO three times weekly (Group 2) and 1.25 mg/kg PO twice weekly for 2 weeks then 1.5 mg/kg PO twice weekly thereafter (Group 3).

Treatment administration and adverse events

KPT-335 was administered orally using whole tablets immediately following feeding. Adverse events (AEs) were reported using the Veterinary Cooperative Oncology

Group- common terminology criteria for adverse events, VCOG-CTCAE v 1.1 [12]. AEs were defined as any expected or unexpected grade 1, 2, or 3 toxicity, whereas a Serious Adverse Event (SAE) was any expected or unexpected grade 4 or 5 toxicity. Dose reductions (0.25 mg/kg) or temporary drug discontinuation not extending beyond 7 days were permitted in dogs experiencing AEs.

Concomitant medications

No concomitant anti-neoplastic therapy (chemotherapy, immunotherapy, radiation therapy) was permitted during the clinical trial. Low-dose prednisone (0.5–1.0 mg/kg/day) was permitted if necessary to treat AEs, and was also permitted in dogs already receiving prednisone that demonstrated PD at study entry. Supportive care medications were administered as clinically needed to treat drug-related toxicities. These included metoclopramide, ondansetron, maropitant, famotidine, ranitidine, omeprazole, metronidazole and loperamide. Other supportive medications permitted included butorphanol, tramadol, fentanyl, diphenhydramine, s-adenosylmethionine and mirtazapine.

Pharmacokinetics analysis

Complete pharmacokinetic (PK) sampling was performed on 8 dogs. Blood samples were collected at 0, 1, 2, 4, 6, 8, 12 and 24 h on day 14, with the exception of one dog who had PK sampling on day 21. A minimum of 2 ml of whole blood was collected in an EDTA tube. The sample was centrifuged at room temperature (3000 rpm for 10 min) and cells were separated from the plasma. Plasma was aliquoted into cryovials and stored in liquid nitrogen within 20 min of collection. Plasma samples were analyzed for KPT-335 using a validated LC/MS/MS method. Parameters evaluated included peak concentration (Cmax), time of observed maximum concentration (Tmax), terminal half-life $t_{1/2}$, Area under the curve (AUC) of analyte vs. time curve from time zero to infinity (AUC_{inf}), AUC of analyte vs. time curve from time zero to the time of the last measurable concentration (AUC_{last}).

Results

Patient demographics

A total of 58 dogs were enrolled and received at least one dose of KPT-335 across 10 study sites. Thirty-five dogs with naïve lymphoma and 23 dogs at the time of their first relapse were enrolled in this clinical trial. Of the 35 naïve cases, 28 dogs had B-cell lymphoma and 7 dogs had T-cell lymphoma. The majority of dogs were classified as having stage III or IV lymphoma ($n = 31$) based on staging tests including physical examination, complete blood count, serum biochemical panel and thoracic radiographs. The mean age of chemotherapy-naïve dogs was 7 years (median 7; range 3–12) and mean weight was 31 kg (median 31; range 6–85). The number of male dogs ($n = 20$, 2 intact) outnumbered female dogs ($n = 15$, all spayed). Of the 23 relapsed lymphoma patients, 14 had B-cell lymphoma and 7 had T-cell lymphoma. Two relapsed lymphoma patients did not have immunophenotyping. The mean weight and age of relapsed dogs was 27 kg (Median 28; range 5–52) and 8 years (Median 7; range 3–13), respectively. As with naïve lymphoma, males ($n = 16$, 2 intact) outnumbered females ($n = 7$, all spayed). Patient demographic data is summarized in Table 1. Of the 58 dogs enrolled in the study, 54 dogs were considered evaluable for responses. Dogs that were considered evaluable for response were dogs that had one baseline assessment and at least one lesion assessment two weeks following the start of therapy. All fifty-eight dogs were evaluated for AEs related to drug administration.

Response to therapy

For all dogs, the ORR was 37% (20/54) in the evaluable patient population. The median DOR was 18 days (range: 7–152), median TTP was 29 days (range: 7–244) and median study duration was 36 days (range: 7–273). Twenty dogs (36%) remained on study for at least 56 days. Of the evaluable patients with naïve lymphoma, the DCR was 33%, ORR 39%, and median DOR was 34 days. The DCR was 29%, ORR of 38% and median DOR was 19 days for dogs with relapsed NHL.

Time to Tumor progression was assessed for all dose groups. The median TTP was 43 days for naïve lymphoma patients ($n = 33$). The median TTP for relapse lymphoma patients was 24 days ($n = 21$). Table 2 illustrates the TTP data for each dosing group and the distinct immunophenotypes, with and without corticosteroid usage. Of note is the median TTP for first relapse dogs with T-cell lymphoma, with a TTP of 43 days ($n = 7$). The median TTP for dogs receiving corticosteroids on or after Day 0 was 73 days compared to dogs on corticosteroids prior to enrollment or not on corticosteroids (24 and 22 days, respectively).

Pharmacokinetics

Seven dogs underwent full PK analysis to determine KPT-335 plasma levels over a 24 h time period post KPT-335 administration on day 14. The dogs received KPT-335 at 1.5 mg/kg ($n = 4$) or 1.25 mg/kg ($n = 4$) on MWF dosing schedule. For all dogs, the mean Cmax was 278 ng/ml with a mean AUC of 1970.6 ng*t/ml, Tmax of 5.3 h and $T_{1/2}$ of 5 h. The mean Cmax and AUC for dogs receiving 1.5 mg/kg were slightly higher than dogs receiving 1.25 mg/kg (312 vs. 244.8 mg/ml and 2346.8 vs. 1576.5 ng*t/ml). Additionally, bioavailability and absorption efficiency of KPT-335 after oral administration is dependent

Table 1 Patient Demographics

	All (*N* = 58)	Group 1 (*N* = 13)	Group 2 (*N* = 35)	Group 3 (*N* = 10)
Median Weight (kg)	30.1	25.2	30.3	33.3
Range (Min, Max)	5, 85	6, 53	6, 85	5, 52
Median Age (yr)	7	7	7	7
Range (Min, Max)	3, 12	4, 12	3, 12	3, 13
Sex				
Female	22	7	11	2
Male	36	6	23	7
Stage				
II	1	0	1	0
III	36	7	21	6
IV	18	5	10	3
V	3	1	2	0
Immunophenotype				
B-cell (Naïve)	28	9	19	0
B-cell (Relapsed)	14	2	6	6
T-cell (Naïve)	7	1	6	0
T-cell (Relapsed)	7	1	3	3
Not Determined	2	0	1	1
Corticosteroid Use				
Prior prednisone	15	1	8	6
Prednisone use after enrollment	25	7	15	3
No prednisone use	18	5	11	1

on feeding, therefore corticosteroid administration to improve appetite in some patients may subsequently promote more consistent plasma drug levels.

Clinical toxicities

The most common AEs across all dose groups related to KPT-335 included: anorexia ($n = 27$, 45%), weight loss ($n = 18$, 31%), vomiting ($n = 15$, 26%), lethargy ($n = 10$, 17%) and diarrhea ($n = 7$, 12%). Most events were considered grade 1 or 2 (73/77, 95%).

No difference was observed in the AE profile when comparing dosing regimens (Additional file 1: Table S1). Of 9 dogs with serious adverse events, three had events attributed to the drug. These include weight loss, weakness and hepatopathy. Other events including hypercalcemia, respiratory distress and hemogram abnormalities occurred in the setting of disease progression and were unlikely to be related to KPT-335. Additionally, protein losing nephropathy was seen in one dog, and did not resolve after discontinuation of KPT-335.

Table 2 Patient Response Evaluation

	All (*N* = 54)	Group 1 (*N* = 13)	Group 2 (*N* = 31)	Group 3 (*N* = 10)
TTP (days)				
Naïve B-cell	44	71	35	–
Naïve T-cell	31	31	32.5	–
Relapsed B-cell	24	19	23	85
Relapsed T-cell	43	43	73	24
Objective Response (n)				
Naïve B-cell	8	4	4	–
Naïve T-cell	5	1	4	–
Relapsed B-cell	4	1	1	2
Relapsed T-cell	4	1	2	1

Discussion

Canine lymphoma is the most common hematopoietic neoplasm diagnosed in dogs [13, 14]. Multi-agent protocols used to treat canine lymphoma typically consist of a combination of prednisone, vincristine, cyclophosphamide and doxorubicin, with response rates > 80% and median survival times of 10–14 months reported [15]. Despite continued research efforts to improve upon patient outcome, the prognosis for canine lymphoma has remained unchanged for over 30 years. Therefore, leveraging novel therapeutic targets is necessary to improve outcomes in patients.

The oral compound, KPT-335, is a selective inhibitor of nuclear export (SINE). Many SINE compounds have been shown to inhibit cell growth and induce apoptosis in human and canine cancer cell lines including pancreatic, melanoma and mammary carcinomas [4, 16–19]. A phase I study of KPT-330 in humans with solid tumors reported stable disease in multiple tumor types including colorectal carcinoma, squamous cell carcinoma, prostatic carcinoma, melanoma and sarcomas [6]. Recently, KPT-335 was evaluated in dogs with cancer, and a dose of 1.5 mg/kg given three times weekly was tolerated and found to have a clinical benefit in dogs with lymphoma [11]. The most common adverse event associated with KPT-335 therapy in dogs was low grade anorexia. Given that the oral bioavailability of KPT-335 is significantly impacted by feeding, maintaining an appetite was important, and prednisone administration at a low dose was previously found to be effective in treating anorexia [11]. This study sought to expand upon the phase I clinical trial results to evaluate the biologic activity and tolerability of KPT-335 in naïve and relapsed canine NHL.

In the current study, KPT-335 was administered orally in three dose groups. KPT-335 was well tolerated across all dose groups with minimal SAEs reported. Consistent with prior publications, the most common AE was grade 1–2 anorexia, with only one dog that experienced severe (grade 3 or 4) anorexia. One dog experienced protein losing nephropathy which was suspected to be related to drug administration and resolved following discontinuation. Hepatopathy was also seen in one dog, and hepatopathies were also documented in the phase I study in several dogs dosed with KPT-335 at 1.5 mg/kg and 2.0 mg/kg [11]. Adverse events typically associated with cytotoxic chemotherapy were seen with this study (anorexia, vomiting, diarrhea), indicating combination therapy with KPT-335 and conventional chemotherapeutic agents may be challenging with agents that have similar adverse event profiles. A single study looking at the combination of KPT-330 with fludarabine and cytarabine in patients with refractory pediatric leukemia found the dose limiting toxicity to be cerebellar toxicity. Dose limiting toxicities previously observed with administration of KPT-330, including weight loss and anorexia, were not seen in this study, supporting further evaluation of standard chemotherapy combined XPO1 inhibitors such as KPT-335 [20].

A limitation of this study includes the variability of concurrent corticosteroid usage in patients. Since study enrollment required disease progression, it is the expectation that these tumors are refractory to corticosteroids, and therefore observed responses were likely due to KPT-335. First relapse and naïve NHL dogs that received corticosteroids after study enrollment to treat drug-associated anorexia received a median dose less than 0.5 mg/kg/day, with therapy initiated an average of 26 days after enrollment. Corticosteroids were initiated in these dogs while in a partial remission or experiencing stable disease, and additional measurable disease response was not noted in these patients, as would be expected if prednisone use was contributing to disease outcome. The prednisone doses used were well below the dose of corticosteroids typically used as anti-neoplastic therapy (1–2 mg/kg/day) and as KPT-335 was administered for several weeks prior to initiation of low-dose corticosteroids, would not be expected to impact disease progression. However, while the longer TTP noted in dogs receiving steroids after enrollment in the clinical trial could reflect inherent variability in sensitivity to KPT-335, a confounding effect of prednisone administration cannot be excluded. Prednisone has been previously shown to abrogate anorexia associated with KPT-335 more effectively than commercially available appetite stimulants at the time this study was completed, and was utilized in the present study for the same purpose. As mild anorexia is a known clinical toxicity of KPT-335, future studies may investigate the utility of novel appetite stimulants (i.e. capromorelin) to limit the confounding effects of oral corticosteroid use in dogs receiving KPT-335.

Consistent with the phase I clinical trial in spontaneous canine cancers, KPT-335 demonstrated biological activity in both relapsed and naïve canine NHL. KPT-330, another SINE compound, has been shown to produce an objective response in patients with refractory or relapsed hematologic malignancies [9, 10]. Taken together, these data support the notion that KPT-335 is effective in both naïve and relapsed lymphoma.

The overall median TTP was 43 and 24 days, which is consistent with expected single agent non-cytotoxic therapy for naïve and first relapse canine lymphoma [15]. Forty percent of patients remained on the study for at least 8 weeks, suggesting a substantial proportion of canine lymphoma patients have a significant, sustained benefit from KPT-335 treatment. The durability of KPT-330 as a single agent cancer therapy has also been demonstrated in refractory/relapsed acute myeloid leukemia patients by lengthening median progression-free survival [9]. Single agent targeted therapies can be associated with favorable initial responses, however combination therapy is often necessary to achieve sustained clinical responses. Combination therapy with XPO1 inhibitors, especially KPT-330, and conventional chemotherapeutic agents has shown promising synergistic effects in a variety of human tumor types [21, 22]. In light of previous studies with SINE compounds in human and canine cancers, the findings of this study may provide opportunities for combined therapy with KPT-335 and cytotoxic agents in human and canine patients that have developed resistance to standard chemotherapeutic agents and protocols across a variety of tumor types.

Conclusions

In summary, this phase II study illustrates the effectiveness and general safety of KPT-335 as a single agent therapy against naïve and first relapse canine lymphoma. Potential future directions include use of combining KPT-335 with cytotoxic chemotherapeutic agents in canine lymphoma.

Abbreviations

AE: Adverse event; AML: Acute myeloid leukemia; AUC: Area under the curve; Cmax: Peak concentration; CR: Complete response; DCR: Disease control rate; DOR: Duration of response; GRP: Growth regulatory proteins; NHL: Non-Hodgkin's lymphoma; ORR: Objective response rate; PK: Pharmacokinetics; PR: Partial response; SAE: Serious adverse event; SD: Stable disease; SINE: Selective inhibitor of nuclear export; Tmax: Time of observed maximum concentration; TSP: Tumor suppressor proteins; TTP: Time to progression; XPO1: Exportin-1

Acknowledgements

The ACI coordinated all aspects of this study, including generation of case report forms, collection of samples, data collation, and quality assurance. The content is solely the responsibility of the authors and does not necessarily represent the official views of the ACI or Karyopharm therapeutics.

Funding

Karopharm Therapeutics provided funding for this clinical trial.

Authors' contributions

CAL designed the clinical trial, assisted in case management, data analysis, and editing the manuscript. ARS wrote the majority of the manuscript. HLG assisted in manuscript editing. HWR, AB, DMV, JL, CM, AT, MKK, AW and AS entered patients into the clinical trial and assisted in case management. All authors read and approved the final manuscript.

Consent for publication

Not applicable.

Competing interests

Karyopharm Therapeutics provided funding and KPT-335 for this clinical trial. CAL has served as a paid consultant for Karyopharm. The authors declare that they have no competing interests.

Author details

[1]Cummings School, Tufts University, Foster Hospital for Small Animals, 200 Westboro Rd, N. Grafton, MA 01536, USA. [2]Sackler School of Graduate Biomedical Sciences, Tufts University, Boston, MA, USA. [3]College of Veterinary Medicine, University of Minnesota, St. Paul, MN, USA. [4]College of Veterinary Medicine, Texas A&M University, College Station, TX, USA. [5]Department of Medical Sciences, School of Veterinary Medicine University of Wisconsin-Madison, Madison, WI, USA. [6]NYC Veterinary Specialists/Blue Pearl Veterinary Specialists, New York, NY, USA. [7]The Oncology Service, The LifeCentre, Leesburg, VA, USA. [8]Veterinary Cancer Group, Culver City, CA, USA. [9]Southern Arizona Veterinary Specialty and Emergency Center, Tucson, AZ, USA. [10]The Oncology Service, Dogwood Veterinary Emergency and Specialty Center, Richmond, VA, USA. [11]The Oncology Service, Friendship Hospital for Animals, Washington DC, USA. [12]Department of Veterinary Biosciences, College of Veterinary Medicine, The Ohio State University, Columbus, OH, USA.

References

1. Turner JG, Dawson J, Sullivan DM. Nuclear export of proteins and drug resistance in cancer. Biochem Pharmacol. 2012;83:1021–32.
2. Nguyen KT, Holloway MP, Altura RA. The CRM1 nuclear export protein in normal development and disease. Int J Biochem Mol Biol. 2012;3:137–51.
3. Gravina GL, Senapedis W, McCauley D, Baloglu E, Shacham S, Festuccia C. Nucleo-cytoplasmic transport as a therapeutic target of cancer. J Hematol Oncol. 2014;7:85.
4. Parikh K, Cang S, Sekhri A, Delong L. Selective inhibitors of nuclear export (SINE)- a novel class of anti-cancer agents. J Hematol Oncol. 2014;7:78.
5. Walker CJ, Oaks JJ, Santhanam R, Neviani P, Harb JG, Ferenchak G, Ellis JJ, Landesman Y, Eisfeld AK, Gabrail NY, Smith CL, Caligiuri MA, Hokland P, Roy DC, Reid A, Milojkovic D, Goldman JM, Apperley J, Garzon R, Marcucci G, Shacham S, Kauffma MG, Perrotti D. Preclinical and clinical efficacy of XPO1/CRM1 inhibition by the karyopherin inhibitor KPT-330 in Ph^+ leukemias. Blood. 2013;122:3034–44.
6. Razak AR, Mau-Soerensen M, Gabrail NY, Gerecitano JF, Shields AF, Unger TJ, Saint-Martin JR, Carlson R, Landesman Y, McCauley D, Rashal T, Lassen U, Kim R, Stayner LA, Mirza MR, Kauffman M, Shacham S, Mahipal A. First-in-class, first-in-human phase I study of Selinexor, a selective inhibitor of nuclear export, in patients with advanced solid tumors. J Clin Oncol. 2016; 34:4142–50.
7. Ranganathan P, Yu X, Na C, Santhanam R, Shacham S, Kauffman M, Walker A, Klisovic R, Blum W, Caligiuri M, Croce CM, Marcucci G, Garzon R. Preclinical activity of a novel CRM1 inhibitor in acute myeloid leukemia. Blood. 2012;120:1765–73.
8. Etchin J, Sanda T, Mansour MR, Kentsis A, Montero J, Le BT, Christie AL, McCauley D, Rodig SJ, Kauffman M, Shacham S, Stone R, Letai A, Kung AL, Look AT. KPT-330 inhibitor of CRM1 (XPO1)-mediated nuclear export has selective anti-leukaemic activity in preclinical models of T-ALL and AML. Br J Haematol. 2013;161:117–27.
9. Garzon R, Savona M, Baz R, Andreeff M, Gabrail N, Gutierrez M, Savoie L, Mau-Sorensen PM, Wagner-Johnston N, Yee K, Unger TJ, Saint-Martin JR, Carlson R, Rashal T, Kashyap T, Klebanov B, Shacham S, Kauffman M, Stone R. A phase 1 clinical trial of single-agent selinexor in acute myeloid leukemia. Blood. 2017;129:3165–74.
10. Kuruvilla J, Savona M, Baz R, Mau-Sorensen PM, Gabrail N, Garzon R, Stone R, Wang M, Savoie L, Martin P, Flinn I, Jacoby M, Unger TJ, Saint-Martin JR, Rashal T, Friedlander S, Carlson R, Kauffman M, Shacham S, Gutierrez M. Selective inhibition of nuclear export with selinexor in patients with non-Hodgkin lymphoma. Blood. 2017;129:3175–83.
11. London CA, Bernabe LF, Barnard S, Kisseberth WC, Borgatti A, Henson M, Wilson H, Jensen K, Ito D, Modiano JF, Bear MD, Pennell ML, Saint-Martin JR, McCauley D, Kauffman M, Shacham S. Preclinical evaluation of the novel, orally bioavailable selective inhibitor of nuclear export (SINE) KPT-335 in spontaneous canine Cancer: results of a phase I study. PLoS One. 2014;9:1–11.
12. Vail DM, Michels GM, Khanna C, Selting KA, London CA, Veterinary cooperative oncology group. Response evaluation criteria for peripheral nodal lymphoma in dogs (v1.0)—a veterinary cooperative oncology group (VCOG) consensus document. Vet Comp Oncol. 2009;8:28–37.
13. Fan T. Lymphoma updates. Vet Clin North Am Small Anim Pract. 2003; 33:455–71.
14. Marconato L. The staging and treatment of multicentric high-grade lymphoma in dogs: a review of recent developments and future prospects. Vet J. 2011;188:34–8.

15. Withrow SJ, Vail DM, Page RL. Hematopoietic tumors. Withrow & MacEwen's Small Animal Clinical Oncology. 5th ed. Missouri: Elsevier Saunders; 2013. p. 608–38.
16. Grayton MT, Wilson-Robles H. *In vitro* evaluation of selective inhibitors of nuclear export (SINE) drugs KPT-185 and KPT-335 against canine mammary carcinoma and transitional cell carcinoma tumor initiating cells. Vet Comp Oncol. 2017;15:1455–67.
17. Breit MN, Kisseberth WC, Bear MD, Landesman Y, Kashyap T, McCauley D, Kauffman MG, Schacham S, London CA. Biologic activity of the novel orally bioavailable selective inhibitor of nuclear export (SINE) KPT-335 against canine melanoma cells. BMC Vet Res. 2014;10:160.
18. Azmi AS, Aboukareel A, Bao B, Sarkar FH, Philip PA, Kauffman M, Shacham S, Mohammad RM. Selective inhibitors of nuclear export block pancreatic cell Cancer proliferation and reduce tumor growth in mice. Gastroenterology. 2013;144:447–56.
19. Gravina GL, Mancini A, Sanita P, Vitale F, Marampon F, Ventura L, Landesman Y, McCauley D, Kauffman M, Shacham S, Festuccia C. KPT-330, a potent and selective exportin-1 (XPO-1) inhibitor, shows antitumor effects modulating the expression of cyclin D1 and survivin in prostate cancer models. BMC Cancer. 2015;15:941.
20. Alexander TB, Lacayo NJ, Choi JK, Ribeiro RC, Pui CH, Rubnitz JE. Phase I study of Selinexor, a selective inhibitor of nuclear export, in combination with Fludarabine and Cytarabine, in pediatric relapsed or refractory acute leukemia. J Clin Oncol. 2016;34:4094–101.
21. Chen Y, Camacho SC, Silvers TR, Razak RA, Gabrail NY, Gerecitano JF, Kalir E, Pereira E, Evans BR, Ramus SJ, Huang F, Priedigkeit N, Rodriguez E, Donovan M, Khan F, Kalir T, Sebra R, Uzilov A, Chen R, Sinha R, Halpert R, Billaud JN, Shacham S, McCauley D, Landesman Y, Rashal T, Kauffman M, Mirza MR, Mau-Sorensen M, Dottino P, Martignetti JA. Inhibition of the nuclear export receptor XPO1 as a therapeutic target for platinum-resistant ovarian Cancer. Clin Cancer Res. 2017;23:1552–63.
22. Kazim S, Malafa MP, Coppola D, Husain K, Zibadi S, Kashyap T, Crochiere M, Landesman Y, Rashal T, Sullivan DM, Mahipal A. Selective nuclear export inhibitor KPT-330 enhances the antitumor activity of gemcitabine in human pancreatic cancer. Mol Cancer Ther. 2015;14:1570–81.

A randomized placebo-controlled trial of the efficacy and safety of a terbinafine, florfenicol and betamethasone topical ear formulation in dogs for the treatment of bacterial and/or fungal otitis externa

S. L. Forster[2], T. Real[1], K. P. Doucette[1] and S. B. King[1*]

Abstract

Background: Treatment of infected otitis externa (OE) relies on the topical application of specific formulations that most often contain an antibiotic, an antifungal and a glucocorticoid. This study is to report the results of a randomized, placebo-controlled field trial evaluating the efficacy and safety of OSURNIA™ (Elanco Animal Health, a division of Eli Lilly and Company, Greenfield, IN), a novel topical ear medication containing florfenicol, terbinafine and betamethasone acetate in an adaptable gel. The study includes 284 dogs with bacterial and/or fungal OE who were randomly assigned to receive two doses of Osurnia or its vehicle, one week apart. Dogs were evaluated at various time points through Day 45, and a total clinical score (TCS) was calculated based on pain, erythema, exudate, swelling, odor and ulceration. The primary outcome measure was the rate of treatment success (RTS), defined as a TCS of 0, 1 or 2 on Day 45. Before and after treatment, a "clap test" was performed to subjectively assess hearing, and blood and urine were collected for routine clinical pathology.

Results: The RTS was significantly higher in ears treated with Osurnia (64.78%) than with placebo (43.42%). There was no significant interaction between efficacy and duration of history, recurrence of otitis or body weight. Adverse events were similar between groups. All dogs treated with Osurnia maintained their hearing, and there were no relevant clinical pathology changes.

Conclusions: The application of two doses of Osurnia, one week apart, is effective and safe to treat microbial otitis externa in dogs.

Keywords: Otitis externa, Otic gel, Clinical efficacy, Clinical safety, Florfenicol, Bethamethasone, Terbinafine

Background

Otitis externa is one of the most common medical conditions affecting dogs. In one epidemiological study of more than 2300 canine general practice consultations, a dermatological problem (21%) was the second most frequent reason motivating owners to consult their veterinarians after preventive veterinary care [1]. Among dogs with skin ailments, OE was the third most common diagnosis given (22% of patients) [1]. Similarly, in a more recent analysis of a random sample of more than 3500 primary care electronic medical records, OE was confirmed to be the most frequently made diagnosis in dogs (10%) [2].

* Correspondence: stephen.king@elanco.com
[1]Elanco Animal Health, 2500 Innovation Way, Greenfield, IN 46140, USA
Full list of author information is available at the end of the article

Otitis externa is a syndrome characterized by inflammation of the external ear canal; it is traditionally attributed to a combination of predisposing (e.g. ear canal conformation, moisture, etc.), primary (e.g. allergic, parasitic, foreign bodies, etc.), perpetuating (e.g. hyperplasia, stenosis, etc.) and secondary (e.g. bacteria, yeast infections, etc.) factors [3]. Indeed, commensal microbes from the external ear canal of normal dogs can proliferate—often because of the underlying factors listed above—and infections with pathogens such as *Staphylococcus pseudintermedius, Pseudomonas aeruginosa, Proteus mirabilis* and *Malassezia pachydermatis* appear to be the dominant problem [4, 5]. The impact of OE is notable, as otitis diminishes the quality of life of dogs and their owners [6].

Although there are no standard guidelines for treatment of canine OE, veterinarians have long used topical formulations developed for this indication; these medications usually include a broad-spectrum antibiotic, an antifungal and a glucocorticoid to reduce inflammation in an attempt to rapidly decrease pain and discomfort [7, 8]. Although it is considered good practice to evaluate results of ear cytology and microbial cultures, which, unfortunately, can yield discordant results [9], the selection of a topical ear formulation in general practice appears more often influenced by subjectivity, prescription habits, and commercial aspects of product supply [7].

The application of topical ear formulations to dogs with OE is fraught with difficulties that can decrease owner adherence to a treatment regimen. The need for once or twice daily drug application into painful and/or stenotic ear canals can be stressful for owners and lead to aggressive behaviours from dogs [6]. Furthermore, in multidose presentations the repeated placement of the tip of the product into infected ear canals could potentially lead to their mutual microbial cross-contamination similar to may be seen with otoscope tips [4]. Failure of compliance can reduce treatment efficacy, but it might also promote the development of bacterial resistance to antibiotics [5]. As a result of these limitations, a one-time use flexible applicator applied less frequently would more than likely improve treatment compliance.

Osurnia (Elanco Animal Health, Greenfield, IN, USA) is a novel topical ear therapy formulated as a pre-measured (1 mL), easy-to-use, single-dose tube with a flexible soft tip; it contains the antibiotic florfenicol (10 mg/mL), the antifungal terbinafine (10 mg/mL) and the glucorticoid betamethasone acetate (1.0 mg mL) in an adaptable gel vehicle designed to coat the ear canal and assist with product remaining where applied.

The objective of this article is to report the results of a randomized controlled trial (RCT) evaluating the efficacy and safety of the novel topical ear product Osurnia, administered twice per affected ear, one week apart, to dogs with bacterial and/or fungal OE. This report aimed at strictly following the 2010 Consolidated Standards of Reporting Trials (CONSORT) guidelines, an evidence-based, minimum set of recommendations for reporting randomized trials.

Methods

Trial design

This trial was a 6-week randomized double-blinded placebo (vehicle)-controlled multicenter parallel trial; the study followed the US FDA's Good Clinical Practices guideline VICH GL9.

Study participants

Dogs of any gender, weight, breed and of at least 8 weeks of age with OE were considered for enrollment after their owner gave informed consent for their dog to participate in this RCT.

To be enrolled in the study, the presence of an active OE was determined by a TCS of 6 or more based on the clinical assessment (including otoscopy) and scoring of the following: pain, erythema, exudate, swelling, odor and ulceration (Table 1).

The OE was characterized as "acute" if the history suggested that the signs of otitis had developed within 6 days of the initial visit, "subchronic" if they had occurred within 7 to 30 days prior to the visit or "chronic" if they had been present for more than 30 days beforehand. The OE was deemed to be recurrent if the dog had been successfully treated for a similar problem (i.e. with no remaining signs of OE post-treatment) in the preceding 3 months. Finally, the otitis exudate was described as erythematous/ceruminous or suppurative.

Importantly, before an ear was considered for treatment, its tympanic membrane had to be visible and assessed to be intact. After scoring on Day 0, exudate was removed using saline in order to allow visualization of the tympanic membrane. Cleaning was not repeated at Day 7.

Exclusion criteria for this RCT included dogs that had been treated beforehand with systemic, topical or otic antibiotics or antifungals within 14 days, systemic or topical anti-inflammatory drugs—including short-acting glucocorticoids—for 14 days, long-acting glucocorticoids for 28 days, cyclosporine for 14 days, otic ear cleaners for 7 days, antihistamines for 14 days and analgesics for 7 days. An *Otodectes cynotis* infestation or an otic foreign body were both considered exclusion criteria. Finally, dogs with known or suspected hypersensitivity to Osurnia's active ingredients (florfenicol, terbinafine or betamethasone acetate), dogs intended for breeding, pregnant or lactating bitches, staff-owned pets and those enrolled in other clinical trials were not considered further.

Dogs were selected from 15 companion animal general practices located in various geographic locations in the USA; this wide selection being done to adequately represent the targeted population for the product being developed. Each site was required to enroll a minimum of 4 dogs (2 evaluable dogs per treatment group) and was not allowed to exceed 30 dogs.

After having been treated with one of the test products, dogs could be removed from the trial for any of the following reasons:

– the presence of a serious adverse event (AE);

Table 1 Total clinical score

Clinical sign	Score '0' descriptor	Score '1' descriptor	Score '2' descriptor
Pain	None noted	Mild/moderate; painful on palpation	Severe: painful when raising pinna
Erythema	None noted	Mild/moderate: barely perceptible to obvious redness visible with an otoscope	Severe: beet or cherry red or erythema extends into pinna
Exudate	None noted	Mild/moderate: small amount to moderate amounts visible in ear canal	Severe: extending out of ear canal and may be crusted
Swelling	None noted	Mild/moderate: minimal occlusion to moderate occlusion of ear canal	Severe: canal completely occluded
Odor	None noted	Mild/moderate: malodor evident when pinna is raised	Severe: malodor evident without raising pinna to expose ear canal
Ulceration	None noted	Mild/moderate: mild abrasions	Severe: abrasions that may be bleeding

- a lack of improvement in TCS on Days 7, 14 or 30, which would justify the need for conventional therapy;
- the perception of lack of test product efficacy at any study day; or
- the administration of, or perceived need for, forbidden concomitant therapy (see below).

In any of these situations, the reasons for withdrawal were documented.

Interventions

Before the first administration of the test products, the ear canals to be treated were cleaned with saline to remove exudate and enable the verification of an intact tympanum. Ears were not flushed prior to the second administration to maintain treatment in the affected ear.

The intervention consisted of the topical application of 1 mL of the active product (Osurnia) or its vehicle (placebo control), once on Day 0 and a second time on Day 7 (±2 days). Either one of the two test products was applied into the ear canal followed by a massage at the base of the ear to allow for its homogeneous distribution. If both ears were affected, treatment was permitted for both, but only the data from the right ear were collected and evaluated for this study, provided that its initial TCS was 6 or greater. The same test product was used to treat both ears.

Concomitant otic medications were not allowed until the exit of the patient from this trial. Additionally, the use of systemic or topical antibiotics, antifungals, anti-inflammatory drugs, glucocorticoids, cyclosporine, analgesics and antihistamines were not permitted until study end. Dogs removed early during the study due to perceived lack of efficacy would be considered as treatment failures, and the investigator would clean the ear(s) with saline and use conventional otitis treatment.

Sample size

Anticipated recruitment was 225 dogs with OE for inclusion to reach a minimum of 150 evaluable cases (i.e. animals which fulfilled the requirements for per-protocol evaluation; assessment of eligibility for inclusion into the efficacy evaluation was determined without knowledge of treatment administered) in a 2:1 ratio of active-versus-vehicle (i.e. 100 dogs treated with Osurnia and 50 administered placebo). Based on prior pilot study results, this number of dogs was calculated to give this study an approximate 85% power to detect a treatment success of 70% with Osurnia and 45% with the placebo.

Randomization

Dogs included in this study were assigned to one of the two treatment groups in a 2:1 ratio according to a randomization sequence generated by computer by the Sponsor's statistician using the STAT version 9 software (SAS, Cary, NC, USA). Each study site had a separate randomization schedule in which dogs were blocked in groups of six.

The original study randomization code was sealed in an envelope and kept by the study sponsor until the end of the study. At each veterinary clinic site, one individual was given the role of "*dispenser*": this person assigned each successively enrolled dog to a letter (A, B, C, D, E or F) corresponding to one of the two treatment groups according to the randomization schedule, and he/she administered the active or placebo ear medications to the patients.

Blinding

At each veterinary clinic, all personnel (including the dispenser) were masked to treatment; the pet owner was also blinded to the intervention. To further preserve this blinding, the dispenser was asked not to disclose any treatment related information to the investigator responsible for grading the effect of treatment. Additionally, the dispenser was not allowed to gather or interpret any data.

Masking was done by placing the active medication (Osurnia) and its vehicle control into identical tubes and packages labeled with one of six code letters (A to F) corresponding to a block of six dogs. Only select study Sponsor personnel knew the treatment associated with each letter code, and it was not made available to study monitors, the statistician and clinical safety representative until the end of the trial prior to final report compilation. There were no reports of unblinding at any participating site.

Participant evaluation

Dogs were examined on Days 0, 7, 14, 30 and 45 or during an exit visit in case of early withdrawal. Clinical examinations included a routine assessment of general appearance and major systems (cardiological, ocular, auricular, gastrointestinal, neurological, respiratory, urogenital, etc.). Pre-existing medical conditions were also recorded. Additional clinical examinations were to be performed in case of a serious AE. Body weights were collected and recorded in pounds rounded to the nearest 0.1 lb.

At each visit, the investigator performed an otoscopic examination and used a standard score to grade the presence or absence of pain, erythema, exudate, swelling, odor and ulceration in the ear canal of the evaluable ear (predetermined as the right ear if both ears were affected and qualified). These observations were then compared to those before treatment, and they were scored as *"no increase in irritation"* or *"increase in irritation"*.

Finally, a subjective evaluation of the dog's ability to hear was measured by a *"clap test"* before treatment (Day 0) and on Day 45 or earlier in case of premature study withdrawal. Personnel at the study site clapped their hands together in a location outside of the dog's field of vision and the ability of the dog to turn its head toward the noise was observed. The following recordings were made: *"dog can hear"* or *"dog cannot hear"* and the dog was then assigned to one of the following four categories:

- Dog could hear at Day 0 and at Day 45 (or study exit)
- Dog could hear at Day 0 and could not hear at Day 45 (or study exit)
- Dog could not hear at Day 0 and could hear at Day 45 (or study exit)
- Dog could not hear at Day 0 nor at Day 45 (or study exit)

Microbial cultures

Before treatment and on Day 45 if a clinical cure (i.e. a TCS of 0, 1 or 2) was not achieved, a swab of the affected ear canal(s) were cultured for bacteria and yeast with testing of their sensitivity to Osurnia's antimicrobial drugs florfenicol and terbinafine. A similar procedure was also done before Day 45 for any dog removed from the trial due to perceived treatment failure. Evaluated (qualifying) pathogens were *Malassezia pachydermatis*, *Candida albicans*, *Staphylococcus pseudintermedius*, *Pseudomonas aeruginosa*, beta-hemolytic *Streptococcus species*, *Escherichia coli*, and *Proteus mirabilis*. To be considered as an evaluable case for efficacy positive growth of at least one of these qualifying pathogens had to be present in the affected ear. Minimum inhibitory concentrations $(MICs)_{50/90}$ were calculated for florfenicol and terbinafine.

Outcome measures of efficacy

Veterinarian investigators were responsible for determining the severity of OE in affected ears before and 7, 14, 30 and 45 days after starting topical ear therapy with the tested products using the scoring system and the calculation of a TCS, as shown in Table 1. In case of premature study exit, a TCS was also assessed at the time of withdrawal.

The primary outcome measure for efficacy was the RTS on Day 45, this being the official end of the study. Treatment success was defined as a TCS of 0, 1 or 2 on a scale of 12 at study end. Cases exiting the study early for reasons related to treatment (i.e. the presence of an AE, a lack of perceived efficacy, etc.) were considered treatment failures regardless of their final TCS.

Safety evaluation

Adverse events were defined as any observation in a study participant that was unfavorable, unintended and that occurred after the use of a test product, whether or not it was considered to be related to the product being administered. A serious AE was defined as one that was considered clinically significant by the investigator and that also required medical intervention. In this RCT, pet owners or study personnel reported all potential AEs as soon as possible to the local investigator; after assessment of the duration, severity, presumed relationship of the event to the administered product and its outcome, AEs were then recorded as *"serious"* or *"not serious"* as defined above. Pre-existing conditions were not considered AEs unless the condition worsened after treatment with the test products.

Before enrollment and on Day 45 or earlier in case of premature study exit, blood and urine were collected for routine hematology, clinical biochemistry and urinalysis (catheterization, free catch or cystocentesis), respectively. Additional samples were collected in case of serious AE occurring during the study.

Statistical methods

Baseline demographic (age, weight, gender, breeds) and OE data (number of ears treated, type of otitis [acute, subchronic, or chronic], recurrent status, exudate type [suppurative or erythematous ceruminous], and hearing status) were first summarized by treatment groups (Osurnia versus vehicle) using SAS PROC FREQ or SAS PROC MEANS, depending on the type of variable. A T-test was used to compare the mean ages at baseline and Fisher's Exact tests were used to compare all other variables except for breed.

For efficacy evaluation, the clinical outcome for each case (*"success"* or *"failure"*) was analyzed using SAS PROC GLIMMIX with the main effects of *"treatment"*, *"site"* and the interaction *"treatment by site"*, with *"treatment"* being a fixed effect and the other two being random effects. A logit link function was employed. The Variance Components (VC) covariance structure was utilized and the Containment method was employed to estimate the denominator degrees of freedom. All efficacy variables (erythema, exudate, odor, pain, swelling and ulceration) were summed on Day 45 (or at study exit if an animal exited early) to obtain a TCS. A case was classified as a "success" if the TCS on Day 45 (study exit) was a 2 or less, otherwise the case was classified a 'failure'; all animals that withdrew from the study early for a treatment related reason were also classified as failures regardless of their TCS.

In addition, TCS and RTS were compared between visits Day 0 and Day 45; dogs that did not return for follow-up visits, those with major protocol deviations or those that did not have positive cultures for qualifying pathogens on Day 0 were not included in such analyses. In this instance, missing data from treated dogs that had to exit the study prematurely were replaced using a *"last observation carried forward* (LOCF)" rule.

The RTS on Day 45 was analyzed using SAS PROC GLIMMIX with the fixed effects of 'Treatment' and one of the following: 'History of Otitis', 'Breed', 'Weight', 'Type of Pathogen' and 'Recurrent Status of Otitis', separately, 'Site' and 'Treatment by site' were included as random effects in each model. The logit link function and VC covariance structure were utilized for each analysis.

Changes in body weight compared to pretreatment values were analyzed using an analysis of variance (ANOVA; SAS PROC MIXED) including the same effects as above. Treatment groups were compared using LSMEANS.

Hematology, serum chemistry, and urinalysis variables were statistically evaluated using an analysis of covariance (ANCOVA; SAS PROC MIXED) with the pre-treatment value used as a covariate. The model included the same effects as for efficacy above. Prior to performing the ANCOVA, Levene's test for homogeneity of variance (SAS PROC GLM) was performed. If the results from the Levene's test were not significant, untransformed data were used in the ANCOVA. In other cases, the data were transformed beforehand (e.g. logarithmic, square root, or reciprocal transformation).

For all statistical analyses, the level of significance was set at $p = 0.05$ for two-sided analyses.

Results

Participant flow

In total, 284 dogs from 49 different breeds were enrolled between April and July 2012. They were randomized to receive either Osurnia (190) or its vehicle control (94). While all randomized cases were included in safety analyses, 49 cases were excluded leaving 235 (159 Osurnia, 76 vehicle) cases for treatment efficacy evaluation. The reasons for exclusion of these dogs included: lost to follow-up ($n = 5$), use of a forbidden concurrent medication ($n = 4$), a negative or non-qualifying culture at enrollment ($n = 31$), an insufficient number of cases enrolled at the site ($n = 4$), a significant delay in presentation for the final visit ($n = 2$), data quality ($n = 1$) and staff-owned pets ($n = 2$). One dog was not evaluated on Day 14; while the missing time point was excluded, the case remained for efficacy evaluation on Day 45 (Fig. 1).

Altogether, 64/284 of the total dogs enrolled (23%) exited the trial early primarily due to lack of efficacy ($n = 51$) followed by adverse events ($n = 8$) and loss to follow-up ($n = 5$). These early exits represented 31/94 (33%) of the dogs with ears treated with placebo and 33/190 (17%) of those with an ear treated with Osurnia. Early exit related to adverse events were similar between the two groups.

Baseline data

On Day 0, before treatment, the two treatment groups had similar descriptive statistics in regards to their age, body weight, gender, number of ears affected, history of otitis, exudate type, and frequency of otitis or presence of subjective hearing loss (Table 2).

In both groups, the range of ages and breeds (not shown) was equally variable and males and females were similarly represented. Dogs with bilateral erythematous and ceruminous OE predominated. The OE was considered recurrent in only 11% of cases. Nearly all dogs (> 96%) were subjectively assessed as hearing properly at baseline.

The prevalence of microorganisms cultured from ear swabs obtained on Day 0 were *Malassezia pachydermatis* (70% of samples), *Staphylococcus pseudintermedius* (46%), *Pseudomonas aeruginosa* (11%), beta-hemolytic *Streptococcus* spp. (10%), *Escherichia coli* (6%) and *Proteus mirabilis* (4%); *Candida* species were not cultured.

Efficacy outcome measures

A total of 235 dogs (159 treated with Osurnia, 76 with placebo) were included in the analysis of efficacy. In dogs from both treatment groups, the mean TCS—as well as that of each of its components (pain, erythema, exudate, swelling, odor and ulceration)—decreased progressively over time until Day 30, and they generally either plateaued or increased slightly between Day 30 and Day 45 (Fig. 2).

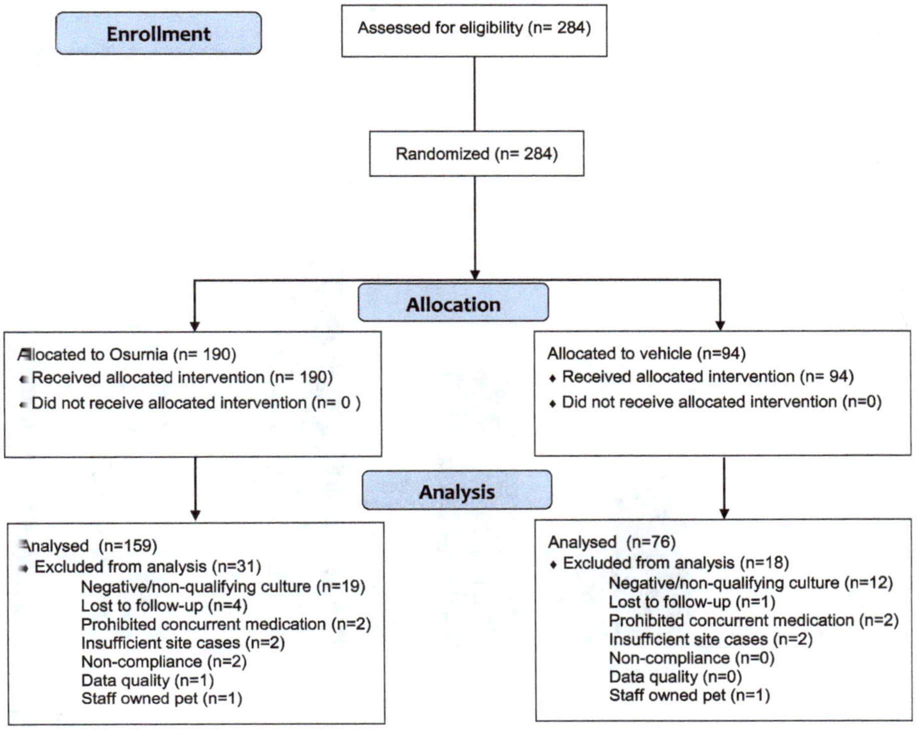

Fig. 1 Case flow diagram

The primary outcome measure of efficacy, the RTS (i.e. a TCS of 0, 1 or 2 on Day 45), was 103/159 (64.78%) for ears treated with Osurnia and 33/76 (43.42%) for ears treated with placebo; this RTS at study end was significantly different between groups ($p = 0.0094$).

The RTS gradually improved after the first dose of Osurnia administered until Day 30, when it plateaued until Day 45 (Fig. 1). In ears treated with the placebo vehicle, the RTS also improved progressively and regularly until the end of the study, but in a proportion always

Table 2 Comparison of treatment groups at baseline

		Osurnia	Placebo	*P*-Value
Number		190	94	
Age	(mean (range); yrs	6.1 (0.3–16.4)	6.1 (0.3–15.8)	0.9097
Body weight	< 40 lbs.; N (%)	78 (41%)	41 (44%)	0.8617
	40–79 lbs.; n (%)	64 (34%)	32 (34%)	
	≥80 lbs.; n (%)	48 (25%)	21 (22%)	
Gender	F:M ratio	90:100 = 0.9	52:42 = 1.2	0.2564
Ears affected	One ear; n (%)	17 (9%)	7 (7%)	0.8217
	Two ears; n (%)	173 (91%)	87 (93%)	
History of otitis	Acute; n (%)	47 (25%)	29 (31%)	0.5436
	Subchronic; n (%)	73 (38%)	32 (34%)	
	Chronic; n (%)	70 (37%)	33 (35%)	
Exudate Type	Erythematous/ceruminous; n (%)	158 (83%)	78 (83%)	1.000
	Suppurative; n (%)	32 (17%)	16 (17%)	
Frequency of Otitis	Recurrent otitis; n (%)	22 (12%)	9 (10%)	0.6894
Hearing Loss	Can hear at Day 0; n (%)	181 (97%)	90 (96%)	0.4846

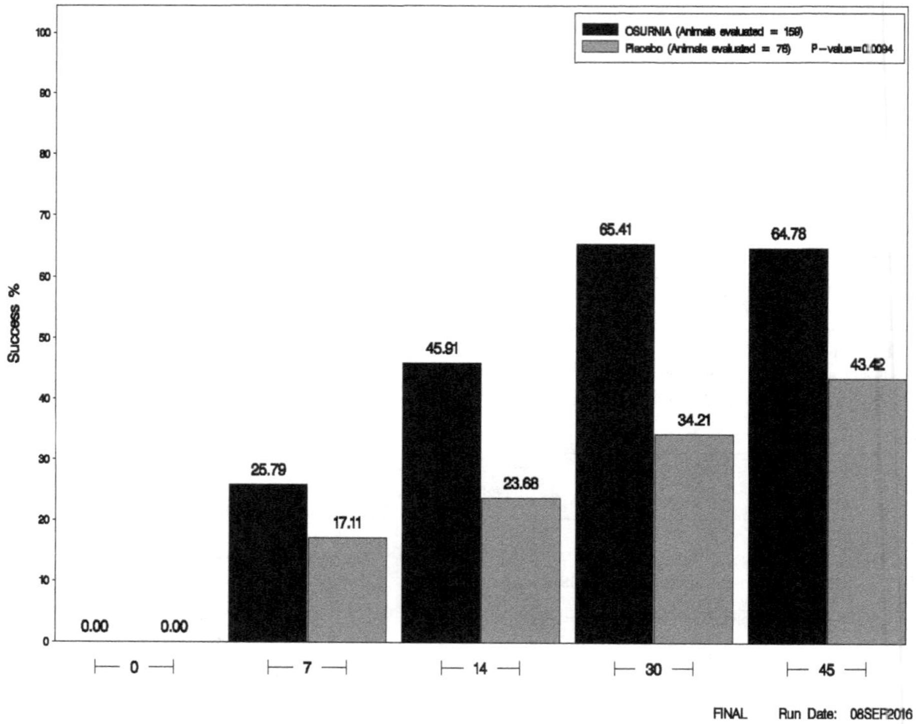

Fig. 2 Treatment success rate by treatment group for each study day

lower to that of ears treated with Osurnia. As would be expected, the RTS decreased with the type of history of OE: ears with acute, subchronic or chronic otitis treated with Osurnia had a respective RTS of 85, 66 and 52% on Day 45. However this was numerically better than those treated with the placebo which had a respective RTS of 44, 52 and 36% on Day 45, respectively.

There was no significant interaction between treatment efficacy and the following variables: duration of history of otitis externa (i.e. acute, subchronic or chronic; $p = 0.208$), recurrence of OE ($p = 0.731$) or body weight ($p = 0.904$). Because of lack of convergence, the statistical model used did not permit the comparison of treatment effect when breed or microbial pathogen types were included as possible cofactors.

Minimum inhibitory concentrations

The minimum inhibitory concentration $(MIC)_{50/90}$ for florfenicol and terbinafine were calculated; a summary of these MICs for pathogens found in at least 10 isolates is detailed in Table 3.

Overall, and including all isolates from all visits, the florfenicol MIC was lowest for *Streptococcus* spp. (MIC_{90} = 2 μg/mL) and *Staphylococcus pseudintermedius* (4 μg/mL), intermediate for *Proteus mirabilis* (8 μg/mL) and *Escherichia coli* (16 μg/mL), and highest for *Pseudomonas aeruginosa* (> 64 μg/mL). The overall terbinafine MIC profile for *Malassezia pachydermatis* isolates ranged from ≤0.004–0.25 μg/mL with an MIC_{90} of 0.06 μg/mL. Importantly, the MIC profiles of baseline isolates were nearly identical to those collected from ears evaluated as treatment failures with only a single doubling dilution change in the MIC_{90} of the yeast.

Safety evaluation

All 284 enrolled dogs (190 Osurnia treated, 94 placebo control) were considered for clinical safety. The most frequently reported adverse reactions with possible relationship to treatment were elevated clinical chemistry values and vomiting. Reported adverse reactions with possible relationship to treatment are presented in Table 4.

However, skin and appendage disorders such as pruritus and dermatitis were the overall most frequently reported AEs noted during the study. These likely represented pre-existing allergic skin diseases.

There was no detectable association between breed, age, gender or number of doses received and the development of AEs. Importantly, there was no evidence of increased irritation (i.e. pain, erythema, swelling or ulceration of the ear canal) associated with dosing of Osurnia.

One dog in each treatment group was reported by the owner as having hearing impairment at the Day 14 visit. In neither case could the hearing loss be confirmed in clinic and all dogs treated with the active product on Day 0 could hear on Day 45, or at the visit scheduled for early study exit.

Table 3 MIC_{50} and MIC_{90}[a]

Bacteria genus/species	# isolates tested	MIC_{50} (μg/mL FFC)	MIC_{90} (μg/mL FFC)
Escherichia coli	25	16	16
Proteus mirabilis	17	8	8
Pseudomonas aeruginosa	52	> 64	> 64
Staphylococcus pseudintermedius	170	4	4
Streptococcus spp	52	2	2
Yeast genus/species	# isolates tested	MIC_{50} (μg/mL TRB)	MIC_{90} (μg/mL TRB)
Malassezia pachydermatis	239[b]	0.015	0.06

[a]These data represent all 392 isolates (284 from Day 0 and 108 from treatment failure cases)
[b]Twenty-one *M. pachydermatis* samples tested did not grow in the MIC plates

Finally, there were no significant changes in body weight, hematology, serum chemistry and urinalysis variables between dogs treated with Osurnia or placebo (data not shown); in all cases, means remained within the normal range.

Discussion

This RCT demonstrates the efficacy and safety of the application of Osurnia, at two doses one week apart, to treat canine OE due to the common microbial pathogens classically seen in this syndrome. The adaptable gel formulation requires less frequent product administration than typically approved OE therapies and, other than cleaning prior to the first administration, does not necessitate the need for additional ear cleaning between treatments which is typically recommended for OE treatment [3, 8].

Generalizability of the results

Overall, the dogs enrolled are representative of general practice patients with microbial OE that are the most likely to be treated with Osurnia. The subjects included exhibited typical characteristics: there was a wide range of breeds, ages and weights and both genders were equally represented. Cases enrolled had an acute and subchronic history more often than chronic OE, and the exudate was more often erythematous and ceruminous rather than suppurative; nearly all dogs appeared able to hear at the beginning of the study. At baseline, microbial cultures most often grew *Malassezia* yeast and *Staphylococcus pseudintermedius*, which are the two most common pathogens isolated in canine OE [3].

The number of patients included was not a source of imprecision, as the results obtained post-trial were compatible with the model estimated at the time of sample size calculation. The efforts made to mask the nature of treatment and to blind personnel and owners proved to be sufficient to avoid unblinding and subsequent bias in treatment efficacy assessments.

In this trial, the clinical assessment scale (TCS) and the primary outcome measure (RTS) were both considered appropriate for assessment of OE as they are based on clinical signs that are relevant to both dog owners and veterinarians. The TCS was established using six classic OE signs/symptoms, each with a maximum of two points, giving a maximum total of 12 points. The RTS, defined as a TCS of 0, 1 and 2, represents an ear canal with no or little residual signs of OE at study end, i.e. an ear likely to be perceived as *"cured"*. Requiring a minimum TCS of at least 6 points for enrollment in the study ensured cases with an OE of at least moderate severity were included in the study. If we take into consideration that the mean TCS of patients at enrollment was 8/12, on average, successful cases had an improvement of at least 6 points (or 50%) over a 12-point scale. Therefore, the primary outcome measure used in this study (RTS) should be considered clinically relevant.

Table 4 Adverse reactions

Adverse reaction[a]	Osurnia		Placebo	
	N	% of total (n = 190)	N	% of total (n = 158)
Elevated Alkaline Phosphatase	15	7.9	3	3.2
Vomiting	7	3.7	1	1.1
Elevated AST, ALT, ALP[a]	2	1.1	0	0.0
Weight Loss (10% BW)	1	0.53	0	0.0
Hearing Decrease/Loss	1	0.53	1	1.1

[a]Aspartate aminotransferase (AST), alanine aminotransferase (ALT), alkaline phosphatase (ALP). Two dogs with pre-existing elevations in ALP were reported to have an increase in liver enzymes (ALP, ALT and/or AST) at study exit. Subsequent clinical chemistries returned to normal

Interpretation of efficacy

In this trial, the effectiveness of Osurnia demonstrated superiority to that of placebo, as the RTS at study end was significantly higher in dogs treated with the active product than those treated with the placebo. In addition, all the individual components of the TCS for the Osurnia treated animals showed improvement over time. It is not surprising that the weakest treatment effect was observed for the parameter *"exudate"*. Exudates need to be differentiated from the ubiquitous cerumen seen in canine ears and in this study, the use of traditionally recommended ear cleaning in cases of microbial OE was not performed thereby potentially impacting this score [8].

For the primary outcome measure, the number-needed-to-treat (NNT, the inverse of the RTS difference between groups) could be calculated as 5 (i.e. five dogs would need to be treated with Osurnia to obtain one more success compared to placebo). This seemingly elevated NNT is not due to the low proportion of RTS in the actively treated group, but due to the unusually high effect of the placebo vehicle. Indeed, the mean TCS and each of its components fell rapidly after the second application of Osurnia and placebo. The return to apparent normalcy in the subjectively evaluated *"pain"* symptom suggests that not only Osurnia, but also the vehicle itself, might have some antalgic effect; this effect might follow, or be concurrent to, the mild anti-inflammatory effect seen on erythema and swelling with both interventions. It can be speculated that ear cleaning to remove debris and exudate prior to treatment administration may be partially responsible for the apparent treatment response in placebo treated dogs, leading to some dogs apparently self healing [8]. However, other possible causes, such as antimicrobial activity of the placebo itself could be considered [10, 11]. This possible activity of the vehicle alone was unexpected, and it is deserving of further evaluation.

In this study, the determination of the MICs for florfenicol confirmed the variability of bacterial susceptibility to this antibiotic, being highest for the Gram negative rods, especially *Pseudomonas aeruginosa*. As a consequence, the efficacy of florfenicol-containing topical ear formulations might be expected to be lower in cases of *Pseudomonas* OE, especially whenever this antibiotic concentration does not exceed the MIC for the organism; however it may be noted that antibiotics, when applied topically rather than given systemically, will more often than not exceed the MICs [12]. Importantly, the bacterial MICs from OE cases failing to respond were not different from those seen at baseline indicating that the treatment failures in dogs administered Osurnia were not due to selection of resistant microbial isolates.

Interpretation of safety

In this RCT, the two doses of Osurnia or its vehicle were well tolerated. Importantly, the overall most commonly reported non-serious AE were pruritus and dermatitis, which likely represented primary factors relating to development of OE rather than resulting from treatment. There were no detectable changes in body weights and clinical pathology parameters (except ALP) during this study and as such would preclude the need for any specific monitoring of these parameters when administering Osurnia. Although a greater number of cases treated with Osurnia had elevated ALP these were not considered to be of clinical significance. These ALP increases were not reported as AEs during the study, remained within normal clinical range and represented less than a 2–3 fold increase. Similarly for vomiting, although a greater number of dogs in the Osurnia treated group vomited, in no case was it considered to be clinical relevant or related to treatment according to the investigators. Importantly, Osurnia used under the conditions of this trial did not lead to any detectable change in response to a clap test, although it is recognised that only Brainstem Auditory Evoked Response (BAER) can truly assess loss of hearing [13]. The post-marketing experience in the EU suggests that deafness or impaired hearing may be a very rare (less than 1 animal in 10,000 treated) event, mainly in elderly animals [14].

Limitations

There were several possible limitations resulting from the design and/or performance of this RCT.

Firstly, there was an initial loss of 49/284 dogs (17%) due to exclusion for a variety of reasons, the main one being the lack of growth of qualifying pathogens at the study onset. Furthermore, one fifth of dogs that began treatment had to exit the study early, mostly due to lack of efficacy. This attrition rate was not likely a source of bias as the early exits for lack of efficacy were higher in placebo (29%) compared to Osurnia (14%) treated animals which would be expected.

Evaluation systems, similar to TCS as an assessment scale and RTS as a primary outcome measure, have been used consistently for approval of other OE treatments with the FDA [15–17], as there are no universally accepted and validated clinical scoring systems for OE. As such use of these could be perceived as not validated which already has been mentioned as a possible source of detection bias in a systematic review of interventions to treat *Pseudomonas* OE [18]. In spite of this limitation, the parameters subjectively evaluated in this study are clinically meaningful and comparable to those mentioned in a recent paper reviewing OE severity scales [19]. Furthermore, the primary outcome measure was chosen to be a near return to normalcy, which should help alleviate any possible detection bias.

The lack of performance of an otic cytology before and after treatment could lead to the perception that not all cases assessed as successfully treated were indeed so. That the main outcome measures focussed on clinical signs rather than cytology was deemed preferable as, even though cytology is perceived to be the *"gold standard"* for OE assessment, it is far from capturing the complex reality of the skin and ear microbiome of normal and allergic dogs [20, 21]. Although cytology and clinical assessment are generally correlated in dogs with OE [22], it has not been possible to establish thresholds with sufficient sensitivity and specificity to allow the use of cytological endpoints in clinical studies [23]. Additionally, in this study, microbial culture was done before treatment, and culture and cytology results have been shown to generally correlate in dogs with either *Malassezia* [23] or microbial OE [9].

Another limitation is that, to be entered in this study, dogs had to have tympanic membranes visible by otoscopy before treatment. This selection criterion, which was proposed as a precaution to limit any potential drug-induced ototoxity, clearly eliminated cases with any hyperplastic ear canals, as seen in dogs with very chronic OE. Even though we did observe that the RTS of dogs with a history of chronic OE was one third lower than that of dogs with acute OE, the factor *"duration of history of OE"* was found not to affect treatment outcome.

The statistical model used did not allow for the determination of any possible influence of the type of microbes cultured and the RTS; this likely reflecting the complexity of OE and its associated microbiome. The study was not specifically designed or powered to answer this question, limiting the determination of which type of microbial OE best responds to the application of Osurnia.

Conclusion

Because of its treatment success rate and minimal clinical safety findings, Osurnia formulated as an adaptable gel, applied twice, one week apart, is a valuable addition in the armamentarium against this common syndrome affecting dogs including first line cases. The ease of use brought by the gel formulation which remains at the site of application and its infrequent dosing are two important additions that should help clients better comply with the veterinarian's prescription.

Abbreviations

AE: Adverse Event; ALP: Alkaline Phosphatase; ALT: Alanine Aminotransferase; ANOVA: Analysis of Variance; ASP: Aspartate Aminotransferase; FFC: Florfenicol; LOCF: Last Observation Carried Forward; MIC: Minimum Inhibitory Concentration; NNT: Number Needed to Treat; OE: Otitis Externa; RCT: Randomized Controlled Trial; RTS: Rate of Treatment Success; TCS: Total Clinical Score; TRB: Terbinafine; VC: Variance Components

Acknowledgements

The authors would like to thank the participating veterinarians and pet owners.

Funding

The study was funded by Novartis Animal Health which is now owned by Elanco Animal Health, a division of Eli Lilly and Company.

Authors' contributions

SBK and SLF were involved in the study design, in-life phase of the study, and interpretation of results and writing of the manuscript. KPD was involved in the interpretation of results and writing of the manuscript. TR was responsible for data analysis, and review of the manuscript. All authors have read and approved the manuscript.

Consent for publication

Not applicable

Competing interests

All authors are employees of Elanco Animal Health, a Division of Eli Lilly and Company.

Author details

[1]Elanco Animal Health, 2500 Innovation Way, Greenfield, IN 46140, USA. [2]Elanco Animal Health Ltd., Lilly House, Priestley Road, Basingstoke, Hampshire RG24 9NL, UK.

References

1. Hill PB, Lo A, Eden CAN, et al. Survey of the prevalence, diagnosis and treatment of dermatological conditions in small animals in general practice. Vet Rec. 2006;158:533–9.
2. O'Neill DG, Church DB, McGreevy PD, et al. Prevalence of disorders recorded in dogs attending primary-care veterinary practices in England. PLoS One. 2014;9(3):e90501.
3. Miller WH Jr, Griffin CE, Campbell KL. Muller & Kirk's small animal dermatology (7th Ed). Philadelphia: Saunders; 2012.
4. Shaw S. Pathogens in otitis externa:diagnostic techniques to identify secondary causes of ear disease. In Practice FOCUS. 2016:12–6.
5. Nuttall T. Successful management of otitis externa. In Practice. 2016;38:17–21.
6. Noli C, Sartori R, Cena T. Impact of a terbinafine–florfenicol–betamethasone acetate otic gel on the quality of life of dogs with acute otitis externa and their owners. Vet Dermatol. 2017; Aug;28(4):386–e90.
7. Bond R. Selecting ear drops for dogs with otitis externa. In Pract. 2012;34:392–9.
8. Forsythe PJ. Acute otitis externa: the successful first-opinion ear consultation. In Practice. 2016;38:2–6.
9. Graham-Mize CA, Rosser EJ Jr. Comparison of microbial isolates and susceptibility patterns from the external ear canal of dogs with otitis externa. J Am Anim Hosp Assoc. 2004;40:102–8.
10. Turcotte P, Saheb S. Antimicrobial activity of phenolic antioxidants. Can J Microbiol. 1978;24:1306–20.
11. Hinton Jr A, Ingram KD. Use of oleic acid to reduce the population of the bacterial flora of poultry skin. J of Food Protection 2000; 63(9): 1282–1286.
12. Ohyama M, Furuta S, Ueno K, Katsuda K, Nobori T, Kiyota R, Miyazaki Y. Ofloxacin otic solution in patients with otitis media: an analysis of drug concentrations. Arch Otolaryngol Head Neck Surg. 1999 Mar;125(3):337–40.
13. Webb AA. Brainsterm auditory evoked response (BAER) testing in animals. Can Vet J. 2009 Mar;50(3):313–8.
14. Osurnia Summary of Product Characteristics EMEA/V/C/003753 -IG/0794/0007 last updated July 2017. http://www.ema.europa.eu/ema/index.jsp?curl=pages/medicines/veterinary/medicines/003753/vet_med_000300.jsp&mid=WC0b01ac058008d7a8.

15. NADA 141–298. United States Food and Drug Administration. Freedom of Information Summary. Surolan Otic Suspension (Miconazole nitrate, polymyxin B sulfate, prednisolone acetate). https://animaldrugsatfda.fda.gov/adafda/app/search/public/document/downloadFoi/862. Accessed 25 Aug 2018.
16. NADA 141–176. United States Food and Drug Administration. Freedom of Information Summary. Baytril® Otic (enrofloxacin/silver sulfadiazine). https://animaldrugsatfda.fda.gov/adafda/app/search/public/document/downloadFoi/686. Accessed 25 Aug 2018.
17. NADA 141–266. United States Food and Drug Administration. Freedom of Information Summary. Posatex Otic Suspension (Orbifloxacin, mometasone furoate monohydrate and posaconazole). https://animaldrugsatfda.fda.gov/adafda/app/search/public/document/downloadFoi/825. Accessed 25 Aug 2018.
18. Nuttall T, Cole LK. Evidence-based veterinary dermatology: a systematic review of interventions for treatment of *Pseudomonas* otitis in dogs. Vet Dermatol. 2007;18:69–77.
19. Nuttall T, Bensignor E. A pilot study to develop an objective clinical score for canine otitis externa. Vet Dermatol. 2014;25:530–7, e92.
20. Tater KC, Scott DW, Miller WH Jr, et al. The cytology of the external ear canal in the normal dog and cat. J Vet Med A. 2003;50:370–4.
21. Hoffmann AR, Patterson AP, Diesel A, et al. The skin microbiome in healthy and allergic dogs. PLoS One. 2014;9(1):e83197.
22. Ginel PJ, Lucena R, Rodriguez JC, et al. A semiquantitative cytological evaluation of normal and pathological samples from the external ear canal of dogs and cats. Vet Dermatol. 2002;13:151–6.
23. Pulido-Vilamarin A, Castaneda-Salazar R, Linares-Linares M, et al. Concordance between otic cytology and culture in diagnosis of external otitis canine by *Malassezia* spp. Revista MVZ Cordoba. 2014;20(3):4720–5.

21

Molecular analysis of the microbiota in hard feces from healthy rabbits (*Oryctolagus cuniculus*) medicated with long term oral meloxicam

David Eshar[1] and J Scott Weese[2*]

Abstract

Background: Analgesia is often indicated in rabbits undergoing surgical procedures or suffering from various painful conditions and the most common adverse effects associated with NSAIDs occur in the gastrointestinal tract (GIT). The objective of this study was to determine the potential effect of long-term (21 days) meloxicam administration on the fecal bacterial microbiota in healthy rabbits.
Samples of hard feces were collected from six rabbits treated with meloxicam (1 mg/kg orally once every 24 h) on days 0,6,14 and 21. Next generation sequencing of V4 16S rRNA gene products was performed.

Results: A total of 2589912 V4 rRNA gene sequences passed all quality control filters. Firmicutes predominated (82.0 ± 6.2%). Sixteen other phyla were also identified but other than Verrucomicrobia (4.4 ± 4.9%), all accounted for less than 1% of the identified sequences. Within Firmicutes, Clostridia was the dominant class, accounting for 76% of operational taxon units (OTUs). In general, there were only few differences observed between time points and different rabbits at the phylum level. A significant change was observed in the relative abundance of Proteobacteria over the 4 time points ($P = 0.02$).

Conclusions: The gastrointestinal tract of rabbits harbors dense and diverse microbiota. Significant alteration of the hard fecal microbiota does not appear to be a considerable adverse effect expected in rabbits treated for 21 days with oral meloxicam at a dose of 1 mg/kg.

Keywords: Microbiome, Rabbits, Gastrointestinal tract, Feces, 16S RNA, Meloxicam, *Oryctolagus cuniculus*

Background

Analgesia is a basic aspect of veterinary medicine, indicated in both laboratory and pet-owned animals undergoing surgical procedures or suffering from various painful conditions [1]. One of the most common classes of drugs used by veterinarians for analgesia is non-steroidal anti-inflammatory drugs (NSAIDs) [1]. Nonsteroidal anti-inflammatory drugs reduce inflammation by inhibiting the action of Cyclooxygenase (COX) enzymes, which convert arachidonic acid into prostanoids and analgesia associated with NSAIDs is mainly due to inhibition of COX-2 [2]. The most common adverse effects associated with NSAIDs occur in the gastrointestinal tract (GIT), and to a lesser degree, impairment of renal blood flow [3,4]. Reported NSAIDs-related GIT pathologies include perforation, ulceration, bleeding and local irritation [3,4]. Because prostaglandins also play a role in the rabbit's GIT motility [5], NSAIDs have the potential to also impair GIT function. To date, several studies have been performed to determine pharmacokinetics and safety of meloxicam in rabbits but none had looked into the potential drug's effect on GIT microbiota [6-8].

The fecal or intestinal microbiota of domestic rabbits has been extensively studied through culture dependent methods, as well as earlier generation culture-independent methods, with a focus on the cecal microbiota [9-13]. However, limitations of these methods for understanding the overall microbial composition are well known. In particular, culture-dependent studies are only able to provide a very superficial (and sometimes misleading) assessment of this complex polymicrobial environment [14-16]. While earlier studies have provided some important information,

* Correspondence: jsweese@uoguelph.ca
[2]Department of Pathobiology, Ontario Veterinary College, University of Guelph, Guelph, Ontario N1G 2 W1, Canada
Full list of author information is available at the end of the article

the ability of next generation sequencing based studies such as this to evaluate millions of bacterial sequences from diverse (and often unculturable) microbial populations is now possible.

This study explores the stability over time of bacterial communities in hard feces in healthy rabbits medicated with oral meloxicam, using high throughput sequencing of the V4 region of the 16S rRNA gene.

Methods

Study population

Ethical approval was obtained from the Institutional Animal Care and Use Committee of Kansas State University. Rabbits enrolled in this study were part of a broader study evaluating long term (29 days) administration of oral meloxicam. Six clinically normal 3-month-old intact female New Zealand White rabbits (body weight range, 2.52 to 2.71 kg) were included in this study. The rabbits were obtained from a commercial source and were specific pathogen (*Pasteurella* sp.) free. The rabbits were housed individually at the research facilities of the Kansas State University College of Veterinary Medicine at a constant temperature (21°C) and humidity (60%), and were exposed to cycles of 16 hours of light and 8 hours of dark per day. Rabbits were fed free choice of timothy hay[a], timothy-based pelleted diet[b] and water was available ad libitum. Rabbits were acclimated to the facility for 5 days after their arrival and were habituated to handling prior to initiation of the study. Immediately prior to the start of the study, each rabbit was determined to be behaviorally normal and healthy based on a thorough physical examination and clinical pathology testing (complete blood count [CBC], serum biochemistry profile and urinalysis), with results compared to published reference ranges [17]. Physical examination, weight and blood testing were repeated weekly in all rabbits enrolled in the study. Fecal production was subjectively monitored for shape, color and consistency, and objectively by weight and fecal pellet size. At the end of the study, all rabbits were humanely euthanatized using pentobarbital[c] (100 mg/kg Intravenous), and necropsy was performed within 15 minutes of euthanasia.

Experimental design and sample collection

Meloxicam[d] (1 mg/kg) was orally administered daily for 29 days to each rabbit via a 3-mL syringe. The rabbits' behaviour, attitude, mentation, level of activity, eating and drinking, and defecation were subjectively assessed daily by the researchers. Hard fecal samples were collected prior to treatment (day 0) and on days 6, 14 and 21 from the start of the meloxicam treatment. At each time point morning (08:00), 10 fecal pellets from a fresh elimination were placed into an individual collection bag. Therefore, four fecal samples were collected from each rabbit during the study period for determination of fecal microbiota. Each sample (10 fecal pellets) was weighed using a digital gram scale and each fecal pellet was measured using hand calipers. All bagged samples were stored at –70°C until analysis.

DNA extraction and quality control

DNA extraction was performed using a commercial kit[e] following the manufacturer's "stool DNA protocol for pathogen detection", which includes an initial bead beating step and proteinase K treatment. DNA quantity and quality were accessed by spectrophotometry using the NanoDrop[f].

16 s rRNA gene amplification and sequencing

PCR amplification of the V4 region of the 16S rRNA gene was designed based on Klindworth et al. [18] using the primers forward S-D-Bact-0564-a-S-15 (5′-AYTGGGYDTAAAGNG-3′) and reverse S-D-Bact-0785-b-A-18 (5′-TACNVGGGTATCTAATCC-3′). The forward and reverse primers were designed containing an overlapping region of the forward and reverse Illumina sequencing primers (TCGTCGGCAGCGTCAGATGTGTATAAGAGACAG and GTCTCGTGGGCTCGGAGATGTGTATAAGAGACAG, respectively) in order to anneal them to primers containing the Illumina adaptors plus the 8 bp identifier indices (forward: AATGATACGGCG ACCACCGAGATCTACAC-index-TCGTCGGCAGCGTC; reverse: CAAGCAGAAGACGGCATACGAGAT-index-GT CTCGTGGGCTCGG). For a final volume of 50 μL, 2 μL of each DNA sample were added to a solution containing 18.7 μL of water, 25 μL of ReadMis[g], 1.5 μL of BSA[h], 0.5 μL of each 16S primer (1000 pmol/μL) and 1 μL of each Illumina primer (1000 pmol/μL). The mixture was subjected to the following PCR conditions, 3 minutes at 94°C for denaturing, and 35 cycles of 45 seconds at 94°C for denaturing, 60 seconds at 50°C for annealing and 90 seconds at 72°C for elongation followed by a final period of 10 minutes at 72°C and kept at 4°C until purification.

PCR products were evaluated by electrophoresis in 2% agarose gel and purified with the Agencourt AMPure XP[i] by mixing 22 μL of amplicon with 72 μL of AMPure on a 96 well plate. After 5 minutes at room temperature, beads were separated and washed twice with 80% ethanol and eluted in 30 μL of water. After purification samples were quantified by spectrophotometry using the NanoDrop[j] and normalized to a final concentration of 2 nM. Sequencing of the library pool was performed at the University of Guelph's Advanced Analysis Centre using an Illumina MiSeq[k] and 2x250 chemistry.

Microbiome assessment

The MOTHUR package of algorithms (v1.30) was used for analysis [19]. Paired end reads were aligned.

Sequences >275 bp and those containing ambiguous base calls or long runs (>3 bp) of holopolymers were removed, as were sequences that did not align with the correct region. Chimeras were detected using uchime [20] and removed. Sequences from chloroplasts, mitochondria, Archaea and eukaryotes were also removed.

Sequences were binned into OTUs at a 3% (0.03) dissimilarity level, and taxonomy was assigned using the Silva 16S rRNA reference database [21].

Coverage was assessed using Good's coverage. Population diversity was described using the inverse Simpson's index. Relative abundances were compared between animals and between timepoints using ANOVA.

Dissimilarity between the two groups was assessed through creation of dendrograms using the Yue & Clayton measure of dissimilarity (a measure of community structure, which considers shared OTUs and their relative abundances) and traditional Jaccard index (a measure of community membership, which considers the number of shared OTUs, not their abundance). Parsimony and unweighted unifrac [22] tests were applied to evaluate the impact of day of treatment on population structure. Principal coordinate analysis (PCoA) was also performed, based on both Jaccard and Yue and Clayton indices. Analysis of molecular variance (AMOVA), a non-parametric evaluation of genetic diversity, was used to evaluate the impact of day.

Results

Meloxicam was easily administered daily to each rabbit, and all of the rabbits seemed to remain healthy during the study. Subjectively, none of the rabbits had changes in behavior, attitude, mentation, level of activity, amount of food or water consumed, or fecal production. Objectively, all participating rabbits continued to gain weight (final body weight range 2.61-2.91 Kg) when compared to the beginning of the study period. Also, all values in the weekly serum biochemistry analysis were within normal limits both before and during the study. No changes were observed in hard feces' shape, color and consistency (no diarrhea or ileus). The mean weight of a 10-pellet fecal sample was 6.75 g (range 6–9 g) and mean measured individual fecal pellet size was 6.2 mm (range 5–8 mm). Post-study gross necropsy and histopathologic evaluation of all participating rabbits did not reveal any major abnormalities.

A total of 3453182 V4 16S RNA gene sequences were obtained; 2589912 of which passed all quality control filters. The number of sequences per sample ranged from 35178 to 250720 (mean 107913, SD 42703). Further analysis was performed on random subsampling of 35178 sequences per sample. Excellent sample coverage was obtained with this subsampled population, as demonstrated by a mean Good's coverage value of 0.972 (SD 0.002, range 0.967-0.975) and rarefaction curves (Figure 1). The number of OTUs ranged from 1814–2525 (mean 2118, SD 170). There was no impact of rabbit (P = 0.16) or day (P = 0.16) on the number of different OTUs that were identified. The overall mean inverse Simpson's value was 73.6 (SD 23.6, range 19.5-119), with no impact of day (P = 0.54) or rabbit (P = 0.07).

The microbiota of all rabbits was dominated at the phylum level by Firmicutes, which accounted for 66.6 ± 6.7% (mean ± SD) of sequences (Figure 2). Sixteen other phyla were identified; however, only Verrucomicrobia (4.4 ± 5.1%) and accounted for greater than 1% of sequences. These other phyla consisted of Actinobacteria (0.18 ± 0.13%), Bacteroidetes (0.38 ± 0.26%), Chlamydiae (0.001 ± 0.00%), Cyanobacteria (0.003 ± 0.003), Deinococcus-Thermus (0.0001 ± 0.0005%), Fibrobacteres (0.021 ± 0.014%), Fusobacteria (0.003 ± 0.002%), Lentisphaerae (0.002 ± 0.002%, Plantomycetes (0.0002 ± 0.0008), Proteobacteria (0.57 ± 0.33%), Spirochaetes (0.043 ± 0.24%), Synergistetes (0.005 ± 0.001%), Tenericutes (0.021 ± 0.017%), SR1 (0.0006 ± 0.001%) and TM7 (0.06 ± 0.07%). Sequences that were unclassified at the phylum level accounted for 27.7 ± 5.5% of sequences.

Within Firmicutes, Clostridia was the dominant class, accounting for 76% of OTUs from Firmicutes, with Ruminococcaceae and Lachnospiraceae being the main families (order, Clostridiales), representing 48 and 20% of sequences from Clostridia, respectively. Unclassified Clostridia were common (24%), followed by smaller numbers of Bacilli (2.9%).

Within Verrucomicrobia, Verrucomicrobiaceae was the predominant (98%) family. Within that family, *Akkermansia* and *Persicirhabdus* were the two identified genera, but they only accounted for 9.9 and 0.2% of sequences from Verrucomicrobia, respectively. The remaining members of that family were unclassified at the genus level.

There were few differences between different timepoints and different rabbits at the phylum level. Rabbit 4 had a significantly higher relative abundance of Verrucomicrobia (12%) compared to the others (2.1-3.5%) (P = 0.03). No other differences between rabbits were evident at the phylum level. There was a significant change in the relative abundance of Proteobacteria over the four timepoints ($P = 0.02$), with day 21 having a significant higher relative abundance than the other three time points. Otherwise, no significant differences between timepoints were identified.

Dendrograms based on Jaccard and Yue & Clayton indices are presented in Figures 3 and 4. There were few differences in microbial population structure. No effect of sampling day was evident by unweighted unifrac (Table 1). A significant difference was noted with parsimony test but only between days 0 and 21 and using the Jaccard index.

Principle coordinate analysis results are presented in Figures 5 and 6. Using AMOVA, there was no difference between days using the Yue & Clayton index ($P = 0.082$),

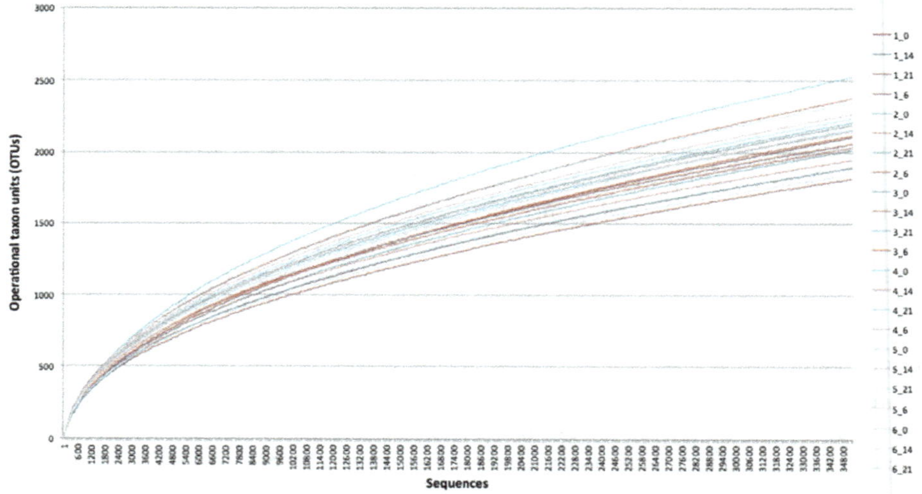

Figure 1 Rarefaction curve demonstrating the change in number of operational taxon units (0.03 level) with increasing sequence numbers in 6 rabbits over 4 different timepoints. Legend: rabbit number_sample day.

but there was a difference using the Jaccard index (P = 0.011), with significant differences between days 0 and 21 (P = 0.002) and days 14 and 21 (P = 0.030).

Discussion

Rabbits enrolled in this study did not show any abnormal clinical signs, hematological values, postmortem evaluation, or physical changes of the hard feces throughout the observed study period, thus suggesting that the tested meloxicam dose can be considered safe for clinical use.

This study identified marked (but perhaps unsurprising) richness and diversity of the fecal microbiome that is incomparable with culture-dependent studies, as an average of over 2000 OTUs were identified. This and the corresponding diversity indices highlight the complexity of the rabbit fecal microbiota, even in rabbits housed under controlled conditions with little or no variation in diet and the need to use broad approaches such as this to understand this environment.

The predominance of Firmicutes was not particularly surprising, as this has been reported in other culture-

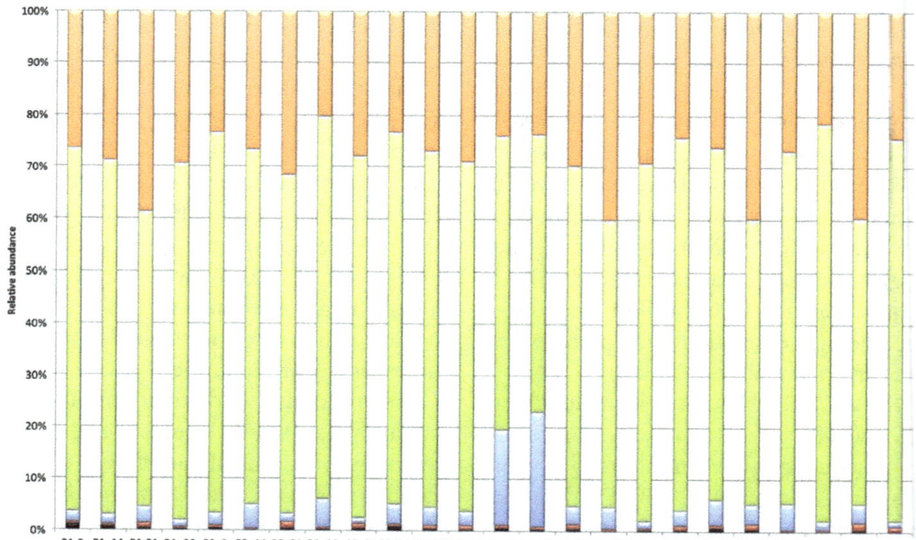

Figure 2 Distribution of the main phyla of the fecal microbiota of 6 healthy adult rabbits (R1-R6) at four different time points (days 0, 6, 14 and 21) after meloxicam treatment.

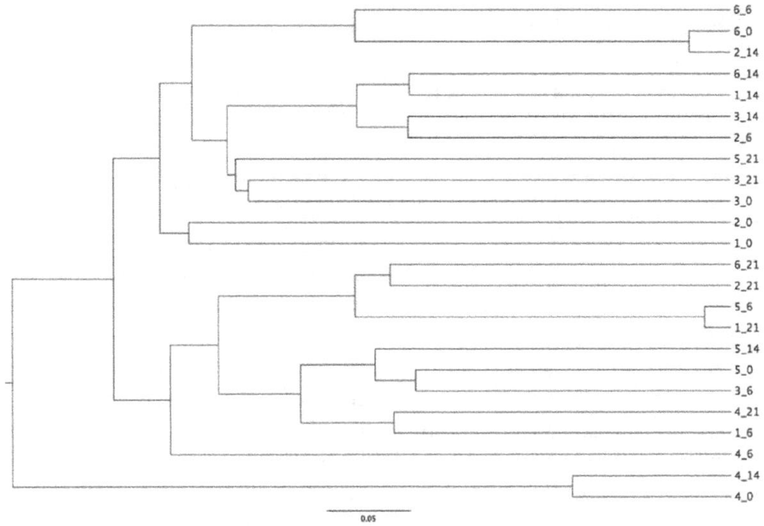

Figure 3 Dendrogram depicting the Yue & Clayton measure of dissimilarity for six rabbits that underwent meloxicam treatment. Legend: identifiers indicate Rabbit_sampling day.

independent studies of the rabbit [13] and can be found in other hindgut fermenters such as the horse [23,24]. It was interesting to observe that Ruminococcaceae and Lachnospiraceae were leading members of this phylum. Those two families are receiving increasing attention in various species as potentially key components of the 'beneficial' microbiota [23,25,26]. There is limited information about these bacteria in rabbits, although they were also reported to be dominant families in a study of 9-week old rabbits [27]. These may be critical components of the rabbit microbiome and groups to study further in terms of gut health and the loosely defined 'intestinal dysbiosis' that is often diagnosed in rabbits with gastrointestinal disease [28].

While the predominance of Firmicutes was not unexpected, the utter dominance of this phylum was remarkable. In studies of the fecal microbiome of most species, while one phylum may be most common, there are typically multiple phyla with relative abundances greater than 5% (or higher) [24,29-31]. Here, only one phylum beyond Firmicutes accounted for greater than 1% of sequences. That was Verrucomicrobia, which accounted for an average of 4.4% of sequences. Verrucomicrobia is a relatively newly described and poorly characterized

Figure 4 Dendrogram depicting fecal microbial community membership of six rabbits that underwent meloxicam treatment based on the traditional Jaccard index. Legend: identifiers indicate Rabbit_sampling day.

Table 1 Comparison of the microbial populations of six rabbits over four timepoints after treatment with meloxicam

	Unweighted Unifrac		Parsimony	
	Jaccard (*P* value)	Yue and Clayton (*P* value)	Jaccard (*P* value)	Yue & Clayton (*P* value)
Day0-Day6	0.48	0.83	0.16	0.56
Day0-Day14	0.71	0.80	0.56	0.57
Day0-Day21	0.17	0.32	0.02	0.58
Day6-Day14	1.00	0.80	0.94	0.57
Day6-Day21	0.73	0.89	0.93	0.93
Day14-Day 21	0.58	0.14	0.53	0.54

phylum. It has been reported in similar relative abundances in other species, including horses [24,32,33], and has been shown to increase in abundance in mice fed type 2 resistant starch [34], perhaps indicating an important role in hindgut fermentation. *Akkermansia* (a member of this phylum) has been shown to be decreased in obese versus lean children and mice [35,36], to be associated with improved glucose homeostasis in metformin treated mice [37], to be associated with reversal of high fat diet induced metabolic disorders in mice [36] and to be reduced in humans with ulcerative colitis [38]. These suggest that this phylum may play an important role in gastrointestinal health in rabbits.

The number of sequences that were unclassified at the phylum level was large, although within the range that has been reported in other fecal microbiome studies and lower than that reported in earlier cloning-based studies of the rabbit cecal microbiota [10,39]. Even within sequences classified as members of the main phyla, Firmicutes and Verrucomicrobia, there were large percentages of sequences that were not identified to lower taxonomic orders. The relevance of these unclassified organisms is unclear. Unclassified sequences are not necessarily unknown phyla. Unclassified could indicate a sequence that does not have any closely related sequences in the reference database, but it could also indicate an inability of the analysis to assign a sequence to known phyla (or lower taxonomic levels) because of similarities in sequences or because of limitations in discriminatory power. Yet, unknown phyla could be present, particularly because of the paucity of knowledge regarding the fecal microbiota. The relevance of these in health and disease is completely unknown but given the high relative abundance, it must be assumed that this unclassified component of the microbiota could be of importance. This underscores our limited understanding of this complex polymicrobial ecosystem and the need for further study to define the microbiota and its individual constituents.

When assessing the microbial composition of these rabbits, there was surprisingly little clustering by individual, as is evident from the dendrograms and PCoA plot. With studies of other species, it is typically reported that there is less intra-individual variation than inter-individual variation [40,41], and if that was the case here, clustering by animal would have been expected. There are a few potential explanations. It is possible that there was enough of an effect of treatment to alter the microbiota of each rabbit, thereby disrupting intra-

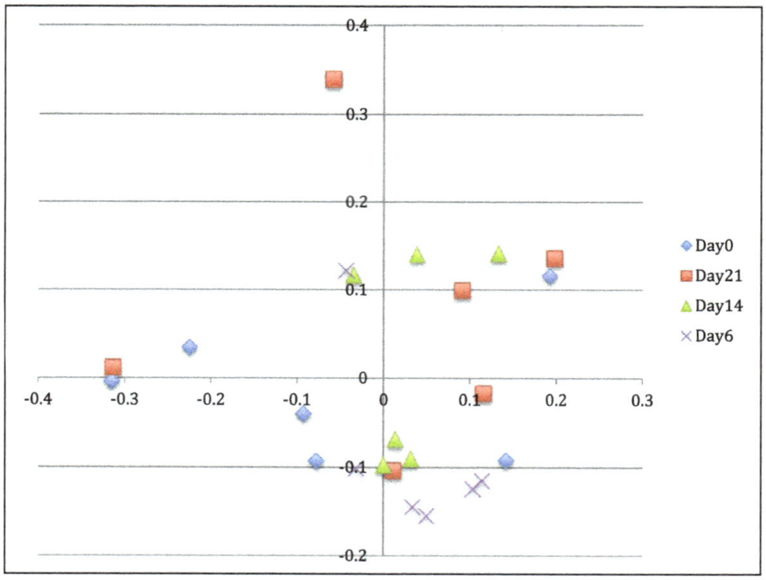

Figure 5 Three dimensional principle coordinate analysis, highlighted by treatment day. Legend: 5a:open box-day0; + = day6; closed circles-day14; x = day 21.

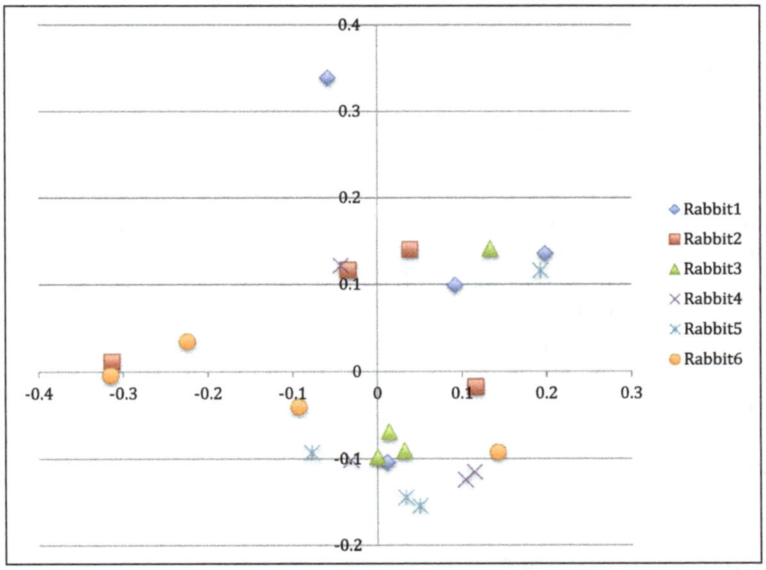

Figure 6 Three dimensional principle coordinate analysis, highlighted by rabbit. Legend: 5b: x: rabbit 1; open box rabbit 2, solid circle rabbit 3; solid triangle rabbit 4; open triangle, rabbit 5; open circle, rabbit 6.

individual consistency, but that the alternation was not in a consistent or strong enough manner to result in a statistically significant effect of sampling day. Another more likely explanation might be the nature of this rabbit population, with similar genetics, housing and diet that resulted in a very homogenous microbiota between individuals. Study of variation in the microbiota of rabbits outside of a research colony would be enlightening. It is also possible that there is more inherent variation in the rabbit microbiota, since a study of rabbits reported similar intra- and inter-rabbit variation [15]. However, that study also involved a homogenously managed group of research rabbits so care must be taken when interpreting the degree of inter- and intra- individual variation from these studies.

Little impact of treatment was identified and there were inconsistent results between different tests. Differences were noted between days 0 and 21 using parsimony test and AMOVA, as well as days 14 and 21 using AMOVA. However, these were only when analysis was based on the Jaccard index. It is important to consider differences between these indices. The Yue & Clayton index is a measure of population dissimilarity based on both microbial presence and abundance, while the Jaccard index compares community membership without assessment of the relative abundance of different members of the community. Thus, differences in Jaccard but not Yue & Clayton indices suggest that changes in the community membership (addition or loss of members) occurred, but that this may have mainly involved low abundance members of community based on a lack of difference when relative abundance is considered. Other than the potential long-term microbiota adjustment to a new diet [42] the accumulated effect of meloxicam should also be considered, and in the absence of clinical or histologic abnormalities, only advanced molecular testing methods had the sensitivity to detect subtle changes in the rabbit's GIT microbiota.

Limitations of the study must be considered. Since there was no untreated control group raised in parallel with these animals and they were all treated at the same time, it is possible that there was some unidentified factor such as a subtle change in diet or stress that accounted for the microbiota change. Additionally, it is known that the fecal microbiome of laboratory raised rabbits is different from rabbits raised under other conditions (e.g. farms, households) [42-44]. As with similar studies, there is always the question of how well the fecal microbiome represents the microbiome in more proximal sections of the gastrointestinal tract. That is an inherent limitation given the inability to easily and non-invasively obtain samples from different areas of the gastrointestinal tract over time. It has been reported that hard feces (which were studied here) are less representative of the cecal microbiota than soft feces [45] but conflicting data have also been reported [15,16]. These data should therefore be interpreted as a description and comparison of the hard fecal microbiota. Optimal approaches for studying the proximal intestinal tract in rabbits are not known. The sample size may also have limited statistical power; however, given the depth of data that are obtained and the similar sample sizes that have been used in other fecal microbiome studies, the sample size was deemed adequate to identify significant changes in the microbiota.

Conclusions

The fecal microbiome of the rabbit is a complex and diverse polymicrobial ecosystem, composed of a wide range of both well-understood and completely unknown bacteria. While there were some noted differences over time, there was no clear and consistent impact of meloxicam treatment on the fecal microbiome. Given the importance of the intestinal microbiome in health and disease, particularly amongst hindgut fermenting species such as the rabbit, it is clear that there is inadequate understanding of the 'normal' microbiota, how it varies within and between rabbits, and how this complex polymicrobial ecosystem influences (and is influenced by) disease, nutrition, management and myriad other factors.

In the absence of adverse clinical, histologic and significant microbial changes observed in rabbits enrolled in this study, it is suggested that alteration of the hard fecal microbiota is not a significant adverse reaction expected with daily oral meloxicam administrated at the tested dose.

Availability of supporting data

The data set supporting the results of this article are available at the MG-RAST metagenomics analysis server (project 8102, http://metagenomics.anl.gov).

Endnotes

[a]Western Timothy Hay, Oxbow Animal Health, Murdock, Neb.
[b]Essentials – Young Rabbit, Oxbow Animal Health, Murdock, Neb.
[c]Vortech Pharmaceuticals, Dearborne, MO.
[d]Metacam 1.5 mg/ml oral suspension, Boehringer Ingelheim Vetmedica, St Joseph, MO.
[e]E.Z.N.A. Stool DNA Kit, Omega Bio-Tek Inc., Doraville, GA.
[f]Roche, Mississauga, ON, Canada.
[g]Invitrogen, San Diego, CA.
[h]Invitrogen, San Diego, CA.
[i]Beckman Coulter Inc, Mississauga, ON, Canada.
[j]Roche, Mississauga, ON, Canada.
[k]Illumina Inc, San Diego, CA.

Competing interests

The authors declare that they have no competing interests.

Authors' contribution

DE participated in fecal collection, data generation and interpretation, and manuscript preparation. JSW participated in data analysis and interpretation, and manuscript preparation. Both authors read and approved the final manuscript.

Acknowledgement

The authors would like to thank Dr. James W. Carpenter for allowing the fecal samples collection from his research rabbits.

Author details

[1]Department of Clinical Sciences, College of Veterinary Medicine, Kansas State University, Manhattan, Kansas 66506, USA. [2]Department of Pathobiology, Ontario Veterinary College, University of Guelph, Guelph, Ontario N1G 2 W1, Canada.

References

1. Wenger S: **Anesthesia and analgesia in rabbits and rodents.** *J Exotic Pet Med* 2012, **21**:7–16.
2. Streppa HK, Jones CJ, Budsberg SC: **Cyclooxygenase selectivity of nonsteroidal anti-inflammatory drugs in canine blood.** *Am J Vet Res* 2002, **63**:91–94.
3. Forsyth SF, Guilford WG, Haslett SJ, Hill PB: **Endoscopy of the gastroduodenal mucosa after carprofen, meloxicam and ketoprofen administration in dogs.** *J Small Anim Pract* 1998, **39**:421–424.
4. Luna SPL, Basilio AC, Steagall PVM, Machado LP, Moutinho FQ, Takahira RK, Brandao CV: **Evaluation of adverse effects of long-term oral administration of carprofen, etodolac, flunixin meglumine, ketoprofen, and meloxicam in dogs.** *Am J Vet Res* 2007, **68**:258–264.
5. Pairet M, Bouyssou T, Ruckebusch Y: **Colonic formation of soft feces in rabbits: a role for endogenous prostaglandins.** *Am J Physiol-Gastrointestinal Liver Physiol* 1986, **250**:G302–G308.
6. Turner PV, Chen HC, Taylor MW: **Pharmacokinetics of meloxicam in rabbits after single and repeat oral dosing.** *Comp Med* 2006, **56**:63–67.
7. Carpenter JW, Pollock CG, Koch DE, Hunter RP: **Single and multiple-dose pharmacokinetics of meloxicam after oral administration to the rabbit (*Oryctolagus cuniculus*).** *J Zoo Wildl Med* 2009, **40**:601–606.
8. Fredholm DV, Carpenter JW, KuKanich B, Kohles M: **Pharmacokinetics of meloxicam in rabbits after oral administration of single and multiple doses.** *Am J Vet Res* 2013, **74**:636–641.
9. Straw TE: **Bacteria of the rabbit gut and their role in the health of the rabbit.** *J Appl Rabbit Res* 1988, **11**:142–150.
10. Abecia L, Fondevila M, Balcells J, Edwards JE, Newbold CJ, McEwan RN: **Molecular profiling of bacterial species in the rabbit caecum.** *FEMS Microbiol Lett* 2005, **244**:111–115.
11. Furet JP, Firmesse O, Gourmelon M, Bridonneau C, Tap J, Mondot S, Dore J, Corthier G: **Comparative assessment of human and farm animal faecal microbiota using real-time quantitative PCR.** *FEMS Microbiol Ecol* 2009, **68**:351–362.
12. Kušar D, Avguštin G: **Molecular profiling and identification of methanogenic archaeal species from rabbit caecum.** *FEMS Microbiol Ecol* 2010, **74**:623–630.
13. Combes S, Michelland RJ, Monteils V, Cauquil L, Soulie V, Tran NU, Gidenne T, Fortun-Lamothe L: **Postnatal development of the rabbit caecal microbiota composition and activity.** *FEMS Microbiol Ecol* 2011, **77**:680–689.
14. Suau A, Bonnet R, Sutren M, Godon JJ, Gibson GR, Collins MD, Dore J: **Direct analysis of genes encoding 16S rRNA from complex communities reveals many novel molecular species within the human gut.** *Appl Environ Microbiol* 1999, **65**:4799–4807.
15. Michelland RJ, Combes S, Monteils V, Cauquil L, Gidenne T, Fortun-Lamothe L: **Molecular analysis of the bacterial community in digestive tract of rabbit.** *Anaerobe* 2010, **16**:61–65.
16. Michelland RJ, Monteils V, Combes S, Cauquil L, Gidenne T, Fortun-Lamothe L: **Comparison of the archaeal community in the fermentative compartment and faeces of the cow and the rabbit.** *Anaerobe* 2010, **16**:396–401.
17. Fiorello CV, Divers SJ: **Rabbits.** In *Exotic Animal Formulary*. 4th edition. Edited by Carpenter JW. St Louis: Elsevier; 2012:517–559.
18. Klindworth A, Pruesse E, Schweer T, Peplies J, Quast C, Horn M, Glockner FO: **Evaluation of general 16S ribosomal RNA gene PCR primers for classical and next-generation sequencing-based diversity studies.** *Nucleic Acids Res* 2013, **41**:e1.
19. Schloss PD, Westcott SL, Ryabin T, Hall JR, Hartmann M, Hollister EB, Lesniewski RA, Oakley BB, Parks DH, Robinson CJ, Sahl JW, Stres B, Thalinger GG, Van Horn DJ, Weber CF: **Introducing mothur: open-source, platform-independent, community-supported software for describing and comparing microbial communities.** *Appl Environ Microbiol* 2009, **75**:7537–7541.
20. Edgar RC, Haas BJ, Clemente JC, Quince C, Knight R: **UCHIME improves sensitivity and speed of chimera detection.** *Bioinformatics* 2011, **27**:2194–2200.
21. Quast C, Pruesse E, Yilma P, Gerken J, Schweer T, Yarza P, Peplies J, Glockner FO: **The SILVA ribosomal RNA gene database project: improved data processing and web-based tools.** *Nucleic Acids Res* 2013, **41**:D590–D596.
22. Lozupone C, Hamady M, Knight R: **UniFrac–an online tool for comparing microbial community diversity in a phylogenetic context.** *BMC Bioinforma* 2006, **7**:371.
23. Costa MC, Arroyo LG, Allen-Vercoe E, Staempfli HR, Kim PT, Sturgeon A, Weese JS: **Comparison of the fecal microbiota of healthy horses and horses with colitis by high throughput sequencing of the V3-V5 region of the 16S rRNA gene.** *PloS One* 2012, **7**:e41484.

24. O'Donnell MM, Harris H, Jeffery IB, Claesson MJ, Younge B, O'Toole PW, Ross RP: **The core faecal bacterial microbiome of Irish Thoroughbred racehorses.** *Lett Appl Microbiol* 2013.
25. Suchodolski JS: **Companion animal's symposium: microbes and gastrointestinal health of dogs and cats.** *J Anim Sci* 2011, **89:**1520–1530.
26. Petrof EO, Gloor GB, Vanner SJ, Weese JS, Carter D, Daigneault MC, Brown EM, Schroeter K, Allen-Vercoe E: **Stool substitute transplant therapy for the eradication of Clostridium difficile infection: 'RePOOPulating' the gut.** *Microbiome* 2013, **1:**1–12.
27. Massip K, Combes S, Cauquil L, Zemb O, Gidenne T: **High throughput 16S-DNA sequencing for phylogenetic affiliation of the caecal bacterial community in the rabbit - Impact of the hygiene of housing and of the intake level.** In *Proceeding of Symposium on Gut Microbiology. Gut Microbiota: Friend or Foe?: 17–20 June 2012.* Clermont-Ferrand, France; 2012:56.
28. Harrenstien L: **Gastrointestinal diseases of pet rabbits.** *Sem. Avian Exotic Pet Med.* 1999, **8:**83–89.
29. Turnbaugh PJ, Hamady M, Yatsunenko T, Cantarel BL, Duncan A, Ley RE, Sogin ML, Jones WJ, Roe BA, Affourtit JP, Egholm M, Henrissat B, Heath AC, Knight R, Gordon JI: **A core gut microbiome in obese and lean twins.** *Nature* 2008, **457:**480–484.
30. Barry KA, Middelbos IS, Vester Boler BM, Dowd SE, Suchodolski JS, Henrissat B, Coutinho PM, White BA, Fahey GC Jr, Swanson KS: **Effects of dietary fiber on the feline gastrointestinal metagenome.** *J Proteome Res* 2012, **11:**5924–5933.
31. Suchodolski JS, Markel ME, Garcia-Mazcorro JF, Unterer S, Heilmann RM, Dowd SE, Kachroo P, Ivanov I, Minamoto Y, Dillman EM, Steiner JM, Cook AK, Toresson L: **The fecal microbiome in dogs with acute diarrhea and idiopathic inflammatory bowel disease.** *PloS One* 2012, **7:**e51907.
32. Steelman SM, Chowdhary BP, Dowd S, Suchodolski JS, Janecka JE: **Pyrosequencing of 16S rRNA genes in fecal samples reveals high diversity of hindgut microflora in horses and potential links to chronic laminitis.** *BMC Vet Res* 2012, **8:**231.
33. Shepherd ML, Swecker WS, Jensen RV, Ponder MA: **Characterization of the fecal bacteria communities of forage-fed horses by pyrosequencing of 16S rRNA V4 gene amplicons.** *FEMS Microbiol Lett* 2012, **326:**62–68.
34. Tachon S, Zhou J, Keenan M, Martin R, Marco ML: **The intestinal microbiota in aged mice is modulated by dietary resistant starch and correlated with improvements in host responses.** *FEMS Microbiol Ecol* 2013, **83:**299–309.
35. Karlsson CL, Önnerfält J, Xu J, Molin G, Ahrne S, Thorngren-Jerneck K: **The microbiota of the gut in preschool children with normal and excessive body weight.** *Obesity* 2012, **20:**2257–2261.
36. Everard A, Belzer C, Geurts L, Ouwerkerk JP, Druart C, Bindels LB, Guiot Y, Derrien M, Muccioli GG, Deizenne NM, de Vos WM, Cani PD: **Cross-talk between *Akkermansia muciniphila* and intestinal epithelium controls diet-induced obesity.** *Proc Natl Acad Sci* 2013, **110:**9066–9071.
37. Shin NR, Lee JC, Lee HY, Kim MS, Whon TW, Lee MS, Bae JW: **An increase in the *Akkermansia* spp. population induced by metformin treatment improves glucose homeostasis in diet-induced obese mice.** *Gut Online First* 2013, **0:**1–9.
38. Rajilic-Stojanovic M, Shanahan F, Guarner F, de Vos WM: **Phylogenetic analysis of dysbiosis in ulcerative colitis during remission.** *Inflamm Bowel Dis* 2013, **19:**481–488.
39. Monteils V, Cauquil L, Combes S, Godon JJ, Gidenne T: **Potential core species and satellite species in the bacterial community within the rabbit caecum.** *FEMS Microbiol Ecol* 2008, **66:**620–629.
40. Lazarevic V, Whiteson K, Hernandez D, Francois P, Schrenzel J: **Study of inter-and intra-individual variations in the salivary microbiota.** *BMC Genomics* 2010, **11:**523–534.
41. Jalanka-Tuovinen J, Salonen A, Nikkilä J, Immonen O, Kekkonen R, Lahti L, Palva A, de Vos WM: **Intestinal microbiota in healthy adults: temporal analysis reveals individual and common core and relation to intestinal symptoms.** *PloS One* 2011, **6:**e23035.
42. Rodríguez-Romero N, Abecia L, Fondevila M: **Microbial ecosystem and fermentation traits in the caecum of growing rabbits given diets varying in neutral detergent soluble and insoluble fibre levels.** *Anaerobe* 2013, **20:**50–57.
43. Bennegadi N, Fonty G, Millet L, Gidenne T, Licois D: **Effects of age and dietary fibre level on caecal microbial communities of conventional and specific pathogen-free rabbits.** *Microb Ecol Health Dis* 2003, **15:**23–32.
44. Abecia L, Rodríguez-Romero N, Yañez-Ruiz DR, Fondevilla M: **Biodiversity and fermentative activity of caecal microbial communities in wild and farm rabbits from Spain.** *Anaerobe* 2012, **18:**344–349.
45. Michelland RJ, Combes S, Monteils V, Cauquil L, Gidenne T, Fortun-Lamothe L: **Rapid adaptation of the bacterial community in the growing rabbit caecum after a change in dietary fibre supply.** *Animal* 2011, **5:**1761–1768.

PERMISSIONS

All chapters in this book were first published in VR, by BioMed Central; hereby published with permission under the Creative Commons Attribution License or equivalent. Every chapter published in this book has been scrutinized by our experts. Their significance has been extensively debated. The topics covered herein carry significant findings which will fuel the growth of the discipline. They may even be implemented as practical applications or may be referred to as a beginning point for another development.

The contributors of this book come from diverse backgrounds, making this book a truly international effort. This book will bring forth new frontiers with its revolutionizing research information and detailed analysis of the nascent developments around the world.

We would like to thank all the contributing authors for lending their expertise to make the book truly unique. They have played a crucial role in the development of this book. Without their invaluable contributions this book wouldn't have been possible. They have made vital efforts to compile up to date information on the varied aspects of this subject to make this book a valuable addition to the collection of many professionals and students.

This book was conceptualized with the vision of imparting up-to-date information and advanced data in this field. To ensure the same, a matchless editorial board was set up. Every individual on the board went through rigorous rounds of assessment to prove their worth. After which they invested a large part of their time researching and compiling the most relevant data for our readers.

The editorial board has been involved in producing this book since its inception. They have spent rigorous hours researching and exploring the diverse topics which have resulted in the successful publishing of this book. They have passed on their knowledge of decades through this book. To expedite this challenging task, the publisher supported the team at every step. A small team of assistant editors was also appointed to further simplify the editing procedure and attain best results for the readers.

Apart from the editorial board, the designing team has also invested a significant amount of their time in understanding the subject and creating the most relevant covers. They scrutinized every image to scout for the most suitable representation of the subject and create an appropriate cover for the book.

The publishing team has been an ardent support to the editorial, designing and production team. Their endless efforts to recruit the best for this project, has resulted in the accomplishment of this book. They are a veteran in the field of academics and their pool of knowledge is as vast as their experience in printing. Their expertise and guidance has proved useful at every step. Their uncompromising quality standards have made this book an exceptional effort. Their encouragement from time to time has been an inspiration for everyone.

The publisher and the editorial board hope that this book will prove to be a valuable piece of knowledge for researchers, students, practitioners and scholars across the globe.

LIST OF CONTRIBUTORS

Jessica Stahl, Katrin Zessel and Manfred Kietzmann
Department of Pharmacology, Toxicology and Pharmacy, University of Veterinary Medicine Hannover, Foundation, Buenteweg 17, 30559 Hannover, Germany

Jochen Schulz
Institute for Animal Hygiene, Animal Welfare and Farm Animal Behaviour, Bischofsholer Damm 15, 30173 Hannover, Germany

Jan Henrik Finke and Christel Charlotte Müller-Goymann
Institut Pharmazeutische Technologie, Technische Universität Braunschweig, Mendelssohnstr. 1, 38106 Braunschweig, Germany

K. J. Wareham, R. M. Hyde, M. L. Brennan and R. S. Dean
Centre for Evidence-based Veterinary Medicine, School of Veterinary Medicine and Science, The University of Nottingham, Sutton Bonington campus, Loughborough LE12 5RD, UK

D. Grindlay
Centre of Evidence Based Dermatology, The University of Nottingham King's Meadow Campus Lenton Lane, Nottingham NG7 2NR, UK

Daniel N. Qekwana
Section of Veterinary Public Health, Department of Paraclinical Sciences, Faculty of Veterinary Science, University of Pretoria, Pretoria, South Africa

Fortune Sithole
Section of Veterinary Public Health, Department of Paraclinical Sciences, Faculty of Veterinary Science, University of Pretoria, Pretoria, South Africa
Ross University School of Veterinary Medicine, Basseterre, Saint Kitts and Nevis USA

Agricola Odoi
Section of Veterinary Public Health, Department of Paraclinical Sciences, Faculty of Veterinary Science, University of Pretoria, Pretoria, South Africa
Biomedical and Diagnostic Sciences, College of Veterinary Medicine, University of Tennessee, Knoxville, USA

James W. Oguttu
Department of Agriculture and Animal Health, College of Agriculture and Environmental Sciences, University of South Africa, Johannesburg, South Africa

Lucy Dorey and Peter Lees
The Royal Veterinary College, Hawkshead Campus, Herts, AL97TA, Hatfield, UK

Domenico Britti and Valeria Maria Morittu
Department of Health Sciences V. le Europa, Campus S. Venuta, Germaneto, 88100 Catanzaro, Italy

Rosalia Crupi, Daniela Impellizzeri, Enrico Gugliandolo, Roberta Fusco and Rosanna Di Paola
Department of Chemical, Biological, Pharmaceutical and Environmental Sciences, University of Messina, Viale Ferdinando Stagno D'Alcontres 31-, I-98166 Messina, Italy

Salvatore Cuzzocrea
Department of Chemical, Biological, Pharmaceutical and Environmental Sciences, University of Messina, Viale Ferdinando Stagno D'Alcontres 31-, I-98166 Messina, Italy
Manchester Biomedical Research Centre, Manchester Royal Infirmary, School of Medicine, University of Manchester, Manchester, UK

Carlo Schievano
Innovative Statistical Research SRL, Prato Della Valle 24, I-35123 Padova, Italy

Maurizio Evangelista
Institute of Anaesthesiology and Reanimation, Catholic University of Sacred Heart, Rome, Italy

Jonathan N. King, Wolfgang Seewald and Gabriele Friton
Companion Animal Development, Elanco Animal Health, Basel, Switzerland

Alessandro Panteri and Melanie Graille
Preclinical, Elanco Centre de Recherche Santé Animale, St-Aubin, Switzerland

Cyril Desevaux
Safety, Elanco Animal Health, Basel, Switzerland

Nolie K. Parnell
College of Veterinary Medicine, University of Leipzig, An den Tierkliniken 23, 04103 Leipzig, DE, Germany

Romy M. Heilmann
College of Veterinary Medicine, University of Leipzig, An den Tierkliniken 23, 04103 Leipzig, DE, Germany
Gastrointestinal Laboratory, Texas A&M University, TAMU 4474, College Station, TX 77843-4474, USA

Jörg M. Steiner and Jan S. Suchodolski
Gastrointestinal Laboratory, Texas A&M University, TAMU 4474, College Station, TX 77843-4474, USA

Nora Berghoff
Gastrointestinal Laboratory, Texas A&M University, TAMU 4474, College Station, TX 77843-4474, USA
Department of Pathobiology & Diagnostic Investigation, College of Veterinary Medicine, Michigan State University, 784 Wilson Rd, East Lansing, MI 48824, USA

Niels Grützner
Gastrointestinal Laboratory, Texas A&M University, TAMU 4474, College Station, TX 77843-4474, USA
Farm Animal Clinic, Vetsuisse Faculty, University of Bern, Bremgartenstrasse 109a, CH, 3012 Bern, BE, Switzerland

Karin Hoelzer, Nora Wong, Joe Thomas, Kathy Talkington, Elizabeth Jungman and Allan Coukell
The Pew Charitable Trusts, 901 E Street NW, Washington, DC 20004, USA

Dong-Hao Zhao, Chang-Liang Ke, Qi Liu, Xu-Feng Wang, Qiang Wang and Liu-Dong Li
Key Laboratory of Aquatic Product Processing, Ministry of Agriculture, Guangzhou 510300, People's Republic of China
Laboratiry of Quality & Safety Risk Assessment for Aquatic Product on Storage and Preservation, Guangzhou 510300, People's Republic of China
Fishery Environments and Aquatic Products Quality Inspection & Testing Center of the Ministry of Agriculture, Guangzhou 510300, People's Republic of China South China Sea Fisheries Research Institute, Chinese Academy of Fishery Sciences, Guangzhou 510300, People's Republic of China

Jeong Woo Kang, Hae-chul Park, Yang ho Jang, Md Akil Hossain, Kyunghun Jeong, Mi young Jeong, Seon-Jong Yun, Sung-won Park, Dae gyun Kim and Kwang-jick Lee
Veterinary drugs & Biologics Division, Animal and Plant Quarantine Agency (QIA), 177, Hyeoksin 8-ro, Gimcheon-si, Gyeongsangbuk-do 39660, Republic of Korea

Stevie O'Keefe
Comparative Biology Centre, Newcastle University, Framlington Place, Newcastle Upon Tyne NE2 4HH, UK

Henri G. M. J. Bertrand
Comparative Biology Centre, Newcastle University, Framlington Place, Newcastle Upon Tyne NE2 4HH, UK
Faculty of Veterinary Medicine, University of Liège, Boulevard de Colonster, Liège 4000, Belgium

Yvette C. Ellen
Comparative Biology Centre, Newcastle University, Framlington Place, Newcastle Upon Tyne NE2 4HH, UK
School of Veterinary Medicine and Science, University of Nottingham, Sutton Bonington Campus, Loughborough LE12 5RD, UK

Paul A. Flecknell
Comparative Biology Centre, Newcastle University, Framlington Place, Newcastle Upon Tyne NE2 4HH, UK
Institute of Neuroscience, Newcastle University, Newcastle Upon Tyne NE1 7RU, UK

Giovanni Widmer and Kevin Huynh
Department of Infectious Diseases and Global Health, Cummings School of Veterinary Medicine at Tufts University, 200 Westboro Road, North Grafton, MA, USA

Lluís Ferrer
Department of Clinical Sciences, Cummings School of Veterinary Medicine at Tufts University, 200 Westboro Road, North Grafton, MA, USA

Claude Favrot
Clinic for Small Animal Internal Medicine, Vetsuisse Faculty, University of Zürich, Winterthurerstrasse 260, -8057 Zürich, CH, Switzerland

Judy Paps and Thierry Olivry
Department of Clinical Sciences, College of Veterinary Medicine, North Carolina State University, 1060 William Moore Drive, Raleigh, NC 27607, USA

Günther Schauberger
WG Environmental Health, Division for Physiology and Biophysics, Department for Biomedical Sciences, University of Veterinary Medicine Vienna, Veterinärplatz 1, A 1210 Vienna, Austria

Johannes Horak
WG Environmental Health, Division for Physiology and Biophysics, Department for Biomedical Sciences, University of Veterinary Medicine Vienna, Veterinärplatz 1, A 1210 Vienna, Austria
Institute of Atmospheric and Cryospheric Sciences, University of Innsbruck, Innrain 52f, A-6020 Innsbruck, Austria

Astrid Haberleitner
Institute of Pharmacology and Toxicology, Department for Biomedical Sciences, University of Veterinary Medicine Vienna, Veterinärplatz 1, A 1210 Vienna, Austria

Ning Ma, Xi-Wang Liu, Ya-Jun Yang, Dong-Shuai Shen, Xiao-Le Zhao, Isam Mohamed, Xiao-Jun Kong and Jian-Yong Li
Key Lab of New Animal Drug Project of Gansu Province, Key Lab of Veterinary Pharmaceutical Development Ministry of Agriculture, Lanzhou Institute of Husbandry and Pharmaceutical Science of CAAS, No.335, Jiangouyan, Qilihe district, Lanzhou 730050, China

Alexandra Trbolova and Igor Capik
Clinic of Small Animals, University of Veterinary Medicine and Pharmacy, Kosice, Slovakia

Masoud Selk Ghaffari
Department of Clinical Sciences, College of Veterinary Medicine, Karaj Branch, Islamic Azad University, Alborz, Iran

Fábio Alessandro Pieri
Departamento de Ciências Básicas da Vida, Universidade Federal de Juiz de Fora, Rua Israel Pinheiro, 2000, Bairro Universitário, CEP: 35020-220 Governador Valadares, Minas Gerais, Brasil
Departamento de Veterinária, Universidade Federal de Viçosa, Av. P.H. Rolfs, s/n, Câmpus UFV, CEP: 36570-000 Viçosa, Minas Gerais, Brasil

Marina Campos de Castro Souza, Ligia Lobato Ramos Vermelho, Marina Lobato Ramos Vermelho, Pedro Griffo Perciano, Andréa Pacheco Batista Borges and Maria Aparecida Scatamburlo Moreira
Departamento de Veterinária, Universidade Federal de Viçosa, Av. P.H. Rolfs, s/n, Câmpus UFV, CEP: 36570-000 Viçosa, Minas Gerais, Brasil

Fabiano Souza Vargas and Valdir Florêncio da Veiga-Junior
Instituto de Ciências Exatas, Universidade Federal do Amazonas, Av. Rodrigo Otávio, 6200, Coroado, CEP: 69.080-005 Manaus, Amazonas, Brasil

Marios Charalambous and Sofie F. M. Bhatti
Small Animal Department, Faculty of Veterinary Medicine, Ghent University, Merelbeke, Belgium

Akos Pakozdy
Clinical Unit of Internal Medicine Small Animals, University of Veterinary Medicine, Vienna, Austria

Holger A. Volk
Department of Clinical Science and Services, Royal Veterinary College, Hawkshead Lane, Brookmans Park, UK

Andrea Cattai, Maurizio Isola and Paolo Franci
Department of Animal Medicine, Production and Health, Agripolis, Università degli Studi di Padova, Padua, Italy

Roberto Rabozzi
CVRS - Policlinico Veterinario Roma Sud, Rome, Italy

Heidi Ferasin
Specialist Veterinary Cardiology Consultancy, Lymington Bottom, Four Marks, Hampshire, UK

Abbey R. Sadowski
Cummings School, Tufts University, Foster Hospital for Small Animals, 200 Westboro Rd, N. Grafton, MA 01536, USA

Cheryl A. London
Cummings School, Tufts University, Foster Hospital for Small Animals, 200 Westboro Rd, N. Grafton, MA 01536, USA
Department of Veterinary Biosciences, College of Veterinary Medicine, The Ohio State University, Columbus, OH, USA

Heather L. Gardner
Sackler School of Graduate Biomedical Sciences, Tufts University, Boston, MA, US

Antonella Borgatti
College of Veterinary Medicine, University of Minnesota, St. Paul, MN, USA

Heather Wilson
College of Veterinary Medicine, Texas A&M University, College Station, TX, USA

David M. Vail
Department of Medical Sciences, School of Veterinary Medicine, University of Wisconsin Madison, Madison, WI, USA

Joshua Lachowicz
NYC Veterinary Specialists/Blue Pearl Veterinary Specialists, New York, NY, USA

Christina Manley
The Oncology Service, The LifeCentre, Leesburg, VA, USA

Avenelle Turner
Veterinary Cancer Group, Culver City, CA, USA

Mary K. Klein
Southern Arizona Veterinary Specialty and Emergency Center, Tucson, AZ, USA

Angharad Waite
The Oncology Service, Dogwood Veterinary Emergency and Specialty Center, Richmond, VA, USA

Alexandra Sahora
The Oncology Service, Friendship Hospital for Animals, Washington DC, USA

T. Real, K. P. Doucette and S. B. King
Elanco Animal Health, 2500 Innovation Way, Greenfield, IN 46140, USA

S. L. Forster
Elanco Animal Health Ltd., Lilly House, Priestley Road, Basingstoke, Hampshire RG24 9NL, UK

Index